£34.99
o5

⚜ Barts and The London
Queen Mary's School of Medicine and Dentistry
WHITECHAPEL LIBRARY, TURNER STREET, LONDON E1 2AD
020 7882 7110

4 WEEK LOAN
Books are to be returned on or before the last date below,
otherwise fines may be charged.

H

H

2 2 SEP 2009

D1422230

Handbook of Outpatient Hysteroscopy
A complete guide to diagnosis and therapy

T Justin Clark MB, ChB, MD (Hons), MRCOG
Consultant Obstetrician and Gynaecologist
Birmingham Women's Hospital, Birmingham, UK

and

Janesh K Gupta MSc, MD, FRCOG
Clinical Senior Lecturer and Honorary Consultant,
Academic Department of Obstetrics & Gynaecology
Birmingham Women's Hospital, Birmingham, UK

Hodder Arnold

A MEMBER OF THE HODDER HEADLINE GROUP

First published in Great Britain in 2005 by
Hodder Education, a member of the Hodder Headline Group,
338 Euston Road, London NW1 3BH

www.hoddereducation.co.uk

Distributed in the United States of America by
Oxford University Press Inc.
198 Madison Avenue, New York, NY 10016
Oxford is a registered trademark of Oxford University Press

Whilst the advice and information in this book are believed to be true and
accurate at the date of going to press, neither the author(s) nor the publisher
can accept any legal responsibility or liability for any errors or omissions
that may be made. In particular (but without limiting the generality of the
preceding disclaimer), every effort has been made to check drug dosages;
however, it is still possible that errors have been missed. Furthermore,
dosage schedules are constantly being revised and new side effects
recognized. For these reasons the reader is strongly urged to consult the
drug companies' printed instructions before administering any of the drugs
recommended in this book.

British Library Cataloguing in Publication Data
A catalogue record for this book is available from the British Library

Library of Congress Cataloging-in-Publication Data
A catalog record for this book is available from the Library of Congress

ISBN   0 340 81651 1
ISBN-13   978 0 340 81651 6

1 2 3 4 5 6 7 8 9 10

Commissioning Editor: Joanna Koster
Development Editor: Sarah Burrows
Project Editor: Naomi Wilkinson
Production Controller: Joanna Walker
Cover Design: Georgina Howard
Copy-editor: Michèle Clarke
Indexer: Laurence Errington

Typeset in 9/12 Rotis Serif by Charon Tec Pvt. Ltd, Chennai, India
Printed and bound in Malta by Gutenberg Press Ltd

What do you think about this book? Or any other Hodder Arnold title?
Please visit our website at www.hoddereducation.co.uk

To our families

Contents

Foreword

Hysteroscopy has become a technique that is now an established part of gynaecological practice. All gynaecologists are able to perform inpatient hysteroscopy although those with an interest in outpatient hysteroscopy are still a minority. The aim of this book is to discuss why outpatient hysteroscopy is essential in any unit, and having justified the case, it informs the gynaecologist of how the service should be set up. The benefits of introducing such a service are justified within the book and also the many conditions that can be investigated and treated effectively. Given that we are in an era of evidence-based medicine, there is also an emphasis on discussing all available data and the clinical trials that have been carried out on any particular topic. This allows the reader to judge the strength of any of the assertions made in the text.

This book tells you everything you need to know about hysteroscopy. It discusses in depth both diagnostic and operative hysteroscopy, and introduces related topics to put the discussion into context. It starts from first principles with simple descriptions of basic anatomy and endocrinology but this is done in such a way as to emphasise the clinical relevance of possessing this knowledge. I feel this section might be particularly useful to undergraduate medical students as well as practising gynaecologists and those in training.

Modern outpatient hysteroscopy no longer needs to be confined to diagnosis but can be used to perform a range of therapeutic procedures. This book is the first of its kind to provide practical, evidence-based guidance on the feasibility and approach to innovative outpatient interventions in benign gynaecology. Clear advice is given on setting up and running an outpatient hysteroscopy service including guidelines and even a business plan. This will be valuable to anybody wishing to set up a new service without 'reinventing the wheel'. There is considerable detail, including figures that are particularly relevant to current practice and I am sure will be easily updated in future editions.

Throughout the book there are good comparative tables allowing the reader to make informed decisions about whether they should use disposable or reusable instruments, for example, and why they might choose one distension media over another. It is also particularly pleasing to see discussion of the most up to date techniques available in order to be fully comprehensive. This is a very clear book with tables and key points and for those with a particular interest, suggestions for further reading. The advice given is sensible and practical. It covers all aspects of the uterus as well as considering the appearance of the cervix and even the vulvo-vagina. It deals with the common problems associated with hysteroscopy such as anxiety and pain and suggests strategies for minimising both.

This book will be useful to all practising gynaecologists, even those who will not be setting up a new service, as it contains much information about common gynaecological conditions.

Professor Mary Ann Lumsden
Professor of Medical Education and Gynaecology
Glasgow Royal Infirmary

Preface

RATIONALE

Hysteroscopy has developed rapidly over the last few years. The technique has moved from being a purely diagnostic 'inpatient' modality to a diagnostic and therapeutic 'outpatient' procedure. Advances in endoscopic technology have driven this paradigm shift. At international, national and local levels, the potential for developing outpatient interventional services in order to help meet healthcare delivery targets is being increasingly recognized. Desired targets include increasing the range, access and quality of services, improving patient choice and user experience, making progress in high priority areas (e.g. cancer) and developing the capacity to deliver these plans. Thus in the context of strategic planning in gynaecology, outpatient hysteroscopic services are likely to become increasingly prominent. The opportunity to meet these needs, by setting up outpatient diagnostic and treatment services ('see and treat' centres), should now to be seized.

AIM AND FORMAT

The purpose of this book is to provide clear, unambiguous information about the capabilities of modern outpatient hysteroscopy and related gynaecological interventions. We have attempted to produce the first complete guide to diagnostic and therapeutic outpatient hysteroscopy, the so-called 'see and treat' approach. Current sources of written information do not deal with the practicalities of outpatient operating and are not generally 'user friendly'. Operating in the conscious patient in an outpatient setting presents many new challenges. We describe strategies and provide tips to overcome these obstacles and thus speed the reader along the 'learning curve'.

This book covers all aspects of modern day outpatient hysteroscopy and is based on our personal experience backed up by the available evidence. The book is divided into three sections. The first describes the fundamental theoretical and practical requirements of outpatient hysteroscopy including diagnosis and details on setting up and running services. The middle section discusses frequently encountered presenting complaints and provides rational approaches for management. The final section addresses operative outpatient hysteroscopy and related interventions. Clinic set-up, pain relief, available technologies and specific operations are described as well as training, safety and medicolegal issues. The book aims to be concise while remaining comprehensive, and a consistent format is presented. An evidence-based approach is adopted throughout the book and summary 'evidence boxes' are provided at the end of each chapter along with key learning points. Where possible, the direction of future practice and research is highlighted in this dynamic field.

AUDIENCE

By providing contemporary evidence-based approaches to managing substantial parts of benign day-to-day gynaecological practice in a concise manner, we envisage that the book will be of interest to a wide audience:

- We anticipate that it will be relevant to all practising gynaecologists with an interest in outpatient hysteroscopy and ultrasound.

- We hope that gynaecologists in training including those preparing for exams will find the essential theoretical as well as practical principles provided in the book invaluable. Once familiar with the equipment, hysteroscopic diagnosis and contemporary management of gynaecological disorders, the trainee with an interest in outpatient interventional gynaecology can progress onto operative work.

- We believe that primary care physicians with a gynaecological bent, community gynaecologists and specialist 'nurse hysteroscopists' should find the book useful because it is about outpatient 'office' procedures, which are not restricted to traditional hospital settings and practice.

We hope that the information contained within this book will aid the reader to set up and develop innovative and successful outpatient hysteroscopic services with the ultimate aim of improving the care that we offer to women with gynaecological conditions.

Good luck!

TJC, JKG (August 2004)

Acknowledgements

Thanks to all those who have trained us in gynaecology, our nursing staff, especially Jan, Linda and 'Frankie' and all the women we have treated in our outpatient hysteroscopy clinic, without whose help we would have been unable to develop innovative outpatient hysteroscopic services.

Abbreviations

ARDS	adult respiratory disease syndrome
BNA	borderline nuclear abnormality
BSCC	British Society of Cervical Cytology
BTB	breakthrough bleeding
CIN	cervical intraepithelial neoplasia
COC	combined oral contraceptive
CSSD	Central Sterile Services Department
CVA	cerebrovascular accident
D&C	dilatation and curettage
DNA	did not attend
DUB	dysfunctional uterine bleeding
EB	endometrial biopsy
ECG	electrocardiograph
ET	endometrial thickness
EVTET	Estrogen in Venous ThromboEmbolism Trial
FDA	Food and Drug Administration
FSH	follicle-stimulating hormone
GIFT	gamete intrafallopian transfer
GnRH	gonadotrophin-releasing hormone
GP	general practitioner
HERS	Heart and Estrogen/progestagen Replacement Study
HIV	human immunodeficiency virus
HPV	human papilloma virus
HRT	hormone replacement therapy
HS	hysteroscopic sterilization
HSG	hysterosalpingography
HSS	hysteroscopic selective salpingography
IMB	intermenstrual bleeding
IVF	in vitro fertilization
IUCD	intrauterine contraceptive device
LH	luteinizing hormone
LLETZ	large loop excision of the transformation zone
LNG-IUS	levonorgestrel intrauterine system
LS	laparoscopic sterilization
MRI	magnetic resonance imaging
NICE	National Institute for Clinical Excellence
NSAIDs	non-steroidal anti-inflammatory drugs

ODA	Operating Department Assistant
ODP	Operating Department Practitioner
OPH	outpatient hysteroscopy
PCB	postcoital bleeding
PID	pelvic inflammatory disease
PMB	postmenopausal bleeding
POP	progesterone-only pill
PTB	proximal tubal blockage
RCA	Royal College of Anaesthetists
RCOG	Royal College of Obstetricians and Gynaecologists
RCT	randomized controlled trial
RF	radiofrequency
SCJ	squamocolumnar junction
SERMs	selective oestrogen receptor modulators
SIS	saline infusion sonography
STI	sexually transmitted infection
SWOT	strengths weaknesses opportunities threats
TC	tubal catheterization
TCU	treatment control unit
TENS	transcutaneous electrical nerve stimulation
TVS	transvaginal ultrasound
USS	ultrasound
WEST	Women's Estrogen for Stroke Trial
WHI	Women's Health Initiative

Part 1

Fundamentals of Outpatient Hysteroscopy

1

Normal anatomy and physiology of the uterus

ANATOMY

Uterus

The uterus is a hollow, pear-shaped pelvic organ with typical dimensions of 8 × 5 × 3 cm (Fig. 1.1). The fundus refers to the rounded upper part of the uterus and the uterine body to the main chamber. The openings of each fallopian tube (*ostia*) are seen where they connect to the upper angles of the uterus (*cornu*) demarcating the fundus from the body. The *isthmus* is the constricted lower part of the uterine body and includes the *internal cervical os* (opening to the uterine body). The *cervix* protrudes into the *vagina*, connecting the uterine

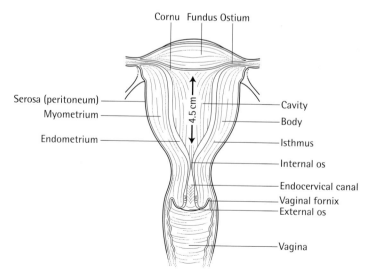

Figure 1.1 *Uterus, cervix and vagina.*

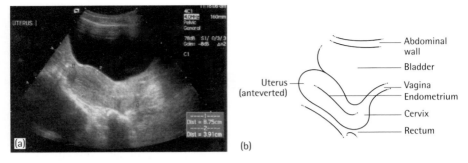

Figure 1.2 *Uterine relations ((a) transabdominal ultrasound; (b) saggital section).*

cavity at the internal os to the vagina at the *external os* (external uterine opening). This forms a sulcus (*fornix*), which is deepest posteriorly and separates the cervix into an intravaginal and supravaginal portion. The ratio of lengths of the uterine body to cervix is 2–3:1 in women of reproductive age and nearer 1:1 in postmenopausal women and prepubescent girls.

UTERINE WALLS AND CAVITY

The uterine body is predominantly made up of layers of ill-defined smooth muscle (myometrium) and the walls are between 1 and 3 cm thick. This dense muscular structure contains a central cavity, lined by smooth glandular columnar epithelium (*endometrium*). The cavity is triangular in shape tapering downwards from the fundus, which appears 'saddle-shaped' as a result of the slightly recessed cornua on either side (Plate 1). The anterior and posterior uterine walls are in apposition so that cavity appears as a cleft on sagittal section (e.g. on ultrasound – Fig. 1.2). The outer, intra-abdominal surface of the myometrium is covered with peritoneum and a thin layer of connective tissue (*serosa*).

UTERINE AXIS

Version of the uterus refers to the longitudinal axis of the uterus, at the level isthmus and cervix, in relation to the vagina. This axis or 'tilt' is commonly around 90° and the lower or cervical part of the uterus is considered to be *anteverted* if it is inclined anteriorly (note that the intravaginal cervix will point obliquely down and back) or *retroverted* if it is inclined posteriorly. *Flexion* of the uterus refers to the axis of the upper part of the uterus at the point where the body and cervix meet (isthmus). Thus the body of the uterus is described as *anteflexed* if it is flexed forwards on itself, or *retroflexed* if it is flexed backwards. The uterus is most commonly anteverted and anteflexed (in 70 per cent of women). In the remainder the uterus takes on an *axial* (mid-position) or retroverted and/or retroflexed position (Fig. 1.3). The sigmoid colon displaces the uterus so that it is usually deviated marginally towards the right side.

RELATIONS

The bladder is situated anteriorly, separated from the uterus by the uterovesical peritoneal pouch (Fig. 1.2). Posteriorly is the rectum, pouch of Douglas and contained small bowel loops and sigmoid colon. The broad ligament is sited laterally.

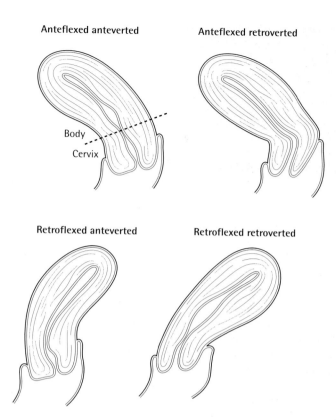

Figure 1.3 *Appreciation of the uterine position and attitude is important when performing hysteroscopy.*

SUPPORT

The uterus is held in the pelvis by several ligaments. These are, from above downwards, the *broad ligament, round ligaments, pubocervical ligaments, uterosacral ligaments* and *transverse cervical* (*cardinal*) *ligaments*. The broad ligament is a folded peritoneal sheet that drapes over the body of the uterus and fallopian tubes and contains loose cellular tissue (*parametrium*) within which reside the ureter and uterine artery. The round ligaments pass laterally from the body of the uterus, below the fallopian tubes, and travel up the sides of the pelvic walls to pass through the inguinal canal and insert into the connective tissue of the labia majus. These pubocervical, uterosacral and transverse cervical ligaments form a cross, which holds the uterus above the vagina, superior to the anterior defect in the levator ani muscle.

CLINICAL RELEVANCE

An appreciation of uterine landmarks, variations in the uterine axis and shape, and an understanding of the effects of hormones on the uterus and endometrium is required in order to optimize feasibility and diagnostic performance of hysteroscopy. The dense myometrium allows the overlying endometrium and associated lesions to be ablated or resected safely without compromising uterine integrity. However, if complications such as perforation do occur, awareness of the surrounding anatomy is needed to direct further investigation and management. Although the condition is beyond the remit of this book, a degree of uterovaginal prolapse is commonly encountered during routine hysteroscopy. Its presence may influence management decisions and so a sound knowledge of uterine structural supports is helpful.

Cervix

The cervix is the cylindrical lower extremity of the uterus and composed mainly of fibrous and elastic tissue with a relatively small amount of interwoven smooth muscle. The external os is circular in nulliparous women and slit-like in parous women. The endocervical canal is approximately 2–3 cm in length and is lined by simple columnar, endometrial-type epithelium that is thrown into oblique and longitudinal mucosal folds (*arbor vitae*) and connects the internal os to the external os (Plate 2). At the external os, this columnar mucosa abruptly meets the thicker, stratified squamous (non-keratinized) epithelium of the intravaginal ectocervix at the *squamocolumnar junction* (SCJ). The position of the SCJ varies according to oestrogen status (puberty, pregnancy, exogenous oestrogen), age and parity. In menopausal women, the SCJ 'retracts' within the canal and may be difficult to see. In women of reproductive age, the red, glandular columnar epithelium is usually seen encroaching onto the ectocervix, surrounding the external os and is correctly termed a cervical *ectropion* or *ectopy*. Throughout life, a transition takes place in the vicinity of the SCJ (*transformation zone*), from columnar to squamous epithelium. This process is known as squamous metaplasia and these epithelial changes predispose this site to premalignant (cervical intraepithelial neoplasia) transformation. The cervical screening programme obtains surface cytological samples of cervical epithelium (cervical smear) in an attempt to detect such changes so that local excisional treatment (large loop excision of the transformation zone or LLETZ) can be performed to prevent progression to overt malignancy.

CLINICAL RELEVANCE
Benign surface lesions

Nabothian follicles are commonly identified on cervical inspection and on ultrasound scanning. These mucoid cysts occur as a result of the squamous metaplasia when invaginated columnar epithelium becomes disconnected from the cervical surface and glandular secretion continues. They are of no significance although extremely large ones can be drained using a large-bore needle. A prominent cervical ectopy may be seen in association with increased circulating oestrogen (e.g. the combined oral contraceptive pill and pregnancy). Exposure of this fragile, glandular epithelium to the acidic vaginal environment may predispose to increased physiological vaginal discharge, intermenstrual and postcoital bleeding. Accessibility of the SCJ can be difficult in oestrogen-deficient women and can render sampling of the transformation zone inadequate. Such issues are important in colposcopy, but are less relevant to hysteroscopy and so will not be discussed further.

Endocervical canal

Traversing the endocervical canal endoscopically requires an appreciation of the cervical axis and the irregular nature of the lining glandular mucosa. In addition, previous excision biopsies of the transformation zone and menopausal state will shorten the intravaginal cervix and narrow the endocervical canal influencing the operative approach (see Chapter 4).

Vagina

The vagina is a 7–10 cm fibromuscular tube (posterior wall 1 cm longer than anterior wall), which connects the vestibule to the cervix, and it is enclosed in highly vascular and richly innervated connective tissue. It is directed up and back at a 45° angle to the horizontal and at 90° to the long axis of the uterus. It is lined by thick, non-keratinized, stratified squamous epithelium, which is continuous with the ectocervix. The epithelium is rich in glycogen in women of reproductive age, which is the substrate acted upon by Doderlein's bacillus to produce lactic acid and a protective acidic vaginal pH of 4.5. The hymen is a thin mucous membrane that closes the vaginal entrance prepubertally and is torn in reproductive life leaving small tag-like remnants (*carunculae myritiformes*).

CLINICAL RELEVANCE

The course of the ureters and uterine arteries are of some clinical importance in relation to administering local anaesthetic blocks and hysteroscopic perforation. The ureters run along the lateral aspects of the vagina, close to the cervix, into the bladder, which sits anteriorly on the vagina. The uterine arteries are located in close proximity to the ureters (i.e. a short distance superior and lateral to the infravaginal cervix). The posterior fornix is covered with peritoneum, situated inferiorly to the pouch of Douglas, facilitating voluntary (or involuntary!) access to the peritoneal cavity.

Vulva

The vulva or external genitalia, is a collective term that comprises the *mons pubis, labia majora, labia minora, clitoris* and *vestibule* of the vagina (Fig. 1.4). The perineum refers to the area below the pelvic diaphragm (levator ani and coccygeus) which contains the external genitalia (anterior) and anal region (posterior).

The labia majora form the lateral boundary of the vulva extending from the mons pubis (subcutaneous mound of hairy skin and subcutaneous fat overlying the symphysis pubis) to the posterior perineum. They consist of stratified squamous epithelium with hair follicles, sweat and sebaceous glands and fat. The labia minora are sited inside the labia majora and are also folds of stratified squamous epithelium that contain sebaceous and sweat glands (*lesser vestibular glands*). They divide anteriorly to enclose the clitoris, and posteriorly they fuse to form the fourchette. The cleft contained within these boundaries (up to the hymen) is known as the vestibule into which opens the vagina, urethra, paraurethral (Skene's) ducts and the ducts of the Bartholin's glands (*greater vestibular glands*). The ducts of the latter mucus-secreting gland open posterior-laterally.

CLINICAL RELEVANCE

A working knowledge of the anatomy and pathology (see Chapter 11) of this region is useful to the hysteroscopist as the area is easily exposed and abnormalities may be contributory to presenting symptoms (e.g. discharge and bleeding). The external, caudal position,

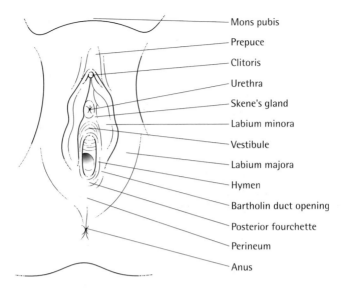

Mons pubis
Prepuce
Clitoris
Urethra
Skene's gland
Labium minora
Vestibule
Labium majora
Hymen
Bartholin duct opening
Posterior fourchette
Perineum
Anus

Figure 1.4 *Vulva and perineum.*

the contained structures and the oestrogen sensitivity subject the vulva to both physiological and pathological processes. These include benign lesions (cysts of various types,
lipomas, vulval varicosities, urethral caruncle or prolapse), infection (bacterial – glandular
abscess; viruses – human papilloma virus and herpes simplex; yeast – candida), skin disorders
(general dermatoses, lichen sclerosis or squamous hyperplasia), senile changes (atrophic vulvovaginitis, urogenital atrophy and inflammation from urinary leakage) and oncological
changes (vulval intraepithelial neoplasia and cancer). The area is richly supplied with
somatic nerves and so gentle manipulation and instrumentation are necessary.

Blood supply and lymphatic drainage of the pelvis and genital tract

The pelvis is supplied by three paired arteries – the *internal iliac, superior rectal* and *ovarian arteries,* and one single artery (the *median sacral artery*). The internal iliac arteries give
off both visceral and parietal branches to the female reproductive tract, which include the
uterine, vaginal, inferior vesical, middle rectal and *internal pudendal arteries.* The main
vascular supply to the uterus comes from the *uterine artery,* which descends on the lateral
pelvic wall, anterior and superior to the ureter, and enters the base of the broad ligament
to reach the lateral margin of the uterus at the level of the cervix, above the lateral
vaginal fornix (Fig. 1.5). It follows a tortuous course to give off numerous anastomosing
branches to the uterus, cervix, vagina and bladder. In addition, the uterus receives a vascular
supply from the ovarian (infra-renal branch of abdominal aorta) and vaginal arteries, which
anastomose with branches of the uterine artery. The vaginal artery passes along the side of
the vagina to supply it as well as part of the bladder and urethra. In addition, the vagina
receives a vascular supply from the inferior vesical and middle rectal arteries. The external
genitalia are supplied by the branches of the internal pudendal artery. The primary mode of

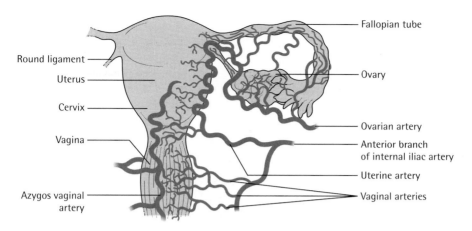

Figure 1.5 *Blood supply to the uterus, cervix and vagina.*

venous drainage is via pelvic venous plexuses that empty into the internal iliac vein. Lymphatic drainage of the uterus, cervix and upper vagina is via lymph nodes sited along the iliac vessels. The lower vagina and vulva communicates with the deep and superficial inguinal lymph nodes and rectal lymphatic plexus.

CLINICAL RELEVANCE

The uterine arteries are located approximately 1.5 cm above the lateral vaginal fornix and give off descending cervicovaginal branches. Care must be taken to avoid direct intravascular injection of local anaesthetic by aspirating prior to injection and avoiding deep paracervical injection.

Innervation of the pelvis and genital tract

The pelvis is innervated by the both the sympathetic and parasympathetic autonomic nervous system (Fig. 1.6). The pelvic sympathetic supply derives from the two *inferior hypogastric (pelvic) plexuses,* which in turn form secondary plexuses to supply the pelvic viscera and vessels. The *uterovaginal plexus* is distributed to the cervix and along the uterine and vaginal arteries. The *ventral rami of the sacral nerves* (S2–4) carry parasympathetic nerve fibres into the pelvis. Afferent (pain) fibres from the upper vagina, cervix and lower uterus travel in these parasympathetic *pelvic splanchnic nerves* to the dorsal roots of the upper sacral nerves (S2–4), while those from the body of the uterus and proximal fallopian tube run along the sympathetic *pelvic/abdominal plexuses* to the lower thoracic and upper lumbar roots (T10–L1). Pain will thus be referred to the corresponding dermatomes. Afferent somatic nerve stimuli are relayed from the lower vagina, vulva and perineum via the *ilioinguinal nerve* (L1), *genitofemoral nerve* (L1–2) and *perineal branch of the pudendal nerve* (S2–4).

CLINICAL RELEVANCE

The concentrated somatic nerve supply to the external genitalia renders this region extremely sensitive so that gentle manipulation and instrumentation are essential prerequisites in

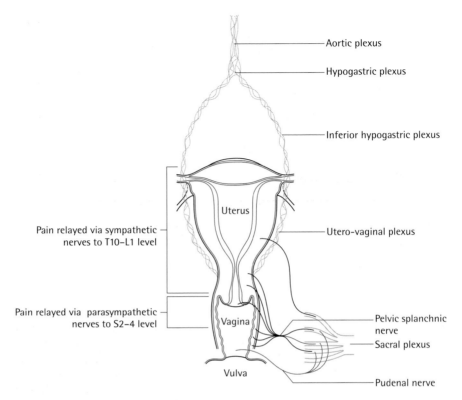

Figure 1.6 *Innervation of the uterus, cervix and vagina.*

order to avoid precipitating discomfort. The sensory nerve distribution precludes complete uterine anaesthesia via local means. Painful stimuli triggered in response to induced uterine contractions, uterine distension and touch at the uterine fundus especially in the cornual regions will be relayed via sympathetic nerves back to T10–L1. This can be a hindrance to the operating office hysteroscopist. However, many of the parasympathetic nerve fibres relaying pain via the pelvic splanchnics back to S2–4 from the lower uterus, cervix and upper vagina can be effectively blocked with local anaesthetic (see Chapter 12). Pain arising from cervical dilatation and torque from hysteroscope movement can thus be eradicated. Outpatient surgery is further facilitated by the relative insensitivity of the uterine body to cutting and heat. Preprocedure administration of simple analgesics, such as non-steroidal anti-inflammatory drugs, will help reduce diffuse visceral pain especially that arising from induced myometrial activity.

ENDOCRINOLOGY AND HISTOLOGY

An understanding of endocrinology underpinning the menstrual cycle, as well as accompanying histological changes within the uterus, enables interpretation of hysteroscopic findings, correlation with symptomatology and a rational basis for treatment.

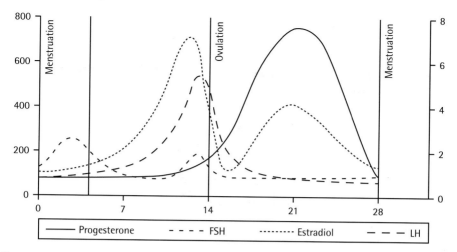

Figure 1.7 *Hormone levels during the menstrual cycle.*

Endocrinology of the menstrual cycle

The endocrine changes of the normal menstrual cycle are shown in Fig. 1.7. Day 1 of the menstrual cycle refers to the first day of menstruation. At this time oestrogen levels are low and follicle-stimulating hormone (FSH) is secreted by the pituitary gland and stimulates follicular development within the ovary. The granulosa cells of the growing follicles produce oestrogen, which acts upon both the hypothalamus (reducing gonadotrophin-releasing hormone production [GnRH]) and pituitary gland. Secretion of FSH from the pituitary is thus inhibited (negative feedback) and circulating FSH levels fall. Only the largest 'lead' follicle possesses enough FSH receptors to continue growth and oestrogen production, the other follicles becoming atretic (days 5–7).

Serum oestrogen concentration rises gradually as the lead follicle matures and eventually crosses a 'threshold' level that releases the pituitary gland from its inhibited state and stimulates it to release luteinizing hormone (LH) and to a lesser degree FSH (positive feedback). This hormonal 'surge' triggers ovulation (day 14) and oestrogen levels fall temporarily so that positive feedback on the hypothalamus and pituitary ceases and is replaced by a negative feedback effect resulting in a fall in FSH and LH. The collapsed postovulatory follicle is transformed into a *corpus luteum*. The granulosa and theca cells of the newly formed corpus luteum produce oestrogen, and more importantly progesterone, so that a stable secretory endometrium is produced in anticipation of conception and ensuing embryonic implantation.

In the absence of pregnancy (trophoblast producing human chorionic gonadotrophin), the corpus luteum cannot be maintained and starts to wane after 7–10 days. Hormone production declines rapidly and it is this progesterone withdrawal that triggers menstruation 14 days following ovulation. Although, a 28-day cycle is illustrated in Fig. 1.7, many women may have longer or shorter cycles. The luteal (secretory) phase is relatively constant (12–14 days) in a regular cycle and so cycle variation is thought to reflects differing lengths of the preovulatory proliferative phase (9–22 days). Thus a woman with a regular 35-day cycle is likely to ovulate around day 21. Normal menstrual cycle parameters are shown in Information Box 1.1.

Information Box 1.1 Normal menstrual cycle parameters

- Cycle duration: 28 days (21–35 days)
- Days of flow: 5 days (2–8 days)
- Estimated blood loss: 35 ml per cycle (20–80 ml)

Histology of the uterus and the menstrual cycle

The uterus is a hollow, muscular organ (*myometrium*) lined by a glandular epithelium (*endometrium*). This is shown schematically in Fig. 1.1 (page 3).

Endometrium

The endometrium can be divided into two layers, the superficial *lamina functionalis* and the deeper *lamina basalis*. During the menstrual cycle, the lamina functionalis goes through a cycle of proliferation, secretion and shedding.

PROLIFERATIVE PHASE (OESTROGEN)

Oestrogen produced by ovarian follicular activity acts upon the thin, raw postmenstrual endometrium causing the epithelium of glands in the lamina basalis to proliferate. Stromal cells expand and grow, thickening the newly formed lamina functionalis, into which blood vessels (spiral arterioles) grow.

SECRETORY PHASE (PROGESTERONE)

Progesterone produced by the postovulatory corpus luteum, converts the proliferative, oestrogen-dominated, endometrium into a secretory, progesterone-influenced one. Glands become tortuous, convoluted and distended with glycoproteins secreted by the lining epithelium. Simultaneously, loosely packed stromal cells increase in size and blood vessels feeding the endometrium become coiled and spiral shaped.

MENSTRUAL PHASE

Regression of the corpus luteum and consequent decline in oestrogen and progesterone levels causes the lamina functionalis to be shed. This arises as a result of constriction of the spiral arterioles, which produces ischaemia, necrosis and bleeding. The glands, connective tissue and blood vessels of the superficial lamina functionalis disintegrate forming menstrual fluid (i.e. sloughed endometrium, mucus and blood). The deeper basal layer (lamina basalis) is able to maintain its blood supply so that epithelium can regenerate from within its embedded glands.

PREGNANCY

Maintenance of the endometrium by the corpus luteum lasts only 14 days unless fertilization and implantation occur. Implantation results in extension of the life of the corpus luteum, a *corpus luteum of pregnancy*, which maintains the decidual, progestinized endometrium.

Myometrium

The myometrium consists of multidirectional smooth muscle bundles held together by connective tissue and pierced by blood vessels and nerves. On average this muscular wall is 12–15 mm thick, but may be 30 mm thick in parts of the body and fundus of the uterus. The myometrium does not undergo structural cyclical alteration, but smooth muscle contractile activity increases during menstruation causing pain. The smooth muscle cells are capable of increase in size (hypertrophy) and increase in number (hyperplasia), as is seen in the gravid uterus.

Serosa (perimetrium)

This is the outer (anterior and posterior) serous covering of pelvic peritoneum and connective tissue.

Cervix

The secretion from glands within the cervix varies in composition during the menstrual cycle. At the beginning of the cycle, cervical mucus is thick, opaque and scant. Mucus production increases during the proliferative phase and peaks around ovulation. The mucus at this time is thin, stretchy and watery so as to promote the passage of sperm (and hysteroscopes!). During the secretory phase, the mucus again becomes thick so as to serve as a barrier to micro-organisms. The glandular columnar epithelium of the endocervix does not generally desquamate during menstruation although some cyclical changes occur.

Endocrinology, histology and abnormal uterine bleeding

Abnormal menstrual cycles fall outside the parameters given in Information Box 1.1. Although various terms have been traditionally used to label abnormal menstrual cycles (e.g. *polymenorrhoea*, *oligomenorrhoea* and *metrorrhagia*), they are better described as frequent, infrequent and irregular respectively. Similarly, excess or heavy or prolonged menstrual bleeding is a clearer explanation than *menorrhagia* or *hypermenorrhoea* and heavy, irregular menstrual bleeding should replace the cumbersome term *menometrorrhagia*. It should be noted that regardless of the pattern of menstrual disturbance, in the absence of serious underlying pathology and anaemia, the need for treatment is dependent upon the impact of symptoms upon a woman's quality of life (see Chapter 10).

Dysfunctional uterine bleeding (DUB)

This is heavy and/or irregular menstrual bleeding in the absence of recognizable pelvic pathology and results from abnormalities in the hypothalamo-pituitary–ovarian–endometrial axis. It is usefully classified as ovulatory and anovulatory.

OVULATORY (80 PER CENT)

- *Inadequate luteal phase.* In the absence of pregnancy, the life of the corpus luteum is relatively constant so that the secretory (luteal) phase of the menstrual cycle is over

10 days (14 days on average). It is believed that inadequate follicular development results in short luteal phase and reduced progesterone levels.

- *Local factors*. The myometrium and deeper layers of endometrium (lamina basalis) are richly supplied by a dense network of outer arcuate and inner radial arteries, which terminate as convoluted spiral arterioles in the lamina functionalis. It is thought that differences in production of locally active, endometrial products, involved in inflammatory and regenerative processes (growth factors, prostaglandins, endothelins, etc.) can precipitate DUB probably because of inadequate vasoconstriction and other haemostatic mechanisms.

ANOVULATORY (20 PER CENT)

Ovulation followed by sex hormone production by the resulting corpus luteum is key to cycle regulation. In the absence of ovulation (e.g. failure of ovarian follicular development), progesterone production by the corpus luteum does not occur and the endometrium is not converted to a stable secretory one, but continues to proliferate in response to unopposed oestrogen. Scheduled and organized endometrial shedding in response to progesterone withdrawal does not occur, resulting in unpredictable and prolonged bleeding. This pattern is most common at the extremes of reproductive life (a reflection of developing or deteriorating ovarian function) and is a common reason for referral to a hysteroscopy clinic. This is because anovulatory bleeding is more often refractory to medical therapy and can be a result of endometrial hyperplasia.

Intermenstrual bleeding

In some women the precipitate mid-cycle, periovulatory fall in oestrogen can stimulate a degree of endometrial shedding (analogous to menstruation). Hormone production by the corpus luteum reinstates endometrial support and such physiological bleeding is consequently light and of short duration. Localized abdominal pain (Mittelschmerz) resulting from peritoneal irritation following ovulation may accompany bleeding of this type.

Menopause

The menopause (cessation of menstruation) is diagnosed retrospectively after a year without a menstrual period (*amenorrhoea*). The climacteric refers to a transitory period (usually 2–5 years) prior to the menopause that is associated with typical menopausal symptoms arising from oestrogen deficiency. Ovarian oestrogen production falls because the number of ovarian follicles are progressively 'used up' with numbers declining throughout reproductive life. Around the age of 50 years there are no follicles remaining capable of responding to gonadotrophin stimulation from the pituitary gland. Follicular oestrogen production stops, menses cease and characteristic symptoms and signs of oestrogen deficiency occur. General atrophy of the whole genital tract occurs. The uterine body shrinks to a greater degree relative to the cervix and the squamocolumnar junction 'retracts' into the endocervical canal.

From an endocrine point of view, oestrogen deficiency releases the hypothalamus and pituitary from inhibition (negative feedback) and FSH and LH levels become markedly elevated in an attempt to stimulate the resistant ovary. This compensatory increase in FSH and

LH can be measured (although absolute levels are of little clinical value unless premature ovarian failure is being investigated) and persists for around 10 years until the pituitary becomes exhausted and levels decline. This hypothalamo-pituitary hyperactivity begins 10 years before the menopause in response to accelerated loss of ovarian follicles after 35–40 years. As the menopause approaches, DUB (and endometrial hyperplasia) often results from anovulatory cycles or a deficient luteal (progesterone) phase.

In women of reproductive age, the predominant circulating oestrogen is β-estradiol produced by the ovary. The less potent estrone, is the main postmenopausal oestrogen and is produced by peripheral conversion of androgens (androstenedione and testosterone) produced by the ovarian stroma and adrenal cortex.

 KEY POINTS

- The anatomy of the uterus, cervix and lower genital tract changes with age and hormonal status.

- Normal production and secretion of hormones by the hypothalamo-pituitary–ovarian axis is key to a woman's menstrual cycle and fertility.

- Physiological or pathological processes that interfere with ovarian production of oestrogen and progesterone, or endocrine responses within the endometrium, explain the majority of abnormal uterine bleeding patterns.

- A sound understanding of anatomy and physiology of the female reproductive system is necessary to interpret symptoms and clinical findings and successfully perform hysteroscopy and related interventions.

FURTHER READING

Jeffcoate SL. In: de Swiet M and Chamberlain G, eds. *Endocrinology in Basic Science in Obstetrics and Gynaecology, 2nd edn.* London: Churchill Livingstone, 1992, Chapter 7.

Last RJ. Abdomen. In: McMinn RMH, ed. *Last's Anatomy, Regional and Applied, 9th edn.* London: Churchill Livingstone, 1994, Chapter 5.

2

Setting up an outpatient hysteroscopy 'diagnosis and treatment' service

INTRODUCTION

It is envisaged that day case outpatient diagnostic and treatment services will dramatically expand in all clinical specialities over the next few years. This change is already in process, driven by many factors including advances in the field of medicine, expansion of patient choice, political influence and economic pressures. The latter part of the twentieth century saw reductions in the length of stay for hospital inpatients across the board. The changing paradigm now involves transferring traditionally inpatient procedures to a day surgery or even further into the outpatient setting.

Outpatient or 'ambulatory' hysteroscopy clinics provide a means of delivering both diagnosis and treatments for many gynaecological conditions. The entire female genital tract can be examined with the use of clinical and relatively non-invasive diagnostic tests such as ultrasound, miniature hysteroscopy and endometrial biopsy. Advances in endoscopy have facilitated access and treatment of benign conditions affecting the uterus and lower genital tract without the need for general anaesthetic or conscious sedation. The outpatient hysteroscopy clinic is thus an ideal environment to deliver a modern 'see and treat' service. This book aims to provide a concise but comprehensive manual for gynaecologists with an interest in participating in outpatient hysteroscopy services.

DEFINITIONS

If you peruse the literature, it quickly becomes apparent that the terms *outpatient, office, ambulatory* and *day case* mean different things to different people. This book is primarily

Information Box 2.1 Definitions

OUTPATIENT OR OFFICE PROCEDURE

Outpatient procedures are performed in an appropriate clinic setting, but without the need for formal operating theatre facilities or general anaesthesia. These clinics are usually within a hospital outpatient department (an *outpatient hysteroscopy clinic*), but contain specific minor operative rooms, other multipurpose facilities or primary care centres. In some parts of the world, particularly the United States, the term *office* is preferred. *True outpatient procedures* will be discharged unaccompanied within the allocated clinic time and do not require a formal recovery period in a hospital bed. However, for the purpose of this book we have included procedures that may require prolonged postoperative recovery times in dedicated ward areas of up to 4 hours.

AMBULATORY PROCEDURE

This term is generally used interchangeably to mean some form of outpatient or day case intervention where the patient is quickly mobilized following surgery without the need for prolonged bed rest. Strictly speaking, ambulatory implies an ability of the patient to mobilize immediately post procedure (i.e. walk out of the operating room). This terminology is probably best avoided.

DAY CASE OR DAY SURGERY

Day surgery is the admission of selected patients to hospital for a planned surgical procedure, and they return home on the same day. *Outpatient* procedures may be considered a subgroup of day case surgery. *True day surgery* patients are day case patients who require full operating theatre facilities with most requiring general anaesthesia. There are now moves to provide dedicated 23-hour services, so that the definition of day case procedures can be expanded to include all hospital stays of under 24 hours' duration.

---

concerned with procedures performed in a hysteroscopy clinic without the use of general anaesthetic. The term outpatient will be used throughout the book for consistency. Definitions are given in Information Box 2.1.

RATIONALE

Is increasingly invasive outpatient diagnosis and treatment justified? To answer this, we need to consider the potential advantages and disadvantages of a move to such services for all 'stakeholders'. This includes patients, healthcare professionals, clinicians, managers, government departments and society at large (Information Boxes 2.2, 2.3).

Over the last few years, outpatient hysteroscopy services have been developed, primarily to provide a diagnostic service. 'Therapy' has been restricted to location and retrieval of intrauterine devices. However, there is an increasing move from an essentially diagnostic

Information Box 2.2 Need for outpatient hysteroscopy? Advantages

PATIENT

- *Choice.* Patients want treatment that is safe, efficient, effective, and one that provides the least possible disruption to their lives. Patients receive treatment that is suited to their needs allowing them to recover in their own home ('patient-centred care'). Most patients report high satisfaction and willingness to recommend this service based on their experience.
- *Convenience.* No need for preoperative general anaesthetic work up or fasting. Rapid postoperative recovery with expectation to return home on the same day. Minimal constraints on activities in contrast to general anaesthesia.
- *Access.* Outpatient surgery provides a means of treating patients faster.
- *Autonomy.* The conscious patient is empowered.
- *Safety.* High-risk medical patients avoid risks of general anaesthesia. Patient feedback to the operator and inherent limitations of extent of surgery reduce the potential for serious morbidity and complications. In addition the risk of hospital-acquired infection is reduced.

CLINICIAN

- *Satisfaction.* Clinicians can provide contemporary, high-quality care for appropriate patients. This enhances job satisfaction, as does the development of a cohesive and motivated team. This field is expanding because of new developments so it is an exciting and stimulating area to be involved in.
- *Autonomy.* It is a 'clinician-centred' service. There is less reliance on other professionals, so that cancellations due to theatre overruns are avoided.
- *Optimize inpatient surgery.* Inpatient beds and formal theatre time is released for more major cases. Planning lists and scheduling surgery is thus optimized.

SOCIETY

- *Cost-efficiency.* Cancellation of patients from emergency pressures in a dedicated out-patient clinic is unlikely. Health resource use is reduced by avoidance of formal theatre facilities and staffing (obviate the need for anaesthetists, nursing staff for preoperative care, theatre and recovery staff, Operating Department Practitioners (ODPs), Operating Department Assistants (ODAs) etc.) and hospital stay (assuming competitive outpatient equipment costs).
- *Delivery of health care.* Health service capacity is increased. Patient throughput is improved and waiting lists are reduced.

service (the viability of which is questionable given the accuracy and usefulness of ultrasound and miniature endometrial biopsy devices) to a comprehensive 'see and treat' service. Many factors have driven this change and the most important of these are illustrated in Fig. 2.1.

Information Box 2.3 Need for outpatient hysteroscopy? Disadvantages

PATIENT

- *Pain.* Inability to completely anaesthetize the uterus in a conscious patient without regional blocks.
- *Complaints.* A minority of women will be dissatisfied with their experience (pain, embarrassment etc.) despite attention to good practice. Prompts from patients should be acted upon.
- *Embarrassment.* This feeling can arise because of the intimate nature of the examination, exposure from the lithotomy position, numbers of personnel present and insensitive comments/behaviour.

CLINICIAN

- *Feasibility.* Outpatient surgery is limited by a number of factors including discomfort, procedure duration, severity of pathology, miniaturization of endoscopic equipment can reduce intra-operative visualization and uterine distension.
- *Additional training required.* Additional operator skills are required and these are often underestimated. Generic skills required include communication, ability to 'multitask', team working, calmness, efficiency and gentle tissue handling.
- *Effectiveness.* Observational series are suggestive of benefit, but experimental data are lacking to support claims (although the same argument can be made for 'established' inpatient procedures).

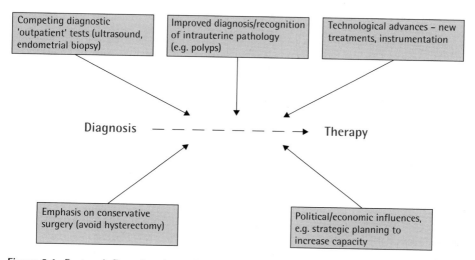

Figure 2.1 *Factors influencing the evolution of 'see and treat' outpatient hysteroscopy.*

SERVICE DEVELOPMENT

Identifying and overcoming obstacles

Outpatient diagnosis and surgery provide a means of treating patients faster and potentially more effectively. Despite the benefits, obstacles to change may need to be identified and overcome. Modernization may require fundamental changes to ingrained and outmoded practices. These may include overcoming clinicians' preferences for inpatient surgery by demonstrating the feasibility and success of outpatient intervention. Clinicians and patients in both primary and secondary care should be made aware of well-organized outpatient services so that appropriate patients are referred. Shorter waiting times, high patient turnover and efficient resource use should be highlighted and championed so that outpatient intervention is recognized as a priority by health service management. Local incentives such as enhanced resources may help facilitate change.

Identifying procedures

It has been recognized that many elective operations are suitable for day surgery, which includes outpatient surgery. It has been suggested that the historical standard, *'Is this patient suitable for day surgery?'* should be replaced by, *'Is there any justification for admitting this case as an inpatient?'* It follows that the standard, *'Is this patient suitable for outpatient surgery?'* should be replaced by, *'Is there any justification for performing this case under general anaesthesia and/or a requirement for full operating facilities?'*

This book identifies and describes all gynaecological procedures suitable for performance in an outpatient hysteroscopy clinic. They are listed in Table 2.1. Advances in medical technologies are likely to mean that, over time, many more procedures will move from inpatient to day case or day case to outpatients, so proscriptive lists of procedures will undoubtedly change.

Infrastructure

A fully equipped treatment room is required. This may be a dedicated hysteroscopy suite or a multipurpose facility (e.g. incorporating other gynaecological procedures such as urodynamics,

Table 2.1 *Outpatient hysteroscopic surgery*

Procedure	Feasibility in outpatients	Limitations
Directed biopsy	√√√	Size of sample
Mirena intrauterine system	√√√	Shape of uterine cavity
Endometrial destruction	√√√	Pain
Myomectomy	√	Grade; size; location
Polypectomy	√√√	Location
Adhesiolysis	√	Extent of pathology
Uterine corrective surgery	√	Extent of pathology
Sterilisation	√√	Visualization and access

Feasibility in unselected patients: √√√ >90%, √√ 80–90%, √ <80%

colposcopy, etc., or other endoscopic procedures). The general set-up, staffing and skill requirements to enable diagnostic and operative outpatient hysteroscopy are listed in Information Box 2.4.

Information Box 2.4 Set-up for operative hysteroscopy

STAFF

- *Receptionist/ward clerk.* Administrative and clerical staff are needed to meet patients and enter details/access case notes.
- *Two dedicated nurses.* Trained in relevant techniques (one should assist the operator and the other act as a 'runner' and stand-by patient advocate).
- *Healthcare assistant/additional nurse.* This person is pivotal to success, staying next to the patient at all times, understanding the procedures and answering questions. Their most important role involves conversing, comforting and supporting the patient. By distracting the patient they are in effect an additional 'local anaesthetist' or 'vocal local'!
- *Operator.* The surgeon should have mastered the relevant procedures and acquired expertise in terms of judgement of feasibility, tissue handling, and efficiency. Good communication skills are paramount.

FACILITIES

- *Reception and administrative facilities.* An area to accommodate and process patients on arrival.
- *Fully equipped treatment room.* This should be a private and patient-friendly environment with a dedicated changing area. It should possess an adjustable operating couch and resuscitation facilities.
- *Hysteroscopy equipment.* Endoscopes, distension media and ancillary instrumentation are discussed in Chapter 3 and in the relevant chapters for specific procedures. The 'stack' should include a monitor, a light source of suitable quality and a camera system. Digital still and moving image capture is a useful adjunct.
- *Information technology.* A computer system with internet access allows data storage in suitable secure databases, which facilitates prospective data collection, and is useful not only in research, but also for ongoing audit as part of clinical governance. More sophisticated programming set-ups can allow the generation of data summaries (with multimedia) for recording within the case notes and letters to primary care physicians – this can be a time-saving resource. Internet access to secure clinic web sites can facilitate booking of appointments via primary care and provide an accessible source of information for patients.
- *Recovery area.* Most patients and relatives will just require sitting accommodation and access to beverages prior to discharge. Access to a formal recovery area with beds (e.g. day case unit) may be necessary if more invasive procedures are undertaken, or in the event of unanticipated patient responses.
- *Equipment maintenance and sterilization.* Decontamination facilities of sufficient standard (see Chapter 3).

Information Box 2.5 Example: referral guidelines for abnormal uterine bleeding

Hysteroscopy can be indicated for investigation of infertility, recurrent pregnancy loss, abnormal glandular cervical smears and for removal of foreign bodies. However, these indications are infrequent and indeed questionable as they are often better investigated by other means. Abnormal uterine bleeding is a common problem and is the main indicator for hysteroscopic evaluation. It can occur in women of all ages. Symptomatic women may harbour serious endometrial pathology, especially postmenopausal women (who should be seen within 2 weeks of referral) and so an effective, efficient service is mandatory. To achieve this requires implementing and disseminating strict evidence-based referral guidelines.

An example of developed and piloted guidelines is shown in Information Box 2.6. The rationale for these guidelines is as follows. Endometrial cancer and premalignant atypical hyperplasia are unlikely causes of abnormal bleeding patterns below the age of 40 years, but become increasingly important after this age. Women under 40 with menorrhagia may require hysteroscopic investigation if intrauterine pathology is suspected on less invasive transvaginal ultrasound scan or if suspected from the severity and persistence of symptoms despite recommended medical treatment. Women can thus be triaged in this way to investigate those most likely to have pathology, preventing the service being overwhelmed and becoming inefficient, and avoiding unnecessary intervention, which in itself can cause undue anxiety and waste resources.

Such guidelines/protocols should be formulated with, and disseminated to, primary care physicians and referring gynaecologists to ensure compliance and improving access for patients to treatment. In Birmingham, this is achieved by providing all general practitioners (GPs) with carbon copies of the referral criteria to avoid the need for traditional referral letters. These guidelines and patient information leaflets are also available on the NHS network to allow on-line booking by GPs who can also print off information sheets for their patients.

Running the service

The purpose and extent of the outpatient hysteroscopy service must be clear and based on local factors (e.g. population, health priorities, resources, etc.) and current best evidence. A recent survey reported that 28 per cent of UK consultant gynaecologists perform, or were in the process of setting up, an outpatient hysteroscopy service. In the main these are diagnostic services, but therapeutic 'see and treat' services are rapidly evolving. Suggested approaches for service development are outlined throughout the book. Here we take the example of a diagnostic service to illustrate the importance of strict referral guidelines to provide a rational basis for investigation and enable efficient service provision (Information Boxes 2.5, 2.6).

Clinical process and development of protocols

The entire patient experience should be anticipated and planned. The development and implementation of explicit management protocols is useful.

> ## i Information Box 2.6 Referral criteria for outpatient hysteroscopy in women with abnormal uterine bleeding
>
> 1   Postmenopausal bleeding.
>
> 2   Persistent ($\geqslant$3–6 months' duration) unscheduled bleeding on hormone replacement therapy (HRT)/tamoxifen treatment.
>
> 3   Persistent ($\geqslant$3–6 months' duration) intermenstrual bleeding in premenopausal women $\geqslant$40 years of age.
>
> 4 $\geqslant$40 years with regular heavy periods (menorrhagia or ovular dysfunctional uterine bleeding (DUB)) who have failed to respond to $\geqslant$3–6 months of medical treatment
>   - tranexamic acid 0.5–1.5 g tds during menses
>   - mefanamic acid 500 mg tds during menses
>   - combined oral contraceptive pill
>   - continuous danazol 100–200 mg daily
>   - progestogens (systemic/local).
>   (If you have ticked this box, **please do not refer,** until one or more of the above treatments has been prescribed for $\geqslant$3–6 months' duration.)
>
> 5   Irregular heavy periods (anovular DUB), failed response to at least 6 months' treatment with progestogens + medical treatment shown above.

PREOPERATIVE ASSESSMENT FOR SUITABILITY AND PATIENT SELECTION

Rigorous preoperative assessment is required prior to any general anaesthetic. As outpatient intervention avoids general anaesthesia, such assessment is not required and furthermore, patients considered high risk for anaesthesia (elderly, obese, cardiovascular and respiratory disease, etc.) present little additional risk with short outpatient interventional procedures. It is tempting to decline outpatient intervention in highly anxious patients, but experience has shown that the ability to predict the minority of patients who turn out to be unsuitable (i.e. unable to tolerate, dissatisfaction with experience, etc.) is poor. In general, a better approach is to offer all patients choice, and provide accurate written and verbal information about the entire outpatient hysteroscopic experience.

OPERATION

Attention to good operative assessment and technique is essential and these are described in the proceeding chapters.

POSTOPERATIVE CARE

Patients should be reassured that in the unlikely event that they are not ready to go home on the same day, they will have the opportunity to stay overnight. The fitness of all patients for discharge should be ascertained and discharge protocols formulated. Patients/carers must understand any constraints on activities following any procedure, particularly if opiate analgesia/sedatives were administered. An adequate supply of postoperative analgesia is essential following certain procedures (e.g. endometrial ablation) along with written infor-mation on how to take it. Written information should also be provided to include information about potential side effects/complications, what the patient should do should a problem arise and an emergency contact number given (ideally 24-hour support, without reliance on primary care, should be provided). Follow-up arrangements are not routinely required, but nurse-led protocols, such as a courtesy phone call the following day, may be useful and reassuring to patients. Good-quality outpatient surgery should have no significant impact on primary or social care services.

Unit management

This should be headed by a lead clinician and day surgery manager/senior nurse who should lead on innovations and development in practice as well as promoting the service in order to prioritize funding. Clear policies and protocols (see above) should be in place and updated to ensure the smooth running of the unit. Two areas that warrant further discussion are staff training and clinical audit.

STAFFING AND TRAINING

Clinicians and nursing staff need to feel confident in their abilities to carry out outpatient hysteroscopic interventions and this is achieved through appropriate training. Specific training is required in outpatient hysteroscopic technique and the advantages for patients. Owing to the practical nature of outpatient intervention, beneficial training might consist of secondment of doctors and nurses to existing units in order to see and experience outpatient hysteroscopy on a first-hand basis. Attendance at theoretical and practical courses in 'see and treat' outpatient hysteroscopic intervention may be useful. All trainees should experience outpatient hysteroscopy during their training.

Investing in training a multiskilled workforce will help develop a cohesive, flexible and motivated team and increase staff retention. Staff will be better able to inform and educate patients and carers if they are familiar with the entire patient experience. Nursing staff should be encouraged to further develop their competencies and thus make a fuller contribution to service provision. The development in the UK of a formalized programme for training of 'nurse hysteroscopists' is such an example of extending traditional roles and modernizing service delivery.

AUDIT

Clinical governance is a priority with emphasis placed on clinical risk management and clinical audit. Outpatient and inpatient activity for selected procedures should be monitored periodically to assess the impact of a 'see and treat' outpatient hysteroscopy clinic. (NB: The UK Department of Health envisages that 75 per cent of all elective surgery will be carried out as day case procedures by 2007). Other outcomes should be audited (e.g. unplanned admissions, 'did not attend' (DNA) rate, appropriate patient selection, adherence to protocols and remedial solutions formulated where practice is deficient).

BUSINESS PLANS

Setting up innovative new services requires the identification of funding sources (e.g. cancer networks, waiting list monies, primary care service developments, payment by results, etc.) obtaining this financial backing and securing managerial support. This is achieved by producing a comprehensive business plan.

Purpose

As clinicians, we are used to conveying information to patients and colleagues. We may be less used to producing business cases to facilitate new or develop existing clinical services. Innovation and patient care can thus be compromised. The production of high-quality business proposals is therefore essential to successfully obtain resources and compete for scarce funding. Guidance on formulation of business plans follows below.

Format

Formulation of business plans involves producing a short, clear and well-illustrated proposal. Remember the simpler and more intelligible the report, the more likely it is that consumers and non-medical managers will understand it. Moreover, the likelihood of a favourable opinion is likely to be higher. The following structure (Information Box 2.7) is commonly used.

1 EXECUTIVE SUMMARY

The key messages need to be clearly conveyed within a short précis of the report. As this section is where critical first impressions are made, the key elements should be emphasized in a concise and compelling way. If the technology has been successfully pilot tested within the base hospital, this should be stated. Estimates of any potential cost or resource savings should be included.

Example

Recent developments in hysteroscopic equipment have enabled many diagnostic and therapeutic interventions that are currently performed as an inpatient under general

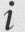

Information Box 2.7 Business plan outline

1 Executive summary
2 Background
3 Description of new intervention
4 Benefits summary
5 Business case
   5.1 Diagnosis/treatment model
   5.2 Tabulated unit costs and resource utilization
   5.3 Comparison with standard/current practice
   5.4 System set up and cost
   5.5 Training requirements
6 Comments/discussion

anaesthesia to be transferred to the outpatient setting under local anaesthesia. Potential benefits of this advance include:

• increased patient satisfaction and outcomes
• increased capacity and cost-efficiency.

It is estimated from the economic models included within this report, that introduction of an outpatient hysteroscopic service could offer a saving of 30 per cent compared with current management pathways. Increased patient satisfaction is anticipated because of shorter waiting times (increased capacity), convenience ('one-stop', 'see and treat' service without the need for hospital admission) and quicker recovery (avoidance of general anaesthesia and reduction in postoperative pain). Advances in instrumentation for diagnosis and treatment and avoidance of general anaesthesia offer potential improvements in patient outcomes in terms of effectiveness and safety.

2 BACKGROUND

This section should succinctly describe the context for the proposal. The importance of the presenting complaint or clinical conditions to be diagnosed and/or treated should be outlined. Local and national prevalence data are useful, as well as information pertaining to disease burden and resource use. Current service provision should be described. A flow diagram (decision model) is a useful way of doing this (Fig. 2.2).

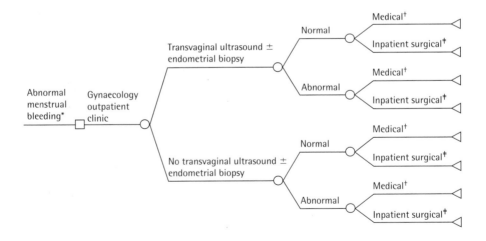

*Abnormal menstrual bleeding refers to excessive, irregular or unscheduled bleeding during the menstrual cycle.
†Medical therapies include reassurance alone, non-steroidal anti-inflammatory agents, antifibrinolytics (tranexamic acid), combined oral contraceptives, progestagens (systemic or local), hormone replacement therapies.
‡Inpatient surgical refers to polypectomy, myomectomy, first or second generation endometrial ablation/resection and hysterectomy.

Figure 2.2 *Example: current practice.*

3 CLINICAL DEVELOPMENTS/NEW SERVICES

The new intervention or service should be described. An explicit service framework or management algorithm is again useful. Comprehensive (and complex) models comparing all available alternate strategies are suitable for use in rigorous health technology assessment incorporating formal economic evaluations. Representative, but simplified decision models are more appropriate when presenting a business case. Such algorithms or 'care pathways', using local data, can be produced for all outpatient interventions described in this book (e.g. diagnostic hysteroscopy, hysteroscopic treatment of uterine pathology associated with abnormal uterine bleeding, infertility and fertility control etc. – see relevant chapters) (Fig. 2.3).

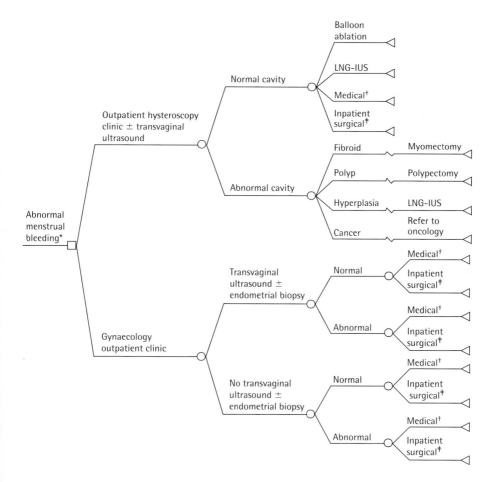

* Abnormal menstrual bleeding refers to excessive, irregular or unscheduled bleeding during the menstrual cycle.
† Medical therapies include reassurance alone, non-steroidal anti-inflammatory agents, antifibrinolytics (tranexamic acid), combined oral contraceptives, progestagens (systemic or local), hormone replacement therapies.
‡ Inpatient surgical refers to polypectomy, myomectomy, first or second generation endometrial ablation/resection and hysterectomy.
LNG-IUS: levonorgestrel intrauterine system.

Figure 2.3 *Example: comparison of current versus proposed practice.*

Information Box 2.8 Example: summary of benefits

BENEFITS FOR THE PATIENT

- Rapid service
- Single hospital visit
- Consultant-led
- Avoid general anaesthetic
- Appropriate referral/scheduling for inpatient surgery*
- Convenience (disruption to family/work minimized)

BENEFITS TO THE EXISTING INPATIENT SERVICE

- Reduced waiting times in general outpatient clinic
- Efficient use of theatre time
- Reduced operation waiting lists
- Increased capacity for service delivery
- Reduced inpatient and day case costs

*Precise scheduling of operating of known pathology and removal of minor/intermediate cases allowing more major surgery.

Any new or novel technology should be highlighted along with personal or external experience with such technology and the impact of similar service introduction in other centres.

4 SUMMARY OF BENEFITS

The anticipated benefits to stakeholders (patients, healthcare professionals, managers, society) of outpatient service delivery should be emphasized (Information Box 2.8).

5 BUSINESS CASE FOR HOSPITAL X

The quantity and spectrum of disease, as well as the amount and patterns of costs, charges, reimbursement, etc., varies between hospitals and healthcare systems. Consequently local data are required, which should include details of referral patterns, clinical activity (inpatient versus outpatient), available infrastructure, resource use and costs. Such clinical data may be available from local hospital sources, but a short audit of activity for defined period is likely to be required.

Cost pressures and resources required to set up and maintain the proposed service need to be identified. Ideally unit costs and resources used should be presented. The degree to which costs and resources are identified and broken down is dependent upon the level of data available, the hospital perspective and practicality. Usually direct costs (equipment, maintenance, staffing, etc.) are sufficient. Local finance departments can provide much of this information, pricing data are readily obtained from medical equipment manufacturers, and published sources relating to procedural and staffing costs are available (see Further reading).

Example

It is proposed that Hospital X set up an outpatient diagnostic and therapeutic ('see and treat') service for abnormal menstrual bleeding. Hospital X sees 2000 women per year in general gynaecological outpatient clinics, referred with abnormal menstrual bleeding. Data available from Hospital X have demonstrated that 800 (40 per cent) of women referred undergo inpatient surgical diagnostic or therapeutic procedures (based on history, clinical findings or failed medical treatments). A recent 3-month audit at Hospital X has shown that 75 per cent of such procedures could potentially be transferred to an outpatient hysteroscopy clinic setting. Furthermore, it is anticipated that overall rates of follow-up will be lower in a 'one-stop' hysteroscopy clinic setting. This is shown schematically in Fig. 2.4 (probabilities shown as decimals).

The anticipated costs and resources used per 100 women referred with abnormal menstrual bleeding are shown in Table 2.2. The chosen denominator will vary according to preference. For example, the total treatment cost can be calculated per patient or per 100 patients treated, or costs per year or per quarter year, etc., assuming a known patient throughput. In the hypothetical example below, per 100 patients is used, as the underlying cause of abnormal menstrual bleeding varies and dictates choice of treatment. Where diagnosis and treatments are assumed to be uniform (e.g. hysteroscopic versus laparoscopic sterilization), cost per patient may be preferred.

Based on these assumptions, introduction of new outpatient hysteroscopy service to replace current service provision is estimated to result in direct cost savings of £17 760 (34 per cent) per 100 women treated for abnormal menstrual bleeding. The outpatient service is likely to have additional benefits to patients, which have not been accounted for here. These include increased patient choice and preference, reduced indirect costs (e.g. patient

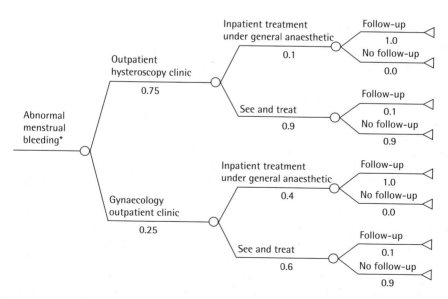

Figure 2.4 *Example: proposed care pathway. Eight possible outcomes modelled. Probability of each outcome derived from multiplication of component branch probabilities.*

Table 2.2 *Example: unit costs and resources*

Resource	Unit cost (£)	Quantity per 100 patients	Total cost (£/100 patients)
Outpatient hysteroscopy service			
Staffing: Staffing levels and hours required will vary, as will grades, need for ultrasonographer, etc. Hourly rates of pay are available (see Further reading).			
Consultant gynaecologist (per hour)	100	80	8000
Nurse F Grade (per hour)	20	80	1600
Auxiliary A grade (per hour)	10	80	800

Equipment: Resource use and costs will vary according to disease prevalence and spectrum, and clinical practice. Costs will also vary according to balance of choice between disposable (e.g. Versacope sheaths, endometrial biopsy devices, cotton wool, gauze, antiseptics) and reusable equipment (tenaculum forceps, Hegar dilators). Anticipated rates of patient agreement and failure rates of outpatient interventions need to be costed. Inpatient surgery will encompass major and minor operating. Capital costs of permanent equipment need to be incorporated (e.g. Thermachoice generators, decontamination units). Decontamination costs and replacement costs need to be estimated and included.

Diagnostic hysteroscopes	1	100	100
Operative hysteroscopes	2	20	40
Versapoint electrodes	150	20	3000
Thermal balloons	300	20	6000
Mirena LNG-IUS	100	20	2000
Disposables	5	100	500
Reusables	2	100	200
Inpatient surgery	1000	10	10 000

Capital and maintenance costs: A cost for maintenance and infrastructure (room heating, cleaning, etc.) needs to be estimated and incorporated.

	20	100	2000
Total per 100 patients			**34 240**

Current (gynaecologic outpatient) service
Aggregate cost: Outpatient costs here are aggregated to include staffing, infrastructure, maintenance, disposables, etc. The main cost drivers of this service are operating theatre usage (staffing) and inpatient/day case hospital stay.

Outpatient clinic (per hour)	200	60	12 000
Inpatient surgery	1000	40	40 000
Total per 100 patients			**52 000**
Net difference in costs	17 760		

This is based on the assumption that 6 patients and 10 patients are seen per consultant-led hysteroscopy clinic and general gynaecology outpatient clinic of 4 hours' duration respectively. Ultrasound is assumed to be performed by clinicians in both services. A single follow-up appointment is assumed to be necessary in 19 per cent of patients going through the hysteroscopy service and 46 per cent of patients going through the general clinics (see Figure 2.4).

transportation, time off work) and intangible costs (e.g. anxiety). Personal development and job satisfaction for involved healthcare professionals is also likely to be enhanced.

Training requirements should also be identified within the business case. Many of the procedures described in this book will have already been mastered by surgeons in the inpatient setting. Translation to the outpatient setting is generally quick and easy in this situation, although it is still often useful to visit another centre experienced in the technique to observe the set-up and delivery of the service. In some cases the technique may be a new one and in this circumstance it is recommended that a short period of supervised training in the technique be undertaken. Professional education and training of support staff may be necessary.

6 COMMENTS/CONCLUSIONS

The rationale for introducing a new intervention or service should be restated and the projected clinical and economic benefits summarized. A clear vision needs to be conveyed, backed up by good science (*evidence-based medicine*) and compliance with current standards and recommendations (regulatory body guidance, e.g. National Institute for Clinical Excellence (NICE), Food and Drug Administration (FDA), etc.) where available. The strengths and limitations of the proposal can be discussed. One approach involves producing a 'strengths, weaknesses, opportunities, threats' (SWOT) analysis (Information Box 2.9).

 Information Box 2.9 Example of SWOT analysis

STRENGTHS

- Rapid access 'one-stop' 'see and treat' clinic providing both a diagnostic and therapeutic service
- Reduced anxiety and waiting time for patients
- Consultant-led
- Evidence-based referral criteria for service
- Reduction on inpatient workload
- Efficient use of inpatient theatre time
- Reduced operation waiting lists
- Increased capacity
- Cost containment

WEAKNESSES

- Initial set-up costs for infrastructure, endoscopic equipment and staff
- Training of medical and nursing staff

OPPORTUNITIES

- Provide evidence-based quality service for patients in a friendly 'one-stop' 'see and treat' environment
- Maximize use of specialist minimal access surgery

THREATS

- The service is developed by another trust and patient referrals are being channelled there
- Inadequate funding/infrastructure may compromise patient access and throughput

FUTURE DEVELOPMENTS

In the UK, health service delivery is to be modernized by the introduction of a 'payment by results' system from 2005 with full implementation by 2008. This will involve cost–volume agreements and single price tariffs for procedures. The idea is to increase competition in an attempt to enhance choice for patients and purchasers (e.g. primary care) thereby improving services, reducing waiting times and containing costs. The cost-effectiveness of outpatient hysteroscopic services will undoubtedly become more attractive in such an increasingly competitive market. Those providers with well-established outpatient hysteroscopic services using a number of possible settings (hospitals, 'diagnostic and treatment centres', primary care and private sector) are likely to do well.

CONCLUSION

Outpatient hysteroscopy units can provide benefits to all involved. They give women choice and provide them with a safe, effective and efficient method for managing many common gynaecological problems, with the least possible disruption to their lives. If outpatient hysteroscopy units are managed efficiently, they can increase capacity and help meet waiting time targets. Clinicians, managers and commissioners should be actively looking to increase outpatient surgery rates. Clinicians should receive adequate training to conduct relevant surgical procedures, backed up by sufficient resources to implement change.

 KEY POINTS

- Outpatient hysteroscopy units provide women with a rapid access, convenient, safe, effective and efficient setting for managing many common gynaecological problems.
- Outpatient hysteroscopic intervention is a cost-effective option for managing common gynaecological complaints without compromising patient care. This should have the effect of better use of inpatient operating lists, increasing health service capacity and patient turnover.
- Implementation of 'see and treat' outpatient hysteroscopy clinics may involve a change in process and culture in order to overcome established inpatient practices and prejudices regarding what represents optimal patient care.
- Routine 'dilatation and curettage' under general anaesthesia is outdated practice and subjects women to unnecessary risks and inconvenience
- A business plan needs to be formulated to acquire necessary funding and support.

FURTHER READING

Clark TJ, Gupta JK. Outpatient hysteroscopy. *Obstetrician and Gynaecologist* 2002;4:217–21; [erratum] 2003;5:37.

Department of Health. *Day Surgery: operational guide, 2002.* [Available at www.publications.doh.gov.uk/daysurgery, accessibility verified 1 May 2004.]

Netten A, Curtis L. *Unit Costs of Health and Social Care.* University of Kent at Canterbury: Personal Social Services Research Unit, 2000. [Available at www.ukc.ac.uk/PSSRU/, accessibility verified September 15, 2004.]

Instrumentation and decontamination

As is true of any type of endoscopic surgery, optimal performance of outpatient hysteroscopic procedures is reliant upon the availability of high-quality equipment. This is not to say that all the latest high-tech developments and gadgets need to be acquired, as an excellent hysteroscopy service can be provided using 'basic', relatively inexpensive equipment of good quality. Choice of instrumentation will be influenced by many factors including manufacturing issues (e.g. quality of product, aftercare, etc.), costs, preference of clinician(s) and the nature of a particular clinical practice. In outpatient work an atraumatic approach is paramount and is achieved by use of finely engineered, diminutive instruments. There is an inherent risk of damage to such delicate instrumentation, especially if a poor technique is employed. Robust design and manufacture will aid reliability and durability of equipment.

This chapter describes the basic hysteroscopic sets required to perform outpatient 'see and treat' hysteroscopy. Additional instrumentation required for specific procedures is detailed in the relevant proceeding chapters.

HISTORICAL BACKGROUND

Hysteroscopy evolved over the last two centuries. The early large, crude optical light-conducting tubes have been replaced by small diameter endoscopes using cold light fibreoptic technology. These microhysteroscopes can be rigid or flexible and provide high-resolution, high-quality video images. The use of outer sheaths with additional instillation ports, enables the continuous flow of distension media, which facilitate the use of finely engineered surgical instruments and energy sources that can be employed down tiny operating channels. Diagnostic hysteroscopies were performed in the outpatient setting over 100 years ago, although safety and acceptability were questionable. General anaesthetic was employed with the more widespread use of hysteroscopy in the latter part of the twentieth century. The miniaturization of modern hysteroscopes has allowed the transition of the procedure from an inpatient back into an outpatient setting. This accompanied the development of outpatient endometrial sampling devices.

GENERIC GYNAECOLOGICAL EQUIPMENT

The hysteroscopist should aim to avoid blind cervical dilatation and so the routine use of a uterine sound or dilators should be avoided. The availability of a 2–3 mm uterine dilator is useful for overcoming the 'pinpoint' stenotic cervix prior to insertion of the hysteroscope. Rigid grasping forceps are required for specimen retrieval and an artery forceps can be useful for retrieving intracervical threads from a 'lost intrauterine contraceptive device (IUCD)' without

Information Box 3.1 Generic equipment

ESSENTIAL EQUIPMENT

- Operating chair/couch (adjustable, ideally electronic) and surgeon's stool
- Dressing pack/vaginal exam pack/sterile instrument tray
- Bivalve speculum
- Sterile cotton wool balls/gauze
- Skin cleanser/non-foaming antiseptic (e.g. aqueous chlorhexidine acetate/gluconate 0.05 per cent, sodium chloride solution 0.9 per cent or sterile water)
- Sterile drapes
- Decontamination and disposal units/services
- Emergency resuscitation and monitoring equipment

STANDBY EQUIPMENT (IMMEDIATELY AVAILABLE ON REQUEST)

- *Local anaesthetic administration*: 10–20 ml syringe; needles, local anaesthetic ± vasoconstrictor agents
- *Mechanical instruments*:
  - vulsellum/tenaculum forcep (single- or double-toothed)
  - set of graded uterine dilators (e.g. Hegar dilators 2–10 mm (7–30 Fr) in 1 mm increments
  - uterine sound/'os finding' malleable cervical probe
  - sponge-holding forcep
  - polyp forcep
  - artery forcep (e.g. Spencer–Wells, straight serrated forcep)
  - uterine curette (miniature, e.g. size 00–1)
  - outpatient endometrial biopsy device (e.g. Pipelle) and specimen pot with preservative
  - range of bivalve specula (small, medium, large)
  - Sims speculum
  - lateral vaginal wall retractor
  - suture scissors
- *Haemostasis*: sutures, Foley balloon catheter
- *Pharmacological agents*: sedatives, analgesics, local oestrogens and antibiotics

the need for dilatation. The use of specifically designed grasping instruments (e.g. Corson myoma extractor) or instruments borrowed from other specialities (e.g. pituitary rongeurs) is advocated by some authorities. Endometrial sampling is best performed with a plastic suction device, although a metal uterine curette can be useful when the uterine cavity is full of distension fluid impeding aspiration of endometrial tissue or to allow retrieval of small focal lesions. The availability of smaller specula aids cervical visualization in women with narrow lower genital tracts (e.g. virgins or vaginal atrophy) and larger specula in obese women. Lateral wall retractors are rarely needed, unless there is considerable vaginal laxity.

Sutures are occasionally required if there is bleeding from cervical trauma and a 30 ml Foley balloon catheter can tamponade uterine bleeding following myomectomy, although this is rare in the outpatient scenario. Emergency equipment should be available primarily for the rapid treatment of vasovagal reactions, but one should be alert for cardiorespiratory events in elderly women and those with associated medical problems. Monitoring equipment is required if conscious sedation is used (see Chapter 12).

HYSTEROSCOPES

Conventional hysteroscopes consist of a rigid telescope with a proximal eyepiece and a distal objective lens that may be angled at 0° to provide direct viewing or offset at 12°, 15°, 25° or 30° to provide a fore-oblique view. The bevelled distal end corresponds to the offset angle of viewing and may aid insertion of the instrument into the uterine cavity. The 0° straightforward telescope provides vision from the normal perspective, thereby facilitating orientation, and is therefore easiest to use. The advantage of a 12–30° terminal lens relates to increased field of view (⩾90°) compared with a 0° lens, with rotation around its axis allowing panoramic viewing of all aspects of the uterus including more inaccessible areas, e.g. tubal ostia. For offset scopes, manufacturing convention has the field of view directed away from the light cord insertion.

Information Box 3.2 Definitions

Endoscope. A slender, telescope-like optical instrument for viewing inside body cavities. Endoscopes can be rigid or flexible and may contain special channels through which ancillary instruments can be passed to perform diagnostic (biopsy) or therapeutic functions.

Hysteroscope. This is a rigid, semirigid or flexible endoscope that has been specifically designed to traverse the vagina and cervix to allow direct visual examination of the uterine cavity. An integral or external outer sheath surrounds the hysteroscope for the passage of distension media. Systems may also include additional sheaths or channels to allow circulation of distension media and passage of ancillary instruments enabling operative procedures.

Hysteroscopy. An endoscopic procedure for direct visualization of the uterine cavity.

Inpatient hysteroscopy. Hysteroscopy performed in an anaesthetized or sedated patient within a formal hospital operating theatre setting.

Outpatient or 'office' hysteroscopy. Hysteroscopy performed in the conscious patient in an appropriate clinic setting without the need for formal operating theatre facilities or general anaesthesia.

The image is conveyed via an integrated fibreoptic system that is contained within the barrel of the telescope and consists of a series of densely packed, small diameter glass (e.g. 'HOPKINS' rod lenses in rigid hysteroscopes) or flexible plastic fibres (e.g. semirigid or flexible hysteroscopes). The hysteroscope provides a panoramic view without magnification (1×) for global observation of the entire uterine cavity. The usual working distance is approximately 30 mm, although the depth of field ranges from infinity to 1–3 mm from the end of the instrument.

Diagnostic hysteroscopy

The standard diagnostic hysteroscope has been 4 mm in diameter enclosed in a 5 mm single flow outer sheath for delivery of distension media, attached to the port site via external tubing. Cervical dilatation can normally be avoided at this diameter in multiparous women and so the instrument is employed in both the inpatient and outpatient setting. Advances in engineering and optical, fibreoptic technology have led to miniaturization of telescopes (1.0–2.9 mm) and, although images are smaller and less bright, there is no significant compromise in image quality. Total working diameters of modern diagnostic system diameters are well under 5 mm (typically 2.5–4 mm) with the addition of the outer single flow examination sheath, increasing accessibility and comfort. These mini systems will normally still block the cervix, preventing rapid escape of distension media, so that adequate cavity distension is achieved (Plate 3).

Operative hysteroscopy

Operative hysteroscopy requires good fluid circulation and this is provided by having continuous flow sheaths surrounding the telescope (Plate 4). These allow both inflow and outflow of distension media, which can be controlled by opening and closing specific ports. The tip of the telescope will be continually flushed, clearing blood and debris from the operative field so that a clear field of view is maintained. Typical continuous flow sheath assembly is shown in Fig. 3.1.

In addition, the sheath system needs to contain one or two working channels for the insertion of ancillary instruments (see below). Standard continuous-flow operative hysteroscopes

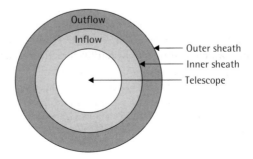

Figure 3.1 *Cross-sectional view of continuous flow hysteroscope assembly. Fluid is instilled via the inner sheath housing the hysteroscope and exits through the outer sheath. The outflow can be attached to suction or allowed to drain by gravity.*

are between 7 and 9 mm in diameter and are unsuitable for outpatient operating because of their size and higher distension pressures. Continuous-flow irrigation sheaths have been miniaturized in keeping with the new generation of small-diameter hysteroscopes. Complete working system outer diameters of 4–5.5 mm have made operative hysteroscopy feasible in the outpatient setting without the need for routine cervical dilatation. Operating channels are usually between 1.6 and 2.0 mm (5–7 Fr). Rigid hysteroscopes are superior to flexible ones for operative outpatient hysteroscopy and a 30° fore-oblique telescope is the most widely used for operative purposes. The operative Versascope (Gynecare) is unusual as it employs a semirigid 0° hysteroscope with peripheral viewing of the operative instruments provided by a deflected (10°) outer sheath (Plate 5). Furthermore, there is no separate outflow channel to allow egress of instilled fluid unless the collapsible operative channel is expanded by insertion of ancillary instruments.

Flexible hysteroscopes

A flexible hysteroscope is shown in Plate 6. Typically they are between 3 and 5 mm in diameter, have working lengths of 230–290 mm, provide a wide field of view (100°–120°) with distal tip deflection of 100°–160°. The operative fibroscopes contain working channels suitable for 3–7 Fr flexible ancillary instruments. There are pros and cons to the use of flexible technology and consideration of these will influence choice of instrument. These are outlined below and summarized in Table 3.1.

ADVANTAGES

Flexible endoscopes have been introduced to hysteroscopy because their design presents three mechanical advantages helpful for hysteroscopy. The first of these relates to the soft, supple shaft, which will adapt to the natural anatomic curvature of the lower genital tract and uterus. Second, the 0° fibroscope has a bendable distal tip, which can be moved 100°–120° (some up to 160°) up or down. This is externally controlled using an angulation lever situated close to the eyepiece of the instrument. The uterine cavity is inspected by using the control lever to steer the distal tip and also by rotating the hysteroscope (see Chapter 4 for technique). Third, the manoeuvrability of the distal tip obviates the need for any lens offset, so the direction of view corresponds to the natural approach. The result is an instrument that can negotiate the endocervical canal, minimizing the need for cervical counter-traction. In addition to atraumatic insertion, fibroscopes provide natural panoramic views of the uterine cavity and can be manipulated to access more remote regions (cornual recesses and tubal ostia), which is attractive in fertility practice as tubal procedures (cannulization and falloposcopy) are facilitated. Completeness of uterine examination may also be enhanced when the cavity is markedly deformed by the presence of large structural defects (polyps, fibroids, adhesions and septae), which necessitates additional manoeuvrability. This is achieved with minimal movement of the hysteroscopic shaft thereby reducing uncomfortable and traumatic torque on the cervix (Fig. 3.2).

DISADVANTAGES

Rigid optics are in far more widespread use than flexible hysteroscopes. This is for a number of reasons. The first reason relates to the optical system and mode of image

Table 3.1 *Rigid versus flexible hysteroscopes*

Factor	Preference	Comment
Visibility	Rigid	Optical properties in terms of image quality (brightness and sharpness), adequacy of panoramic view and operator confidence in formulating diagnosis superior with a rigid hysteroscope
Manoeuvrability	Flexible	Steerable flexible 0° hysteroscopes facilitate viewing of less accessible areas, e.g. cornual recesses and tubal ostia, while maintaining the orientation advantages of a 0° objective lens
Diagnostic accuracy	=	No significant difference in diagnostic accuracy for endometrial pathology
Length of procedure	Rigid	Duration of diagnostic procedure increased although still short (<5 min) so any difference is probably clinically unimportant
Failure rate	Rigid	Higher failure rate with flexible hysteroscopes attributable to inability to negotiate the cervical canal and inadequate views. Overall failure rates are approximately double those of rigid hysteroscopy (4 versus 7 per cent respectively)
Surgical intervention	Rigid	Directed biopsies and removal of IUCDs possible with flexible hysteroscopes. Substantive operative flexible hysteroscopy is not feasible with delicate flexible instrumentation
Safety	=	Neither associated with serious adverse effects
Perioperative pain	Flexible	More discomfort on entry and during the procedure with rigid compared to flexible hysteroscopes (cervical torque). This difference may be relate to the fore-oblique (offset) angle employed (0° flexible versus 30° rigid) rather than type of scope. If any difference is real it is of marginal clinical significance as overall reported discomfort is low and procedures short
Convenience	Rigid	Maintenance and sterilization more complex and awkward with flexible hysteroscopes
Cost	Rigid	Higher costs associated with flexible hysteroscopy because of higher equipment, sterilization and maintenance costs in addition to the higher failure rates, compared with rigid hysteroscopes. However, flexible may be cost-effective if preferred by women

transmission. The fibreoptics contained within flexible endoscopes provide lower image quality with the optical fibre pattern apparent in the image (grid-like picture). Compared with rigid hysteroscopes with their densely packed rod lens system, image resolution is inferior with fibroscopes (the fibreoptic bundles carry both the light and the image) and a shallower depth of field is obtained (1–50 mm, fixed focus). However, further recent

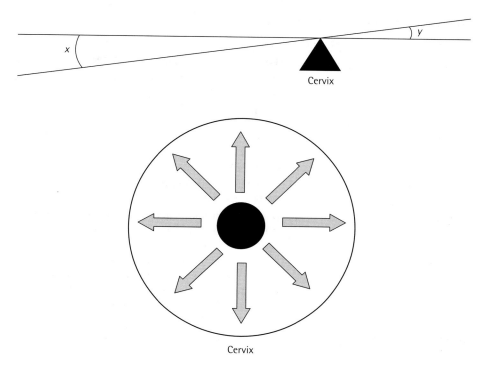

Figure 3.2 *Hysteroscopy and cervical torque. The cervix acts as a fulcrum around which the hysteroscope is 'levered'. During hysteroscopy, the majority of the hysteroscope is outside the uterine cavity (in contrast to laparoscopy) so that a greater degree of external movement is required to manipulate the distal tip of the instrument (angle x > y). This can produce painful torquing pressures on the cervix.*

advances in fibreoptics and digital image processing are likely to provide images of an increasingly comparable quality.

The second reason relates to their limited versatility. Although modern flexible designs incorporate working channels for insertion of flexible ancillary instruments, they are of limited therapeutic use. This is because the small operating channels can only accommodate small, but flexible and consequently rather fragile, forceps, loops and cannulas (diameter 3, 5 and 7 Fr). Such delicate instruments are inferior for operative hysteroscopy compared with the heavier instruments that can be passed down a variety of differently configured rigid systems.

The third reason is in regard to maintenance and sterilization. Although modern fibroscopes are durable, fully immersible in chemical disinfecting media and can withstand gas sterilization, this is generally more complex and awkward with flexible hysteroscopes. Finally, flexible endoscopic technology is generally more expensive to purchase.

SUMMARY

Flexible hysteroscopes provide good vision and exposure of the uterus and possibly greater patient comfort. However, the cervical canal is short (1–4 cm) and easily traversed with rigid instruments. Furthermore, the uterus is a firm, usually small and regular, fibromuscular cavity amenable to complete panoramic inspection with rigid instruments which are well tolerated. The advantages gained as a consequence of the superior manoeuvrability of flexible endoscopes are not fully realized in such an environment compared with other areas with longer, more diverse and tortuous anatomy (e.g. the gastrointestinal tract), where fibroscopes are invaluable.

ANCILLARY INSTRUMENTS

Continuous flow hysteroscopes contain one or two auxiliary ports, often with rubber seals, connected to working channels down which ancillary instruments can be passed, facilitating operative procedures. Varied types of instruments are available. The miniaturization of hysteroscopic systems suitable for outpatient work means that the integral working channels are narrow, typically 1.6–2.0 mm (5–7 Fr) in diameter (a limited range of 3 Fr instruments is also available). Accommodated instruments are thus diminutive, and this mechanical disadvantage places substantial limitations upon their operative use. Only the smallest intrauterine pathology can be grasped or biopsied and manoeuvrability is restricted, limiting access. Most mechanical instruments are 'semirigid', manufactured using surgical steel alloys to improve flexibility and torsional strength, employing spring-loaded handles to optimize manoeuvrability and containing integral cleaning or 'flush' ports to prevent blockage. The geometry of the distal tips of scissors and grasping forceps varies in an attempt to optimize particular functions (Plate 7). Despite fine engineering, they remain subject to damage and their use is limited, especially if intrauterine bleeding ensues. This applies even more so to the delicate 'flexible' instruments designed for use down flexible hysteroscopes.

Mechanical instruments are used mainly for obtaining directed focal uterine biopsies, excising or removing very small polyps, dividing filmy adhesions or thin septae and

 Information Box 3.3 Ancillary instruments

MECHANICAL
- Grasping forceps
- Biopsy forceps (toothed, spoon, cup, punch)
- Scissors (blunt or sharp tip, hooked, etc.)
- Myoma fixation instruments ('screw')
- Retraction loop ('snare')
- Aspiration cannulae/suction catheters

ELECTRICAL
- Needle electrode (straight or hooked)
- Retraction loop ('snare')
- Laser fibres (KTP, Nd:YAG, argon)

SPECIFIC THERAPEUTIC DEVICES
- Essure permanent birth control system (Conceptus, Inc. – see Chapter 19)

retrieving the threads of a lost IUCD. Punch biopsy forceps are also available for the biopsy of more resistant tissues (e.g. fibroids, myometrium or atrophic tissue). Particulate debris can be aspirated using specifically designed catheters. Heavier, rigid instruments are required for hysteroscopic metroplasty and are suitable for use with larger diameter inpatient operating hysteroscopes. To some degree the restrictions placed upon outpatient hysteroscopic surgery because of miniaturization have been overcome by the advent of relatively cheap and safe bipolar electrodiathermy systems (see Chapter 14) and specific therapeutic devices (e.g. Essure sterilization device, Conceptus, Inc.).

DISTENSION MEDIA

Hysteroscopic diagnosis requires adequate visualization of the uterine cavity. Clear and consistently maintained intrauterine visualization is necessary if surgical procedures are to be successfully performed. The outpatient setting, with its dependence upon smaller diameter hysteroscopes, can present challenges to this, which need to be overcome. Selection of the optimum medium is the first step to address such challenges.

The uterus can be expanded using gas (carbon dioxide – CO_2) or fluid. Fluids can be high viscosity and immiscible with blood (dextran) or low viscosity and miscible with blood. Low viscosity fluids can be subdivided into physiologic isotonic solutions (normal saline, Ringer's lactate, water) or hypotonic solutions (glycine 1.5 per cent solution in water, sorbitol, mannitol). Although visualization with dextran is excellent, it is no longer recommended because it is expensive and associated with problems (fluid overload/pulmonary oedema, anaphylaxis, blood dyscrasias and instrument damage from carmelization). Non-isotonic media remain popular for inpatient hysteroscopic procedures, despite their propensity for causing hyponatraemic fluid overload, as the media are non-conductive (electrolyte free) and thereby suitable for monopolar electrosurgery. As fluid balance is harder to accurately record in the outpatient setting, and monopolar diathermy rarely employed, safer isotonic solutions (0.9 per cent normal saline) or CO_2 are the media of choice.

Choice of distension media: CO_2 versus saline

CO_2 and saline are both effective and safe media for distension. CO_2 is a cheap, colourless, non-volatile gas that is rapidly absorbed and has the same refractive index as air, which produces uterine views of great clarity. However, views are compromised if there is bleeding. Saline is an aqueous solution and provides good visibility in the presence of clots, mucus and debris. However, it becomes turbid as it mixes with blood and debris. This does not pose a problem provided that irrigation of fluid takes place, with outflow provided anatomically (through the cervix or fallopian tube) or with the use of a continuous hysteroscopic flow system. Saline is a widely available electrolyte-containing media and so is an effective conductor for use with the newly developed bipolar intrauterine electrosurgical systems. It also offers the advantage of reducing the risk of plasma electrolyte disturbance from absorption. CO_2 has been traditionally more widely used in diagnostic hysteroscopy, but with advancing technology facilitating operative outpatient hysteroscopy, the balance is favouring the use of saline. A detailed comparison of CO_2 and saline distension media is shown in Table 3.2.

Table 3.2 *Distension media: saline versus carbon dioxide (CO_2)*

Factor	Preference	Comment
Convenience	=	CO_2 is easy to infuse but does require use of a more complex delivery set-up (electronic hysteroscopic insufflator). Although automated pumps are available for delivery of saline, gravity/syringe feed or pressure pump normally suffice. However, uncontrolled fluid spillage compromises accurate input/output measurement and is untidy
Cervical dilatation	Saline	CO_2 may require cervical dilatation more often than saline when larger (>4 mm) diagnostic sheaths are used
Visibility	=	CO_2 has the same refractive index as air and produces views of optimal clarity, but any difference is academic and of no clinical significance. Bubble formation is more common with CO_2 (50 per cent) compared to saline (10 per cent). CO_2 may have to be converted to saline if bleeding occurs, although increased light refraction and fluid turbulence can still impair viewing without adequate irrigation
Length of procedure	Saline	CO_2 takes longer to expand the uterine cavity, prolonging the procedure compared with saline, although of minimal clinical significance as duration of both procedures are short
Failure rate	=	No difference
Feasibility of bleeding	Saline	CO_2 gives an unsatisfactory view with active bleeding compromising diagnosis. Special care is required to avoid damage to the fragile endocervical mucosa on hysteroscope insertion when CO_2 is used. Saline is compatible with continuous flow fluid systems, which overcome minor to moderate bleeding
Feasibility of operative procedures	Saline	CO_2 is not practical for operative purposes because of problems with gas leakage from the uterus and limited visibility owing to the build up of blood, debris and bubble formation
Feasibility of electrosurgery	Saline	Saline as a conductive electrolyte medium, which cannot be used with monopolar electrodes, but is the ideal medium for bipolar intrauterine surgical systems. Monopolar electrodes can be used with CO_2, but bleeding compromises view
Vasovagal reactions	Saline	Apparently increased occurrence of vasovagal reactions with CO_2 insufflation, although there are many confounding factors, e.g. uterine distension pressure employed
Dissemination of pathology	=	No strong evidence to support higher likelihood for dissemination of infective organisms or malignant cells with a fluid medium
Shoulder tip pain	Saline	Referred shoulder tip pain (from diaphragmatic irritation) may be greater postoperatively with CO_2. Saline is rapidly absorbed from the peritoneal cavity following transtubal leakage

(Continued)

Table 3.2 (*Continued*)

Factor	Preference	Comment
Safety	=	Saline is a physiological (isotonic) medium and so hyponatraemic hypervolaemia is avoided. Low viscosity fluids are rapidly reabsorbed from the peritoneal cavity after transtubal leakage. CO_2 under controlled, low pressure is very safe
Perioperative pain	=	No difference. Both methods associated with minimal abdominal discomfort. The need for local anaesthesia is the same
Postoperative pain (immediate)	=	There is higher postoperative pelvic discomfort with CO_2, but any difference is of minimal clinical significance. It has been suggested that analgesic requirements may be greater postoperatively after using CO_2
Postoperative pain (delayed)	=	There is no difference in pain prior to discharge. Both methods are associated with minimal discomfort
Patient satisfaction	Saline	Marginally increased satisfaction with saline distension, although difference of questionable clinical significance
Cost	=	Comparable low cost for diagnosis, although initial outlay for CO_2 insufflation apparatus to control the flow rate and pressure is higher. Saline is more versatile and cost-effective for operative work than CO_2

Delivery of distension media

CARBON DIOXIDE

Liquid and gas media are potentially hazardous if used under high pressure for prolonged periods and will trigger uterine smooth muscle contraction and pain. CO_2 delivery requires the use of an electronic insufflator that can provide a preset flow rate and insufflation pressure that cannot be exceeded. If intrauterine pressure is kept steady between 40 and 50 mmHg of pressure (25–50 ml/min flow rate), painful uterine contractions are minimal and the view with contemporary hysteroscopes usually adequate. It should be noted that the intrauterine pressure achievable is limited by the tube and hysteroscope diameters. Generally it is recommended that the flow rate should be restricted to $\leqslant 100$ ml/min and the maximum inflow pressure should not exceed 100 mmHg. Higher pressures (maximum 200 mmHg) are associated with more transtubal insufflation into the peritoneal cavity (tubal passage at 70 mmHg) and shoulder tip pain from diaphragmatic irritation. Many operators start at a lower insufflation pressure (30–50 mmHg) to reduce bubble formation and patient discomfort, and increase as needed. It is reassuring to note that no CO_2 embolism has been reported in a non-anaesthetized patient to date.

SALINE

Prolonged procedures under high pressure are not going to be tolerated in the conscious patient and consequently plasma electrolyte disturbances from fluid overload are highly unlikely when isotonic saline is used in the outpatient setting. Strict fluid balance is not therefore required, but procedures should be abandoned if >2 l of fluid are required to complete a procedure (pulmonary oedema can still occur, but occurs with much higher fluid volumes and is much easier to treat than hyponatraemic overload). Saline can also be delivered at a predefined flow rate using automated devices, which also electronically monitor irrigation and suction pressures (if suction is required). However, simple syringe delivery or gravity feed (<1.2 m above uterus) is perfectly adequate for diagnostic procedures. For operative procedures, the inline fluid pressure can be increased by simply increasing the bag height, using a manually operated pressure cuff connected to a manometer, or reverting to electronic automated devices. To obtain around 50 mmHg of intrauterine pressure, irrigation pressures should start at 75–120 mmHg (200 ml/min if automation used) for ≤5 mm diameter hysteroscopes. Higher inflow pressures (150–250 mmHg) can be safely used for short periods to increase uterine distension if required. The outflow port of continuous flow systems should be connected to a collection bag to minimize spillage onto the floor and aid estimation of fluid absorption.

Additional considerations

Lower starting pressures should be considered in nulliparous and postmenopausal women who are more likely to experience pelvic discomfort from uterine stimulation. For safety reasons, older patients and those with cardiovascular compromise may require lower pressures and more conservative procedures of shorter duration.

Troubleshooting

POOR VIEW

The occurrence of suboptimal visualization will vary, dependent upon population characteristics, but should not generally exceed 5 per cent of procedures once the endometrial cavity has been entered. If inflow is poor, a check of the tubing and connections will usually identify inadequate connections or debris blocking the inflow/outflow channels.

INTRAVASCULAR INFUSION

Rapid intravascular infusion is more likely in the following circumstances:

- when a false passage is created
- with use of large diameter hysteroscopes (>5 mm), which allow higher flow rates
- when intrauterine pressure exceeds the mean arterial pressure/static venous pressure.

Thus atraumatic entry, miniature hysteroscopes and low infusion pressures are recommended.

ILLUMINATION AND IMAGING

An external, high-intensity 'cold light' source provides illumination: 150–300 W xenon or halogen bulbs transmit light down a fibreoptic cable, which is connected to the proximal part of the hysteroscope through which light is transmitted via rod lenses and fibreoptics to the distal end. The field of view and brightness are reduced in small diameter micro hysteroscopes and so an efficient light source is mandatory. The hysteroscopic image is transmitted via a proximally attached light-weight camera to a colour video monitor, which provides magnification, improves visualization and is ergonomically advantageous. Camera equipment consists of a video camera with its coupling lens, which converts the optical image into an electrical one. This is attached via a camera cable to a camera control unit and onto a television monitor that converts the image back to an optical one. A multitude of electronic equipment and software is now on the market for digital still and video image capture (e.g. DVD image capture systems, colour photographic paper, etc.). Most standard systems provide excellent picture quality in terms of image resolution and colour. More sophisticated systems further improve picture quality (e.g. three-chip cameras, digital signal processing, flat screen monitors), but inevitably costs are higher and the advantages are often only marginal.

It is important to emphasize two further points regarding illumination and imaging:

- light cables are fragile and must be handled with care to prevent breakage of the delicate component glass fibres

- there is no place for performing hysteroscopy without video relay.

ENERGY SYSTEMS

The use of bipolar intrauterine electrodiathermy systems (Versapoint) is dealt with in Chapter 14. Resectoscopes and laser fibres are unsuitable for use in the outpatient setting because of instrument diameter and costs respectively. Although miniature point and snare electrodes using monopolar current for use in non-conducting media are available, they have been rendered redundant by the advent of safer bipolar systems for use in saline.

SPACE MANAGEMENT, DOCUMENTATION AND DATA CAPTURE
Stack

Attention to space management in the treatment room is important to improve the ergonomic environment and facilitate equipment set-up, operator comfort and room turnover. All equipment (external light source, camera control unit, video monitor, electrosurgical generators, and automated distension media delivery systems) is best mounted on an appropriate mobile trolley or 'stack'. Miniaturization of equipment (e.g. mobile multifunctional documentation terminals – MEDI PACK), the development of adjustable flat screen panels and integral data capture systems have further reduced space occupation.

Information technology

Digital image capture, processing and printing has revolutionized data recording for clinical, research, audit, teaching and medicolegal purposes. The ability to display still or moving images may also enhance patient understanding and satisfaction with consultation. The use of computers, printers and associated software all housed in an appropriate, unobtrusive work station, allows standardized recording of information, construction of databases and generation of appointments and patient letters (see also Chapter 4).

Information Box 3.4 Hysteroscopic equipment: summary of basic set-ups

DIAGNOSTIC OUTPATIENT HYSTEROSCOPY

- *Hysteroscope and sheath system*
    - rigid hysteroscope (standard or miniature 1.0–4 mm) or flexible (3.6–4.9 mm)
    - diagnostic sheath (rigid, 2.5–5.5 mm, single flow)
- *Distension media*
    - carbon dioxide or fluid medium
    - automated units (e.g. Hysteroflator/Endomat) or manual set-up (gravity feed versus pressure cuff with pump and manometer)
    - inflow tubing
    - pressure cuff (1 l and 3 l), with pump and manometer or Micro Hysteroflator
- *Illumination and imaging*
    - cold light source 150–300 W power (halogen)
    - flexible fibreoptic light cable
    - video system including camera, fibreoptic cable, camera control unit and colour monitor
    - stack for housing (i.e. mobile videocart)
- *Information technology*
    - image/video capture and storage, computerized data recording and appropriate software

OPERATIVE OUTPATIENT HYSTEROSCOPY – AS FOR DIAGNOSTIC EXCEPT:

- *Hysteroscope and sheath system*
    - continuous flow operative sheath inflow and outflow channels, working channel (1.2–2.0 mm)
    - passive versus suction outflow and calibrated collection system (collecting drapes and receptacle)
- *Ancillary instruments (1.2–2.0 mm)*
    - mechanical
    - electrical (e.g. Versapoint bipolar intrauterine system or Storz bipolar vaporization electrode)
    - Procedure-specific (e.g. Essure permanent birth control system)

NB: A continuous flow system can be routinely employed for diagnostic purposes if desired, to facilitate directed biopsies and seamless conversion to therapeutic procedures ('see and treat').

DECONTAMINATION OF SURGICAL INSTRUMENTS

Decontamination is a process that removes or destroys contamination, thereby preventing infectious agents or other contaminants reaching a susceptible site in sufficient quantities to initiate infection or any other harmful response. In the clinical arena, effective decontamination is essential to minimize the risk of transmitting infection and so render reusable surgical instruments safe for further use. It requires the implementation of a number of procedures, as shown in Fig. 3.3.

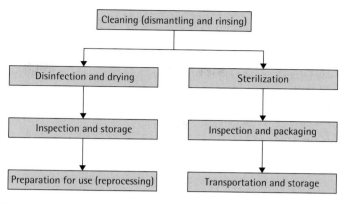

Figure 3.3 *Decontamination process.*

Decontamination process

OVERVIEW

Within endoscopy, different levels of disinfection are used: cleaning followed by disinfection or cleaning followed by sterilization. All facilities must comply with current legal requirements, published standards (both European and UK) and Department of Health best practice guidance. Decontamination should begin as soon as possible after endoscopes and their accessories have been used.

Cleaning

Effective cleaning (with warm water and a neutral or enzymatic detergent) is an essential prerequisite to disinfection and sterilization and is vital to ensure removal of debris (blood, mucus, infectious agents or biofilm). Thorough manual or automated cleaning ensures adherent infectious agents are largely removed and better contact between the disinfectant and any remaining infectious agents in subsequent stages of decontamination. Failure to remove deposits may result in infection, misdiagnosis or instrument malfunction. The head of the light cable should be wiped clean with 70 per cent isopropyl alcohol.

Disinfection

This is a process used to reduce the number of viable infectious agents (micro-organisms, viruses and other transmissible agents, e.g. prions), but this may not necessarily inactivate some microbial agents such as viruses and bacterial spores. Disinfection may not achieve the same reduction in microbial contamination levels as sterilization.

Immersion in a suitable liquid chemical disinfectant is the most widely used procedure for the decontamination of flexible and heat-sensitive rigid endoscopes. A high level of disinfection is achievable assuming adequate contact time and temperature, but is a difficult process to control. Automated endoscope reprocessors are available, which have a disinfection phase and may also include a washing phase. As an alternative to the use of liquid chemicals, rigid endoscopes may be disinfected at a high level using various other methods (e.g. moist heat). Boiling water is not recommended, as there are difficulties in ensuring that the required temperature is maintained, and it does not kill spores. A wide variety of disinfectants are available (e.g. alcohols, aldehydes, chlorine dioxide, peroxygen compounds and quaternary ammonium compounds). Although gluteraldehyde is widely used, it is a powerful irritant and sensitizer and so alternative agents should be considered on health and safety grounds. Tap water contains microbes, including *Pseudomonas* spp. and *Mycobacterium* spp., and so sterile or pretreated water is recommended for the final rinsing required to remove any deposited toxic chemical residues.

Sterilization

This is a process used to render an object free from viable infectious agents including viruses and bacterial spores. Steam under pressure is preferred to the use of liquid chemical disinfectants for the disinfection of all invasive or surgical endoscopes. It is unsuitable for heat-sensitive instruments. Sterilization is the preferred process for rigid endoscopes. Many are now heat tolerant and all components, including the telescope, are autoclavable. Porous load autoclaves that sterilize at 121–124°C for a minimum of 15 minutes or 134–137°C for a minimum of 3 minutes are suitable for processing autoclavable rigid endoscopes and accessories.

The choice of endoscopic equipment and reprocessing method will depend upon several considerations, as listed in Table 3.3.

Decontamination of hysteroscopes and the outpatient setting

The rapid turnover of hysteroscopic procedures in an outpatient setting, as well as the design, complexity and fragility of the instruments, present particular problems to decontamination procedures. It is imperative that all decontamination procedures be in accordance with manufacturers instructions (establishing heat, chemical, pressure and moisture tolerance of instruments) minimizing risk of damage to the endoscope. Single-use (i.e. disposable) accessories should be used where feasible. As technology advances, endoscope design is likely to further impact on options for reprocessing and instrument durability. For example, the development of fibreoptic hysteroscopes that can be used in association with disposable sheaths will reduce the amount of decontamination required. The arguments for disposable or reusable devices are presented in Table 3.4. The most sensible policy, which is adopted by most units and takes into account both cost and safety considerations, appears to be employment of a combination of single use and reusable devices.

The infection risk is increased in relation to the invasiveness of the procedure. Endoscopes that are passed into normal sterile body cavities are deemed invasive (e.g. laparoscopes) and should be sterilized prior to use. Hysteroscopy is somewhat less invasive and equipment can be decontaminated by high-level disinfection. Increasing mucosal trauma will increase the risk of uterine infection and bacteraemia (Information Box 3.5).

Table 3.3 *Decontamination process: disinfection versus sterilization*

Factor	Disinfection	Sterilization
Effectiveness	Effectively reduces the number of viable infectious agents, but may not achieve the same reduction in microbial contamination compared to sterilization	Recommended method as it eradicates viable infectious agents including viruses and spores
Damage – process	Heat and some disinfectants are tissue fixatives and may cause lumens or the taps and moving parts of the hysteroscope to block. During drying, lensed instruments should not be immersed in alcohol for prolonged periods (>5 min) as this causes damage to the lens cements	Heat and some disinfectants are tissue fixatives and may cause lumens or the taps and moving parts of the hysteroscope to block. Steam-sterilized endoscopes should not be rapidly cooled as this may stress component parts and shorten the life of the instruments
Damage – transport	Completed on site. Little risk of damage related to transportation	It is recommended that a Central Sterile Services Department (CSSD) should carry out all reprocessing of autoclavable equipment, which is usually off site. Delicate endoscopes and accessories can be easily damaged during handling and transportation without due care and attention
Cost	Cost associated with on-site chemical disinfection likely to be lower as long as high standards of decontamination observed	Most CSSDs provide 24-hour turn around service. However, more equipment and hence capital outlay is required to maintain a smooth service without access to onsite reprocessing. Costs are likely to be higher with contracted CSSD
Versatility	Some chemical disinfection regimens possible for even the most delicate and compound instrumentation	Flexible and heat-sensitive hysteroscopes cannot be sterilized under pressure
Practicality	Increased availability of equipment allows increased flexibility in service provision, especially when unforeseen circumstances and heavy workloads arise	Equipment may be unavailable unless department is well stocked
Safety	Health and safety considerations resulting from exposure of both users and patients to chemical substances potentially harmful to their health	Not applicable if dedicated CSSD used as recommended

Table 3.4 *Disposable versus reusable instrumentation*

Factor	Disposable	Reusable
Cross-infection	Infection risk minimal. Reassuring to users and patients	Rigid endoscopes are relatively simple to clean, disinfect and sterilize, and so the availability of disposable single use telescopes may not be an attractive option. Decontamination of miniature hysteroscopic equipment is problematic because instrumentation is delicate, often constructed from a wide range of materials and contains long, narrow lumens where debris can be hard to remove and air cannot be readily displaced. Risk of infection transmission is, however, very low
Damage	Avoids damage related to decontamination processing and age. Effectiveness and safety of equipment optimized as a result	Effective decontamination requires robust decontamination procedures, which may damage equipment (stressed component parts, corrosion, blocked moveable parts, lens/optic damage, e.g. condensation and fogging)
Quality of equipment	Assuming high-quality manufacture, equipment should be reliable. Cheap, light-weight materials subject to malfunction. Convenience and quality generally preferred by clinicians	In addition to infection risks, failure to remove deposits could potentially result in misdiagnosis or morbidity from instrument malfunction. The decontamination process may compromise instrument function (e.g. stiffened taps and other moveable parts)
Environment	Non-degradable	Agents used potentially toxic, energy used in all aspects of processing (heating, transportation, etc.)
Costs	Replacement purchasing costs higher, but may be cost-effective from putative benefits (e.g. enhanced safety, quality, etc.)	Cheaper instrument costs per case, but this may not translate into increased cost-effectiveness

Storage and preparation of endoscopes

Disinfected endoscopes and other non-autoclavable components should be dried by purging with compressed air or by using 70 per cent alcohol. A local policy should be developed for the storage of endoscopes in conjunction with the device manufacturer's instructions. Sterilized endoscopes must be stored sealed in the container or packaging in which they were sterilized. Hysteroscopes that have been subjected to high-level disinfection should be reprocessed again in accordance with manufacturers' instructions, depending upon the time elapsed since the previous disinfection procedure.

Information Box 3.5 Endometritis

Endometritis is a polymicrobial disease involving a mixture of gram positive and negative, aerobic and anaerobic organisms. In the majority of cases, it arises from an ascending infection from organisms found in the normal indigenous vaginal flora. Commonly isolated organisms include *Streptococci, Staphylococci, Ureaplasma urealyticum, Klebsiella pneumoniae, Enterobacter aerogenes*, coliforms and anaerobes (e.g. *Peptostreptococcus, Gardnerella vaginalis* and *Bacteroides bivius*). *Chlamydia trachomatis* and *Neisseria gonorrhoea* may also occur. Treatment requires the use of broad-spectrum antibiotics with appropriate microbial coverage (e.g. amoxycillin and clavulonic acid, cephalosporin plus metronidazole, etc.).

KEY POINTS

- Advances in optical technology, image processing and auxiliary instrumentation have enabled miniaturization of hysteroscopic systems suitable for both diagnostic and operative work in the outpatient setting.

- Miniature hysteroscopes can be rigid, semirigid or flexible in design. Choice between systems will depend upon clinician preference and practice.

- Carbon dioxide and normal saline are suitable uterine distension media for use in outpatient hysteroscopy. Isotonic saline is preferred for operative work.

- The advent of bipolar intrauterine electrosurgery has overcome many of the limitations of mechanical ancillary microinstrumentation.

- Bipolar electrosurgery in saline has facilitated operative hysteroscopic procedures without the risk of electrolyte imbalance arising from hyponatraemic fluid overload.

- Decontamination is a combination of processes, including cleaning, disinfection and/or sterilization, used to render reusable surgical instruments safe for further use.

- Effective decontamination is a key component in provision of high-quality hysteroscopic services.

- The overall incidence of infection following hysteroscopic procedures is very low.

- The susceptibility of the patient to infection and type of procedure will influence the risk of infection transmission in addition to the effectiveness of method used to reprocess the hysteroscope.

- The rise in incidence of variant Creutzfeldt–Jakob disease, hepatitis B and human immunodeficiency virus (HIV) has put decontamination services under scrutiny. To date, the endoscopic transmission of HIV has not been reported.

- Disposable 'single patient use' or reusable equipment is available and a policy employing both is probably the most cost-effective.

FURTHER READING

Brill AI. Energy systems for operative hysteroscopy. *Obstet Gynecol Clin North Am* 2000;**27**:317–26.

Cicinelli E, Schonauer LM, Barba B, Tartagni M, Luisi D, Di Naro E. Tolerability and cardiovascular complications of outpatient diagnostic minihysteroscopy compared with conventional hysteroscopy. *J Am Assoc Gynecol Laparosc* 2003;**10**:399–402.

Medical Devices Agency. Decontamination of endoscopes. Device Bulletin MDA DB2002(05) 2002. [Available at www.medical-devices.gov.uk, accessibility verified July 30, 2004.]

Shankar M, Davidson A, Taub N, Habiba M. Randomised comparison of distension media for outpatient hysteroscopy. *Br J Obstet Gynaecol* 2004;**111**:57–62.

Unfried G, Wieser F, Albrecht A, Kaider A, Nagele F. Flexible versus rigid endoscopes for outpatient hysteroscopy: a prospective randomized clinical trial. *Hum Reprod* 2001;**16**:168–71.

4

Outpatient hysteroscopy: how to do it successfully

If outpatient hysteroscopy is to be judged as successful, it needs to provide the clinician with useful diagnostic information that influences subsequent management. Patient outcomes should be optimized and women satisfied with their overall experience. The outpatient setting can present many challenges, with the conscious patient being generallyless forgiving of induced discomfort or prolonged procedures arising from poor hysteroscopic technique. It is therefore essential that the fundamentals of good diagnostic technique are mastered. Once diagnostic competence is established such that manipulation and orientation of the hysteroscope becomes second nature to the operator, then outpatient hysteroscopy can be taken to the next level with operative procedures being routinely undertaken.

This chapter addresses the essentials of the hysteroscopic approach along with potential pitfalls and strategies to help overcome them.

PRE-HYSTEROSCOPY

Patient selection

The main indications for hysteroscopy are problems relating to abnormal uterine bleeding and reproduction (Information Box 4.1). Specific indications and contraindications for diagnostic and therapeutic outpatient hysteroscopy are detailed throughout this book. Indications have evolved since the introduction of hysteroscopy because of changing clinical practices and the advent of competing technology such as transvaginal ultrasound. Traditional indications such as assessment of uterine scar integrity/thickness, diagnosis and removal of retained products of conception and heterotopic bone are now no longer valid or required indications. There are few absolute contraindications to outpatient hysteroscopy in a well-equipped outpatient treatment room (Information Box 4.2). The majority of elderly patients and those with cardiorespiratory, orthopaedic (positioning), mental health and other chronic medical conditions are suited to hysteroscopy in the outpatient

Information Box 4.1 Indications for diagnostic hysteroscopy

PRIMARY – ABNORMAL UTERINE BLEEDING

- Postmenopausal bleeding
- Unscheduled bleeding on hormone replacement therapy
- Unscheduled bleeding on tamoxifen
- Excess or erratic menstrual loss
- Intermenstrual bleeding
- Postcoital bleeding

SECONDARY

- Infertility
- Recurrent pregnancy loss
- Abnormal glandular cervical smears
- Locating (and removing) foreign bodies within the genital tract

SCREENING/SURVEILLANCE – CONTENTIOUS

- Tamoxifen therapy
- Hormone replacement therapy
- Endometrial hyperplasia

 Information Box 4.2 Contraindications for outpatient hysteroscopy

- Active pelvic inflammatory disease
- Severe vaginitis
- Pregnancy
- Profuse uterine bleeding (likely to impair vision)
- Absence of informed consent

setting because the procedure is short, safe, well-tolerated and does not require general anaesthetic.

Cervical stenosis, extensive intrauterine adhesions and blood dyscrasias (including anti-coagulation) were previously considered to be relative contraindications to hysteroscopy. This is no longer the case following miniaturization of hysteroscopes, as an atraumatic approach is the rule. There is no convincing evidence that hysteroscopy results in dissemination of malignant cells and worsening prognosis. Established malignancy of the uterus should not therefore be considered a contraindication to hysteroscopy, but its use in advanced management (e.g. treatment planning, staging) needs to be considered carefully and fully justified.

Preoperative psychological support and patient preparation

Suggested strategies to reduce pain and anxiety and provide psychological support are outlined in Chapter 12. The key is to ensure that a well-informed patient arrives to a relaxed,
private and friendly environment, is offered choice and is involved in decision making. In
this way co-operation can be anticipated. Although procedural audits report high satisfaction
rates for outpatient hysteroscopy, women invariably report 'embarrassment' as the main
negative aspect of their experience. These more simple details of process are easily overlooked. It is therefore important to have preoperatively informed the patient about needing
to remove undergarments (a separate and connecting private changing area should be used
and gowns provided as necessary) and likely staffing presence including their respective
roles. They should be aware of the need for lithotomy positioning and resulting exposure,
which will be minimized as far as possible. As is the case when conducting any intimate
examination, anxiety and self-awareness is reduced further by adopting an expeditious,
matter of fact, but sensitive approach. Women should be encouraged to empty their bladder prior to the examination so that comfort is increased. There is no need to catheterize
the bladder, especially as this can cause urinary tract infections.

Patient history

An efficient, but thorough and relevant history should be obtained. A systematic approach
is to be encouraged and also facilitates subsequent research and audit if information is
recorded in a standard fashion (see 'Recording information', page 71). In particular the
woman's age, menopausal status and use of exogenous hormones should be ascertained.
Potential contraindications (Information Box 4.2), medical risk factors for hysteroscopy,
and drug allergies should be enquired about. It is important to exclude pregnancy in premenopausal women and obtain the date of the first day of the last menstrual period. This
information will also help interpretation of endometrial appearances.

Prophylaxis against infection

Uterine instrumentation has the potential to cause endometritis, ascending pelvic infection
and, rarely, life-threatening septicaemia. As the incidence of infection is low, routine
antibiotic prophylaxis is not necessary, but is reserved for those patients at risk of endocarditis (prosthetic heart valves and past history of endocarditis only for gynaecological
procedures). The recommended regimen is i.v. amoxicillin 1 g plus i.v. gentamicin 120 mg
at induction followed by oral amoxicillin 500 mg 6 hours later. Women with diabetes mel-
litus, joint prostheses or immunocompromise do not require antibiotic prophylaxis.

The most commonly encountered infection resulting from uterine instrumentation is a
mild endometritis giving rise to lower abdominal discomfort and persistent watery, often
blood-stained discharge. This can be easily treated with a 7-day course of augmentin or
erythromycin and metronidazole after genital tract swabs have been taken for microbiology. Cervical preparation may reduce the possibility of ascending infection, although there
is no strong evidence for this. Sterile water, saline or non-foaming aqueous antiseptics (e.g.
chlorhexidine, povidone-iodine) can be used to clean the cervix.

Uterine instrumentation is contraindicated in the presence of active genital tract or pelvic infection. Where genital tract infection is suspected from symptoms or a past history, intervention should be deferred and genital tract swabs taken for chlamydia and gonorrhoea in women of reproductive age. A suggested regimen for treatment of suspected pelvic inflammatory disease is doxycycline, cefotoxin and metronidazole for 14 days. The presence of intrauterine pus at hysteroscopy warrants treatment with broad-spectrum antibiotics.

Timing

Diagnostic hysteroscopy should be postponed if the appointment coincides with days of heavy menstrual flow for the patient, as visualization may be poor and the procedure is more likely to be perceived as unpleasant by the woman. The secretory phase is traditionally considered to be a less favourable time than the proliferative phase of the menstrual cycle. This is because secretory endometrium is thicker and so diagnostic accuracy may be impaired. Some authorities advocate the early proliferative phase when the endometrium is at its thinnest. Others recommend the late proliferative phase near to ovulation, so that the cervical canal can be traversed more easily. In reality, timing of procedures to coincide with non-menstrual phases of the cycle is unnecessary with modern, small diameter, continuous flow hysteroscopic equipment. Diagnostic and therapeutic procedures can be successfully carried out at any time with appropriate experience. This is not only an evidence-based approach, but also a practical one, in terms of scheduling clinical practice and patient convenience.

Set-up of equipment

Anticipate what equipment is likely to be required and have it all easily accessible and ready for use (see instrumentation in Chapter 3) prior to positioning and exposure of the

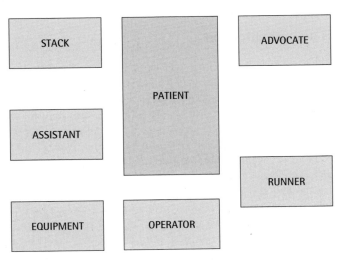

Figure 4.1 *Outpatient hysteroscopy: schematic representation of a standard set-up.*

patient. All staff should know where equipment is located and be familiar with its use. It is often when procedures are more difficult than expected that rapid and smooth access to additional equipment is most needed. (e.g. cervical dilators, cervical manipulators, miniature curettes, biopsy forceps, endoscope with working channels, etc.). Note that a video camera and monitor must always be used. A standard room set-up is shown in Fig. 4.1.

PATIENT PREPARATION

Positioning the patient

Adequately positioning is vital. This is aided by electronically operated, tilting couches, which are suitable for operative and electrosurgical procedures. Problems in accessing the uterine cavity most commonly arise when there are acute degrees of uterine displacement (anteversion/retroversion) or in obese patients. To overcome potential access problems, the patient should be positioned in the dorsal lithotomy position with her buttocks at the end or slightly overhanging the end of the bed. Her hips should be well flexed and abducted, with her legs supported by comfortable padded behind-the-knee stirrups, to keep her legs from shaking during the procedure. Her abdomen, genitalia and legs should be covered with a blanket to reduce exposure. The couch should be tilted down slightly (15°) to help retain instruments within the genital tract. The operator sits between the patient's legs and the couch height is adjusted so that the operator is comfortable, able to manipulate equipment freely, has easy access to the operating tray and instruments, and is able to see the video monitor without straining. The procedure should not start until adequate, comfortable positioning has been obtained and confirmed with the patient. A gown, sheet or drapes should be used to minimize patient exposure and consequent embarrassment.

This position will facilitate external hysteroscopic manoeuvrability, which should be kept to a minimum to reduce patient discomfort, but is often required to visualize the entire uterine cavity and perform surgical procedures. Particular care should be exercised with older or disabled patients, where mobility may be limited and musculoskeletal problems likely (e.g. osteoarthritis, hip replacements, osteoporosis), in order to avoid causing pain and joint damage.

Attending to the patient

It is important to ensure that the patient is as relaxed as possible before beginning the procedure and that this is maintained throughout. A dedicated nurse or nurse assistant (the so called 'nurse anaesthetist' or 'vocal-local') is the best person to help here by conversing with the patient. Any request by the operator to nursing staff for equipment should be made quietly. It is a good idea to prewarn the patient of any sensations likely to be experienced in relation to particular surgical manoeuvres (e.g. initial speculum insertion, fluid irrigation), especially potentially painful ones (e.g. application of vulsellum, hysteroscopic endometrial thickness assessment, endometrial biopsy). Many patients may want to observe the procedure on the video screen. However, any desire to do this should be established beforehand as otherwise it can be counterproductive by inducing anxiety.

Clinical examination

Prior to invasive testing, it is good practice to perform a thorough clinical examination. To facilitate hysteroscopy, the vulva, vagina and cervix are all exposed and easily inspected. If using a 0° hysteroscope then a bimanual examination is not mandatory in the absence of any lower genital tract abnormality, and if an earlier gynaecological examination (performed in response to the current presenting complaint) has been performed. Although a preliminary bimanual examination or pelvic ultrasound scan will help define the uterine shape, size and position, safe entry into the uterine cavity is invariably feasible with experience without prior palpation and by following the correct technique described below. If you are using an offset distal lens (30° most common), then prior knowledge of the uterine position can aid insertion of the hysteroscope by orientating the bevel of the lens in order to guide the endoscope through the cervix into the uterine cavity (see Fig. 4.2).

Local anaesthetic

Routine use of preoperative analgesics and sedatives and routine application of local anaesthetic to the cervix is not necessary for standard diagnostic hysteroscopy or endometrial

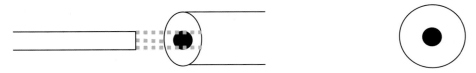

(a) Correct technique: forward facing distal lens (0°). When the 0° hysteroscope is aligned with the long axis of the endocervical canal, represented by a dark circle, it is located centrally on the monitor. This alignment should be maintained whilst traversing the canal and internal os and is achieved by adhering to the principle of strict visual control. If the correct view is lost, the instrument should be withdrawn very slightly and fine adjustment made to the angle of approach to relocate it before further advancement. On entering the cavity, the distal lens is moved in an upward direction if the uterus is anteflexed by moving the shaft of the endoscope downwards, and vice versa if the uterus is retroflexed.

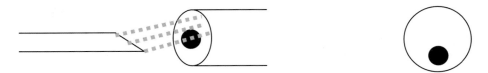

(b) Correct technique: offset, 30° fore-oblique distal lens. Most operators position the 30° hysteroscope with the bevel of the lens and light source lowermost (if endoscope is manufactured according to convention), so that the viewing angle of the distal lens is pointing in a upward direction. Furthermore, this orientation is useful for the more common anteverted/anteflexed uterus. When the hysteroscope is aligned with the long axis of the endocervical canal, the dark circle representing it is located at the bottom (6 o'clock position) of the monitor. This is the alignment that should be maintained whilst traversing the canal and internal os. If the internal os is narrow and the uterus anteverted, then the hysteroscope can be rotated and inverted at this point so that the bevel aids upward deflection of the instrument into the uterine cavity.

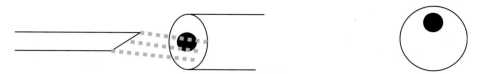

*(c) **Correct** technique: offset, 30° fore-oblique distal lens (inverted). When a 30° hysteroscope is inverted so that the viewing angle is pointing downward (the bevel of the lens and light source are uppermost), the endocervical canal will be located at the top (12 o'clock position) of the monitor. This orientation can be useful in guiding the instrument into the cavity when a retroverted/retroflexed uterus is encountered. If the internal os is narrow and the uterus retroverted, then the hysteroscope can be rotated at this point (as it appears in [b]) so that the bevel aids downward deflection of the instrument into the uterine cavity.*

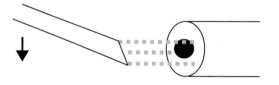

*(d) **Incorrect** technique: misalignment of an offset, 30° fore-oblique distal lens (central). The natural tendency is to adjust the hysteroscope so that the endocervical canal appears centrally, however, this is incorrect with an offset lens as the instrument is then no longer aligned with the axis of the endocervical canal. Damage to the cervical mucosa will occur and this trauma will cause pain.*

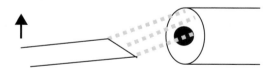

*(e) **Incorrect** technique: misalignment of an offset, 30° fore-oblique distal lens (eccentric). Here the hysteroscope is misaligned with the cervical canal such that it will impinge upon the anterior wall of the endocervical canal. The dark circle denoting the cervical canal is only partially visualized on the monitor, appearing eccentrically at the 6 o'clock position.*

Figure 4.2 *Practical hysteroscopy: difference in approach between 0° and 30° hysteroscopes.*

biopsy (Information Box 4.3). This is because the procedure is short, does not usually require cervical dilatation and is associated with minimal discomfort. Access to local anaesthetic should however, be available. Local anaesthetic indications are listed in Information Box 4.4 and techniques are described in Chapter 12.

Information Box 4.3 Drawbacks from routine use of local anaesthetic

- *Vasovagal attacks.* Administration may paradoxically provoke such episodes, especially in high-risk patients (e.g. cardiac arrhythmias, ischaemic heart disease).
- *Pain.* In addition, some patients are averse to injections – 'needle phobia'. Pain from injections at the start of the procedure may be counterproductive if patient distress results.
- *Anaphylaxis.* Allergic reactions to the anaesthetic agent are rare.
- *Cardiovascular collapse.* Direct intravascular injection can lead to life-threatening sequelae, especially in high-risk patients (e.g. elderly, ischaemic heart disease).
- *Effectiveness.* Conflicting evidence from clinical trials. Aids cervical dilatation, but pain experience influenced by many factors, including hysteroscopic technique.
- *Interference.* Visualization can be reduced with transcervical infusion of topical agents. Bleeding from injection sites can obscure cervical views and complicate uterine instrumentation.
- *Haemorrhage.* Simple tamponade usually stops minor bleeding from cervical injection sites. More serious bleeding from uterine vessels possible with deep paracervical infiltration techniques.
- *Cost.* In the absence of convincing cost-effectiveness data, routine administration of local anaesthetic is not justified.

Information Box 4.4 Indications for administering local cervical anaesthetic during hysteroscopic procedures

- *Cervical dilatation.* When necessary to overcome cervical stenosis, retrieve uterine specimens or foreign bodies.
- *Application of vulsella.* Local anaesthesia is not essential if patient prewarned and vulsellum applied gently without full ratcheting – the injection of local anaesthetic itself may be more uncomfortable.
- *Cervical cautery.* When cauterizing cervical lesions (ectopy, granulation tissue, sessile polyps).
- *Hysteroscopic surgery.* When anticipating specimen retrieval requiring cervical dilatation.

PROCEDURE

Insertion of hysteroscope

SPECULUM–ASSISTED

A warmed metal or disposable laterally opening ('Cusco's') speculum is inserted gently into the vagina and opened to expose the cervix, which is then gently cleaned with sterile water, saline or a non-foaming antiseptic. A Sims' speculum should be avoided, as the cervix will need to be routinely grasped with a vulsellum or tenaculum forceps, which is often uncomfortable. The hysteroscope should be connected to the light source and insufflation line, the monitor turned on and the video camera fixed in the correct vertical

Information Box 4.5 Distension media: delivery techniques

- Syringe
- Gravity feed
- Pressure bag
- Automated pump

Information Box 4.6 Indications for vaginoscopic approach to hysteroscopy

- *Vaginal laxity.* Poor pelvic floor tone may result in expulsion of the vaginal speculum or an obscured view of the cervix.
- *Virgin.* Narrow introitus making pain and trauma from speculum insertion more likely. Psychosexual factors may also be relevant. Juveniles should have such procedures under a general anaesthetic.
- *Atrophic lower genital tract.* Narrow introitus making pain and trauma from speculum insertion more likely.
- *Vulvar dermatoses.* Namely architectural destruction typical of advanced lichen sclerosus.
- *Limited hip mobility.* This may preclude insertion of a vaginal speculum.
- *Endometrial biopsy not indicated.* Vaginoscopic approach may be associated with less discomfort by avoiding the need for mechanical vaginal distension using a speculum, and is the technique of choice.

orientation, focused and balanced. The hysteroscope is supported and held by the light cable and/or camera (if in a sterile drape). The ergonomic handling of different hysteroscopes varies slightly according to design features and will influence the individual operator's approach. The hysteroscope should be inserted vaginally and the distension media inflow released once immediately adjacent to the cervix, to avoid excess vaginal loss of fluid unless a vaginoscopic approach is used. See Information Box 4.5 for delivery of distension media.

NO−SPECULUM OR 'VAGINOSCOPIC' APPROACH

The hysteroscope is introduced into the vagina without a speculum or cervical forceps. The labia minora are closed manually and the table tilted downwards slightly to limit the exit of CO_2 or normal saline, thus achieving a satisfactory distension of the vagina. The hysteroscope is advanced in order to visualize the cervix and identify the external cervical os, which is traversed, and the hysteroscope slowly introduced into the endocervical canal. Although this approach can lead to unwanted fluid spillage, it is associated with less discomfort by avoiding speculum insertion. Furthermore, the range of external hysteroscopic movement is increased, aiding visualization within the entire uterine cavity. Use of this technique is however, limited because most women undergoing hysteroscopy will require a global endometrial biopsy, which necessitates the use of a speculum. Indications for vaginoscopy are listed in Information Box 4.6.

Intracervical advancement of hysteroscope

This is potentially the most difficult part of the procedure. The technique varies slightly according to the angle of viewing (usually 0° or 30°) provided by the chosen hysteroscope. The key principle is to avoid trauma to the fragile endocervical mucosa, as this stimulates pain, can lead to poor views from bleeding and predisposes to false passage formation (Information Box 4.7).

Trauma and obscured visualization from bleeding is avoided by prohibiting routine blind dilatation of the cervical canal and instead advancing the hysteroscope under direct vision. This skill takes a short time to acquire for most trainees, as it contrasts with how many have been trained to dilate blindly and insert larger diameter instruments used in conventional, inpatient hysteroscopy under general anaesthesia. Such an approach is wholly inappropriate for outpatient work. Routine cervical dilatation is unnecessary in over 90 per cent of patients using the standard 5 mm diagnostic sheath and is even less frequently required with modern smaller diameter hysteroscopes <4 mm, which are being increasingly employed for diagnostic work. Indications for cervical dilatation are given in Information Box 4.8.

The initial inspection of the most proximal portion of the cervical canal is vital. If the cervical canal cannot be definitively seen, it is crucial not to push on blindly in the hope that the canal will materialize, for the reasons outlined above. The endocervical canal appears as a 'black spot' and this should be identified before further advancement of the hysteroscope. This

Information Box 4.7 False passage

A false passage is an blind-ending channel or passage within the myometrium that is artificially created when a uterine instrument (dilator, hysteroscope, curette), inserted through the external cervical os, traumatizes and perforates the endocervical canal. The artefactual appearance produced can compromise diagnosis because disturbed endometrium can resemble hyperplasia and the blind-ending channel can be confused with uterine anomalies or atrophic postmenopausal cavities. Serious complications can arise from rapid intravasation of distension media (fluid overload, CO_2 embolism) and from bleeding and visceral injury if complete uterine perforation into the peritoneal cavity occurs.

Information Box 4.8 Indications for cervical dilatation for hysteroscopic procedures

- *Cervical stenosis.* To enable access to the uterine cavity.
- *Uterine outflow.* May improve visualization with single flow diagnostic systems when fluid outflow is inadequate.
- *Uterine drainage.* Release of intrauterine chronic fluid collections (debris, pus or blood) secondary to cervical outflow obstruction.
- *Uterine instrumentation.* For example, introduction of polyp forceps, endometrial ablation devices/catheters, insertion of intrauterine coils.
- *Uterine specimen retrieval.* For example, polyps, 'lost' coils.

dark circle is produced by light absorption from the distant uterine fundus. When the long axis of the hysteroscope is aligned with the cervical canal, the black spot will appear centrally with a 0° 'end-on' rigid or flexible hysteroscope. A 0° distal lens permits direct visualization and it is much easier to master orientation as the direction of view corresponds to the natural approach so avoiding tissue trauma. This is in contrast to a 30° forward oblique hysteroscope, where the dark circle will appear eccentrically (i.e. at the 6 or 12 o'clock position depending upon which way up the endoscope is held) when the hysteroscope is in alignment with the axis of the cervical canal. The degree of distal lens offset needs to be appreciated when you are manipulating the hysteroscope. These principles are illustrated in Fig. 4.2, page 58.

Tenaculum forceps should not be routinely used, but may be necessary if there is a 'pinpoint,' fibrous (usually from previous cervical biopsy) or stenotic external cervical os. Other indications are given in Information Box 4.9. The tenaculum should be placed on the anterior cervical lip at 12 o'clock and gentle counter-traction applied, with the distal lens in the external os, to straighten the cervical canal and help overcome any resistance, in order to enter the canal. Local anaesthetic is not required if only a small amount of the relatively insensitive ectocervical tissue is grasped very slowly and the patient prewarned of an impending sharp sensation. Asking the patient to cough immediately prior to application may dull any induced discomfort. If tenaculum application is necessary to assist formal dilatation of the cervix, then local anaesthetic will be necessary.

Systematic panoramic inspection of the proximal cervix, with small back and forth motions, will usually identify the cervical canal and characteristic endocervical folds by allowing the distension medium to open the cervix, creating a 'microcavity'. If a stenosed cervical canal is encountered (Information Box 4.10), gentle forcible advancement of the hysteroscope with the aid of counter-traction provided by a cervical tenaculum will often safely overcome minor degrees of stenosis. If this fails then gentle cervical probing with a semiflexible graduated 'os-finding' uterine probe or formal dilatation with graduated cervical dilators will be necessary under local anaesthetic. Additional techniques to overcome cervical stenosis and help identify the cervical canal are listed in Information Boxes 4.11 and 4.12.

Information Box 4.9 Indications for cervical application of vulsella/tenaculum forceps

- *Cervical stenosis.* Allows counter-traction to be applied when the hysteroscope is being inserted to overcome cervical stenosis.
- *Cervical dilatation.* Counter-traction necessary.
- *Uterovaginal prolapse.* Allows the cervix to be stabilized, so that the hysteroscope can be inserted more easily.
- *Vaginal laxity.* Facilitates identification of the external cervical os, when obscured by lax vaginal walls. Uterine instrumentation thus aided.
- *Patulous cervical os.* Application of one or two vulsella to occlude the cervix prevents retrograde loss of media when adequate uterine distension cannot be maintained.
- *Acute flexion/version of uterus.* May help straighten the cervical canal or bring the uterus more proximal thereby easing hysteroscopic entry and inspection of the uterine cavity.
- *Uterine fibroids.* May help straighten the cervical canal when deviated or compressed by the presence of uterine or cervical tumours, usually fibroids.

Information Box 4.10   Factors predictive of cervical stenosis or atresia

- Postmenopausal women (hypo-oestrogenic/senile changes)
- Nulliparity
- Previous cervical biopsy
- Previous uterine surgery (ablation, D&C and Caesarean section)
- Uterine fibroids (deviation and/or compression)
- Previous uterine infection (adhesions)
- Treatment with gonadotrophic releasing hormone (hypo-oestrogenic changes)

Information Box 4.11   Interventions to overcome cervical stenosis

- *Cervical countertraction.* A single-toothed vulsellum or tenaculum may be applied to the anterior cervical lip. A 'pin-point' cervix or a cervix flush with vault (following cone biopsy) can then usually be overcome.
- *Cervical dilatation.* Mechanical dilatation using graded dilators after application of local anaesthetic to the cervix is effective in most circumstances.
- *Local oestrogen.* Rescheduling hysteroscopic examination after administration of local or systemic oestrogen for 1–2 weeks may help in postmenopausal women (rarely required).
- *Prostaglandins.* Oral, sublingual and vaginal prostaglandins have been tested in randomized trials to prime the cervix and reduce resistance, facilitate cervical dilatation and minimize risks of cervical and uterine trauma. Results are conflicting and any benefit is probably related to operative inpatient hysteroscopy with large diameter endoscopes. In addition to a lack of proven efficacy, the additional costs and side effects preclude their routine use.

The hysteroscope should be advanced slowly up to the level of the internal cervical os, making fine adjustments as necessary, if resistance is encountered so that the objective lens can be redirected into the axis of the cervical canal, so keeping it in view (Fig. 4.2, page 58).

Intrauterine advancement of hysteroscope

The internal cervical os is generally the narrowest portion of the cervical canal and this, combined with its more fibrous composition, can obstruct entry into the uterine cavity when hysteroscopic sheaths >4 mm diameter are employed. A slight pause at this point allows the inflowing medium time to further distend the uterine isthmus and assist pain-less entry into the cavity. The hysteroscope is then advanced under direct vision, and care taken when the uterine cavity is entered to steer the hysteroscope correctly, in keeping with the axis of the uterine body, thereby avoiding touching the uterine wall. If a 30° hystero-scope is used, then the beginner may experience some difficulty, as the telescope will not be advancing in the direction that appears on the monitor. In addition, rotation of a fore-oblique

> ## ⓘ Information Box 4.12 'I can't find the cervical canal': Techniques to overcome this problem
>
> - *Careful initial inspection.* Patient, panoramic inspection of proximal cervix using small back and forth motions. Inflow of the distension medium will normally distend the cervical canal, making its presence obvious.
> - *Consider false passages.* Occasionally the proximal cervix has a 'Swiss cheese'-type appearance, where a few potential 'cervical canals' are visualized. Gentle back and forth movements will help to identify which are false. If a blind-ending passage has been iatrogenically created, then gently withdraw the scope and perform a panoramic inspection as outlined above. The true cervical canal can usually be identified.
> - *Consider anatomic anomalies.* When acute degrees of anteversion or retroversion are not immediately apparent, the operator should consider these and therefore pay particular attention to the extreme anterior and posterior aspects of the proximal cervix, as the cervical canal can often be found here. Congenital or acquired uterine anomalies should also be considered. The uterine axis and cervix may also be deviated by the presence of fibroids or other pelvic masses. A bimanual pelvic or ultrasound examination is helpful to identify such scenarios. The acutely displaced uterus may then be overcome, altering the patient tilt and angle of inspection accordingly. Consideration should be given to use of angled rigid, semirigid or flexible scopes.
> - *Apply a cervical vulsellum.* Deviation of the cervical canal or acute degrees of ante/retroflexion can sometimes be corrected by application of gentle cervical counter-traction.
> - *Probe the cervix blindly.* This should be performed in a controlled fashion with the aid of a vulsellum to provide counter-traction to the gentle advancement of the hysteroscope. The canal will usually become quickly visible where flimsy adhesions had been co-apting the cervical walls.
> - *Look for mucus.* Gently advance the hysteroscope following the mucus stream into the cavity.
> - *Dilate the cervix.* Cervical probing with small diameter dilators should be performed if hysteroscopic probing fails. Blind cervical dilatation should only be performed after a bimanual examination to determine the uterine axis. If dilatation is not achieved easily or if it causes patient discomfort, then it should be abandoned and consideration given to performing cervical dilatation under ultrasound guidance or under general anaesthetic.
> - *Use a zero degree lens.* Orientation is more difficult with an offset lens and so a 0° hysteroscope may be preferable for the inexperienced.

hysteroscope when a narrowed isthmus is encountered may aid entry into the cavity by directing the 'sharpened' bevelled end towards the axis of the uterine body (Fig. 4.2, page 58).

The hysteroscope should be kept still for a few seconds within the uterine body to allow the cavity to distend and allow adequate panoramic visualization of the entire uterine cavity. In obese patients or when the uterine cavity is large and deviated, a complete panoramic view may be difficult to obtain. Correct positioning of the patient is essential in these circumstances and should be checked when difficulties arise. In addition, if a bi-valve speculum is in situ, its removal will increase the range of external hysteroscopic movement.

Inspection of the uterine cavity

Standard panoramic hysteroscopy refers to global observation of the entire uterine cavity and close inspection of the endometrial surfaces and is described here. In contrast to 'contact' hysteroscopy (see page 70) the technique does not involve image magnification by the optical lenses contained within the telescope, although the hysteroscopic image relayed to the video camera is magnified when displayed on the video monitor.

The entire uterine cavity should be examined using a systematic approach. Our approach starts with an initial panoramic view of the cavity obtained with hysteroscope at the level of the uterine isthmus. Uterine landmarks (cornua, tubal ostia, fundus) should be identified to confirm cavity entry and so that the hysteroscope is correctly orientated. This allows a general structural assessment with attention drawn to any focal lesions (e.g. polyps, fibroids, adhesions) or congenital uterine anomalies. The next step is to inspect the endometrium closely by advancing the distal end of the instrument to within a few millimetres of the mucosal surface, in keeping with the depth of field (fixed focus) provided by the particular hysteroscope (usually from ⩾1–3 mm).

We begin with a detailed inspection of the endometrium overlying the fundus, followed by examination of both cornual recesses and tubal ostia. There is considerable variation in the depth of the cornua and the appearance of the ostia, which may or may not be recessed behind an incomplete circular membrane. The ostia appear slit-like if closed, and circular when opened by the flow of the distension medium. The remaining endometrial surfaces are inspected usually beginning with the anterior, followed by both lateral and finally posterior surfaces (Fig. 4.3).

Modern hysteroscopes have a wide (75–120°) forward viewing angle. Complete inspection is accomplished by simple rotation of a hysteroscope with a 30° fore-oblique lens on its axis, so enlarging the field of view to the relevant areas (note that the camera must remain fixed in position to maintain orientation). A 0° hysteroscope requires slight side-to-side, up-and-down and back-and-forth movements of the distal lens to view the entire endometrial surface. This produces a degree of torque on the cervix, which can be uncomfortable for the patient, if movements are excessive. Zero degree hysteroscopes have been developed to counteract such problems. These are either flexible, steerable instruments (see page 69) or miniaturized semirigid hysteroscopes housed within a distally curved 10° outer sheath which can be rotated through 360° to enable fuller peripheral viewing and visualization of more inaccessible areas of the uterus such as the tubal ostia.

If the endometrium appears inappropriately thickened, then this can be assessed either by pressure (to produce a surface imprint) or by gently probing a furrow into the endometrium with the tip of the instrument. The patient should be prewarned that they may experience some discomfort and this is why such manoeuvres should be reserved until the visual inspection is terminated. Once inspection of the uterine cavity has been completed, the hysteroscope is slowly withdrawn into the cervical canal, which is inspected again as the instrument is withdrawn. A more detailed inspection of the cervical canal is often possible at this time.

A summary of hysteroscopic techniques aimed to minimize patient discomfort is presented in Information Box 4.13. Tips to optimize hysteroscopic visualization are given in Information Box 4.14 (page 70).

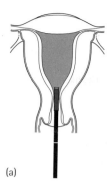

(a)

(a) Panoramic view. Advancement of the hysteroscope should cease at the level of the uterine isthmus once the internal cervical os has been traversed. This allows time for the cavity to distend and focal lesions to be identified. Dual chamber uteri and large submucous fibroids may be overlooked if the instrument is advanced rapidly into the uterine body. Visualization of both tubal ostia confirms that the uterine cavity has been reached.

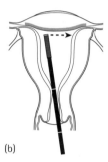

(b)

(b) Fundus and cornual regions. The hysteroscope is advanced and the cavity systematically inspected. A suggested technique is to move under high magnification from the right tubal ostia across the uterine fundus to the left tubal ostia. The hysteroscope should then be withdrawn and the fundus inspected once more.

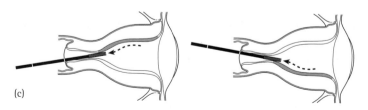

(c)

(c) Anterior and posterior uterine walls. The anterior wall is inspected from distal to proximal followed by the posterior wall.

Figure 4.3 *Hysteroscopic technique: systematic inspection of the uterine cavity.*

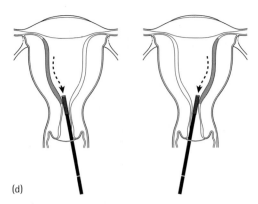

(d)

(d) Lateral uterine walls. The right and left lateral walls are inspected from distal to proximal. Note that appropriate up–down and side-side movements are required with a 0° hysteroscope whereas a 30° instrument, with its increased field of view, can survey most of the uterine cavity with rotational movements alone.

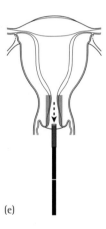

(e)

(e) Endocervical canal. The hysteroscope is slowly withdrawn, again obtaining a panoramic view of the uterine cavity. Although the endocervical canal has been visualized whilst the hysteroscope is introduced, it is better inspected in detail on withdrawal, as the canal has been nicely expanded by inflowing distension media. Once the external cervical os has been reached, the instrument is removed.

Figure 4.3 (*Continued*).

Endometrial tissue sampling

OUTPATIENT (BLIND) ENDOMETRIAL BIOPSY

If the indication for hysteroscopy is abnormal uterine bleeding, then an endometrial biopsy will be required if the woman is over 40 years of age or has other risk factors for serious endometrial disease. Although a polyp or myoma may occasional be exposed after suction

Information Box 4.13 Techniques to minimize discomfort during outpatient hysteroscopy

- *Avoid painful manoeuvres.* These include routine application of vulsella, cervical dilatation, speculum insertion (if global biopsy not required).
- *Minimize hysteroscope movement.* Less instrument manipulation required with 30° terminal lenses (increased field of view) or steerable and flexible endoscopes.
- *Do not touch side walls* . By meticulously avoiding contact with the cervical or uterine side walls, painful stimuli are minimized. This requires a patient, hysteroscopic approach, keeping the cervical canal and uterus under direct vision at all times.
- *Vaginoscopy.* Avoids excessive instrumentation (speculum or tenaculum).
- *Minimize distension pressure.* Distension pressures should be titrated to their minimum effective levels. Syringe delivery of fluid is the best way to achieve this.
- *Operator approach.* Communication with the patient and expediency are essential.

curettage, we do not believe this possibility warrants a routine check hysteroscopy. This is because the yield from such a policy will be low (especially when poor visualization following endometrial abrasion is taken into account) and the clinical significance of such findings is likely to be minimal.

HYSTEROSCOPICALLY DIRECTED ENDOMETRIAL BIOPSY

The principal concerns over blind endometrial sampling are that it is:

- non-representative as only a small proportion of the endometrial surface is sampled (estimated to be between 4 and 40 per cent depending on technique), and
- focal lesions are missed.

These drawbacks may be overcome to some degree by taking hysteroscopically directed biopsies. Small studies comparing such an approach with traditional dilatation and curettage, has shown panoramic hysteroscopy with selective sampling to have higher accuracy and provide more diagnostic information. Limitations of such an approach relate to the small amount of tissue obtained from small ancillary instrumentation (typically 1.6–2.0 mm biopsy forceps). This, along with crush artefact, can impair histological assessment and necessitate the need for multiple biopsies.

Flexible hysteroscopy

Flexible hysteroscopes are discussed fully in Chapter 3. From a practical viewpoint, the technique for hysteroscopic examination of the uterine cavity is slightly different for flexible hysteroscopes. The 0° fibroscope is advanced with the rounded distal point straight ahead as for a rigid endoscope with no lens offset. The uterine cavity is then inspected by rotation of the hysteroscope and by bending the distal end up and down (100–160° in either direction) using the angulation control lever close to the eyepiece of the instrument (Fig. 4.4).

> ### *i* Information Box 4.14 Tips to obtain an optimal view at hysteroscopy and rectify a poor view
>
> - *Avoid menstruation.* There is no evidence to support the view that diagnostic accuracy is influenced by cycle phase. It is sensible, however, to avoid procedures during the initial heavy days of menstruation, as views are likely to be compromised as a result of bleeding and sloughing menstrual endometrium.
> - *Check hysteroscope is focused.* This should be done ideally along with a white balance prior to starting the procedure. However, intraoperative focusing is easy if required.
> - *Ensure adequate distension pressure.* Check that fluid/gas is inflowing (e.g. check that the inflow tubes are attached, unkinked and all taps are open). Higher rates of inflow are required to distend large uterine cavities (which appear darker owing to increased absorption of light – use maximum intensity) and so insufflation pressure should be increased. Unwanted leakage of distension media from patulous cervical canals or an 'overdilated' cervix can be corrected by apposing the cervical lips with the vulsella placed anteriorly and posteriorly, or using larger diameter scopes in addition to closing the outflow channel of a continuous flow system. A slight downward Trendelenburg tilt may also help to retain intrauterine fluid. If cervical dilatation required, avoid overdilatating the cervix.
> - *Avoid bleeding.* Perform the whole procedure under careful *direct* endoscopic vision. Avoid cervical dilatation and traumatizing the cervical or uterine side walls. Avoid touching intrauterine abnormalities (e.g. vascular submucous fibroids) or endometrial lesions (e.g. hyperplastic areas) until the end of the procedure, if at all. Avoid unduly high distension pressures, which may stimulate endometrial bleeding. Use miniature hysteroscopes (2.5 mm diameter) to minimize inadvertent tissue trauma or the need for cervical dilatation. Check that blood is not on the lens if a 'red circle' is all that can be seen. Saline may be better than CO_2 as blood may be washed away and bubble formation is generally not a problem. Plan the procedure, so that repeated reinsertion of the hysteroscope is avoided.
> - *Avoid tissue trauma.* Fragments of endometrial tissue may become trapped over the lens obscuring visualization unless the hysteroscope is removed and the lens cleaned.
> - *Ensure adequate outflow.* For diagnostic procedures, visualization problems more commonly arise from inadequate distension pressures. However, tight cervical canals may preclude adequate outflow, and hence fluid circulation (inflow and outflow) is suboptimal and collected endometrial debris or blood cannot be cleared. Check that the outflow tap on the hysteroscope is open (if an outflow channel is present). Cervical dilatation is required under these circumstances.

Contact hysteroscopy

Microscopic examination of the endometrial epithelium at cellular level, containing blood vessels and glands, necessitates direct contact with the mucosal surface and high magnification ($\times 20$ to $\times 150$) with a specially designed microcolpohysteroscope (properties of a telescope and a compound microscope). This technique does not require uterine distension and is called 'contact' hysteroscopy. It has limited use in clinical practice and consequently the

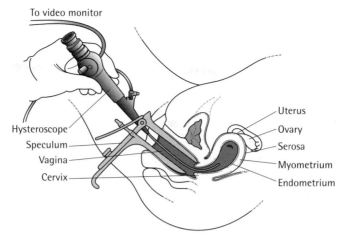

To video monitor

Hysteroscope
Speculum
Vagina
Cervix

Uterus
Ovary
Serosa
Myometrium
Endometrium

Figure 4.4 *Flexible hysteroscopy.*

technique has not gained widespread popularity and has been replaced by panoramic hysteroscopy, so will not be considered further.

RECORDING INFORMATION

An accurate record of diagnostic findings needs to be archived. A combination of descriptive prose, dictated letters and diagrammatic representations is normally employed. Information and findings should be recorded in a systematic way using standard terminology to aid understanding and form the basis for research and audit. Findings from the clinical examination should be recorded along with the following hysteroscopic findings:

- clinical findings from pelvic examination (standard)
- description of the endocervical canal
- description of the uterine cavity
  - size
  - shape
  - endometrium
  - structural pathology.

A recommended practical nomenclature for recording diagnostic information is described in Chapter 5.

Line drawings can be produced free-hand, using preprinted forms or with the aid of suitable computer software (Fig. 4.5). Digital still and moving image capture, processing and printing have added another dimension to recording clinical data. Data are computerized and summary sheets can be included within the case notes. Such formats can also help to convey information to patients and also be used for clinical, research, audit, teaching and medicolegal purposes.

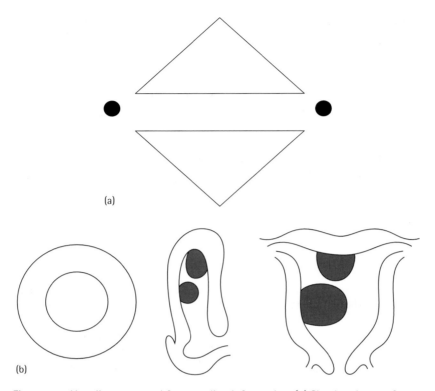

Figure 4.5 *Line diagrams used for recording information. (a) Simple schema of a normal uterine cavity. (b) Cervical, saggital and coronal views of the cervix and uterine cavity. Polyps are indicated in the central-fundal and posterior-left lateral positions.*

POSTOPERATIVE CARE

Minimal postoperative care is required following diagnostic outpatient hysteroscopy. It is good practice to offer patients refreshment and observe them for a period of 30 minutes in a sitting recovery area. This allows patients to reflect on their experience and allows them to air any outstanding questions or residual concerns. Verbal and written information should be given so that women will not be alarmed if postoperative spotting, discharge and pain from uterine cramping is experienced. Simple analgesics may be required. In the unusual situation where women receive narcotic analgesia or conscious sedation, they should not be allowed to drive home, leave unaccompanied or drink alcohol for 48 hours because of possible induced drowsiness.

Women should be given a unit contact number in the event of untoward symptoms such as fever or severe and persisting bleeding or pelvic pain, which may suggest infection or an unrecognized operative complication. Women should be informed of the necessity of any follow-up arrangements for discussing laboratory results, undertaking repeat proced-ures or for the assessment of treatment response. A summary of the essential procedural steps involved in outpatient hysteroscopy is given in Information Box 4.15.

DECONTAMINATION

Cleaning, disinfecting and sterilization issues are dealt with in Chapter 3.

AUDIT

Auditable standards for diagnostic performance include the need for cervical dilatation and local anaesthesia, mean time to complete the procedure, failure rates and diagnostic accuracy. Although the need for cervical dilatation will vary according to the population and diameter of the diagnostic sheath used, evidence and experience suggest that cervical dilatation should be required in <5 per cent of cases when hysteroscopes <5 mm diameter are used. As a result the average diagnostic procedure time, measured from insertion to removal of the hysteroscope, should be <5 minutes. Failure rates, should be ≤5 per cent and are defined as:

- inability to enter the uterine cavity
- poor visualization precluding diagnosis, or
- patient intolerance of the procedure

Accuracy of endometrial assessment can be evaluated by comparison with histology and clinical follow-up. The positive and negative predictive values for endometrial cancer are approximately 80 per cent and 99 per cent at a 5 per cent disease prevalence and endometrial hyperplasia 60 per cent and 96 per cent at a 10 per cent disease prevalence, although the actual values will depend upon local disease prevalence, which should be determined. Complications should be recorded, although these will depend upon the case mix and type of procedure. As a rule, vasovagal reactions should occur in <3 per cent of hysteroscopic procedures if miniature (<5 mm diameter) instruments are used, and uterine perforation rates are <0.2 per cent.

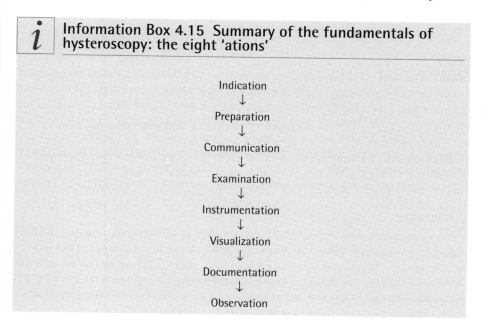

i Information Box 4.15 Summary of the fundamentals of hysteroscopy: the eight 'ations'

Indication
↓
Preparation
↓
Communication
↓
Examination
↓
Instrumentation
↓
Visualization
↓
Documentation
↓
Observation

COMPLICATIONS

Diagnostic outpatient hysteroscopy

Table 4.1 lists the complications likely to be encountered with diagnostic outpatient hysteroscopy along with suggestions for management. A systematic review reported only eight major complications (five perforations) in over 25 000 diagnostic procedures. In the conscious outpatient, positional complications including nerve, back and soft tissue injuries as well as deep vein thrombosis are avoided. Potentially more serious adverse events can occur with operative work and these are discussed in detail below with tips on avoiding, recognizing and managing such complications. The inherent limitations of surgical hysteroscopy in an outpatient setting, combined with the use of isotonic normal saline for operative work and the avoidance of general anaesthesia, make the occurrence of serious side effects rare. However, it is still important that the operator can recognize and manage complications if they do occur, in order to avoid serious long-term morbidity.

Operative outpatient hysteroscopy

FLUID OVERLOAD
Avoidance

High rates of fluid inflow and procedures >20 minutes are unlikely to be tolerated in the conscious patient and so problems with significant fluid overload (resulting from excessive intravasation of fluid) are unlikely, even with saline-free low viscosity fluids (e.g. dextrose). Furthermore, outpatient electrosurgical procedures are only feasible using a bipolar intrauterine system, which requires the use of saline as a conducting and distension medium. Physiological media can lead to fluid overload and pulmonary oedema, but not hyponatraemia or problems with hypo-osmolality.

Recognition

Infusion pressures should be kept low (between 60 and 100 mmHg, not to exceed mean arterial pressure), operating time minimized and fluid volumes monitored. Fluid overload should be suspected when procedures are prolonged and associated with a substantial fluid discrepancy (>1000–1500 ml). A discrepancy of 1500 ml should result in cessation of the procedure. Older patients with cardiovascular compromise are particularly sensitive to sequelae of electrolyte imbalance. Classic symptoms are nausea, vomiting, headache, lethargy or agitation, followed by bradycardia and hypertension ('TURP syndrome'). Untreated pulmonary and cerebral oedema can develop, leading to cardiovascular collapse.

Management

Measure serum urea and electrolytes. If plasma sodium is <125 mmol/l, then institute fluid restriction (800 ml/day) and use diuretics (e.g. 40 mg frusemide i.v.) and consider supplemental oxygen. Plasma sodium >120 mmol/l will require hypertonic saline infusion (70 mmol sodium/h). Physiological media (normal saline) can lead to fluid overload and pulmonary oedema, but not hyponatraemia and problems with hypo-osmolality). Pulmonary oedema is much easier to treat in these circumstances.

Table 4.1 *Recognizing and managing complications associated with diagnostic hysteroscopy*

Complication	Recognition	Management
Vasovagal attacks	The woman may report feeling sick and faint. Clinical signs are easily detected – pallor, sweating, bradycardia, hypotension and reduced conscious state. Such episodes may be minimized by avoiding unnecessary uterocervical manipulation, excess uterine distension, prolonged procedures and excess pain.	Most affected women will respond rapidly to (a) stopping procedures and removing all instrumentation and (b) simple, supportive measures which include putting the woman in the supine/recovery position, giving fluids (oral ± i.v), cool fanning and reassurance. Atropine may be required in some cases.
Cervical trauma	Application or removal of instrumentation may result in bleeding from traumatized cervical tissue, which is easily visualized.	Tamponade with a 'swab-on-a-stick' or ring forceps will stop bleeding from puncture sites. Partially torn or avulsed tissue may require a haemostatic suture.
Uterine perforation	Penetration of the serosal uterine surface often gives a filmy, 'areolar' tissue appearance. Perforation is diagnosed when contents of the peritoneal cavity are seen (adipose tissue, bowel) and the hysteroscope can be advanced beyond the distance of the uterine cavity.	In the absence of heavy bleeding from the perforation site, broad spectrum antibiotics should be prescribed and the patient observed for 2–4 hours. Admit if there is persistent pain or shock. When the woman is discharged, instructions should be given to contact the unit if symptoms of pain or bleeding ensue.
Haemorrhage	Bleeding obscuring hysteroscopic visualization or profuse/persistent bleeding is observed following withdrawal of instruments.	See operative complications below. Postoperative observation for a short period is mandatory because bleeding may increase when the intrauterine pressure is reduced.
Cardiovascular collapse	The woman may complain of feeling unwell or, breathless and appear clammy followed by sudden catastrophic loss of consciousness in association with absent respiration and pulse. Direct intravascular injection of local anaesthetic or anaphylaxis to agents/media (e.g. high molecular weight dextran) may be causative. Be vigilant in women with cardiac disease.	Cardiopulmonary resuscitation protocols should be followed in conjunction with a 'crash' resuscitation team if available. A cardiac defibrillator, and 'crash' trolley containing adrenaline, atropine and anti-arrhythmics, should be immediately available.
Infection	Endometritis is rare following diagnostic hysteroscopy (approx. 1 in 500 general population). Can be associated with operative procedures such as endometrial ablation (approx. 1 in 200).	Infection risks are minimized if (a) a sterile and efficient approach is adopted, where repeated uterine re-instrumentation is avoided and (b) hysteroscopy is postponed and genital tract swabs taken if an abnormal vaginal discharge is seen. Prophylactic antibiotics are only indicated if there is a proven past history of pelvic infection (oral antibiotics) or for cardioprophylaxis (parenteral antibiotics). Give oral broad spectrum antibiotics for delayed endometritis.

UTERINE PERFORATION
Avoidance
See Table 4.1. This complication is avoidable if the hysteroscope is passed under direct vision at all times.

Recognition
See Table 4.1. Persistent or worsening abdominal pain, especially if associated with pyrexia and shock, is suggestive of faecal peritonitis, which can present up to 10 days after the original insult.

Management
See Table 4.1. Exploration of the peritoneal cavity is indicated when perforation occurs with the use of thermal energy or is initially unrecognized following sharp mechanical instrumentation. Laparotomy is indicated in the presence of continuous bleeding or hypotensive shock (especially if lateral perforation has lacerated the uterine vasculature). In such circumstances, patient resuscitation and correction of coagulopathy will be necessary with the use of intravenous plasma expanders and blood products.

HAEMORRHAGE
Avoidance
Bleeding can often arise from inadvertent trauma such as cervical tears from placement of tenaculum forceps, forceful cervical dilatation, false passage creation and accidental contact with the uterine wall. High uterine distension pressures can initiate bleeding from abnormal endometrial vasculature. Special care is required in women on warfarin or with known bleeding diatheses.

Recognition
See Table 4.1. Perform intrauterine instrumentation and surgery under direct vision at all times. If blind cervical dilatation is required (Information Box 4.8), then use local anaesthetics with vasoconstrictors (e.g. vasopressin, adrenaline) to minimize bleeding. Patient tolerability will limit surgery in the outpatient setting and so procedures likely to precipitate major haemorrhage should be rare. However, the operator should give careful consideration to procedure selection and feasibility and be alert to possible complications. Bleeding is most often a problem when surgery involves deep myometrial penetration (resection of uterine septae, adhesions, fibroids). Hysteroscopic view can be rapidly obscured if bleeding occurs because of the limited circulation of distension media associated with small-diameter endoscopes.

Management
If obvious bleeding vessels are visible, then coagulate using electrodiathermy. Otherwise, consider bladder catheterization and bimanual uterine compression initially. If bleeding is still a problem then insert a 10–30 ml Foley catheter or balloon catheter (e.g. Rusch

balloon) to facilitate intrauterine tamponade. Gradual deflation (50 per cent at 1 hour) and removal of the catheter can usually be done within 2 hours. However, the catheter may need to be kept *in situ* for longer (24 hours) if bleeding continues on deflation. Uterine perforation (requiring laparoscopy/laparotomy) and/or coagulopathy (requiring correction with blood products) should be considered in cases of continued bleeding or hypotensive shock.

ELECTROSURGICAL COMPLICATIONS
Avoidance

The development of intrauterine bipolar electrodiathermy systems means that outpatient surgery using this modality is inherently safer electrically than standard inpatient monopolar systems. It is possible, however, to go inadvertently into the underlying deep myometrium using miniature bipolar electrodes if the tip is not kept under direct endoscopic vision at all times. The tip should not be too far away from the focal length of the imaging system, as distance is much harder to judge and risk of unwanted contact higher. Measured systematic movements, avoiding prolonged and concentrated periods of high-power electrical discharge, are essential to prevent thermal injuries. The operator should be especially cautious using thermal energy near the uterine cornu, where the myometrium is thinnest, or when the cavity is distorted by fibroids or other uterine anomalies.

Recognition

Systematic inspection of the uterine cavity at all stages of the intervention will identify any areas of inadvertent myometrial penetration. Inspection at high magnification is required where suspicious areas are identified in order to exclude uterine perforation. This is done by visualizing the white appearance of deep, intact layers of myometrium. The Versapoint electrodes are only 1–3 mm in length and so full thickness damage is unusual. However, full thickness penetration should be suspected where no reflected light from the underlying myometrium is seen, or more obviously when filmy areolar or adipose tissue or bowel is seen. The most feared complication is thermal injury to the bowel following inadvertent uterine perforation (see Uterine perforation, page 76).

Management

See Uterine perforation, page 76. Laparotomy is indicated with appropriate antibiotic prophylaxis.

AIR EMBOLISM (SEE ALSO CHAPTER 14)
Avoidance

Ambient air or pressurized gas can potentially enter the circulation through open endometrial venous channels. It is thought that this is more likely if the level of the uterus is above the heart so that negative pressure occurs during diastole, thus sucking air through the open venous sinuses. However, this complication is unlikely in the outpatient setting where low rates of inflow and distension pressure are used. Traditionally associated with CO_2, it is now recognized that bipolar electrodiathermy can cause air emboli following intravasation of air created from vapour pockets. This complication appears to be associated with prolonged myomectomy and has not been reported in the outpatient setting.

- Avoid acute reverse Trendelenburg positioning.
- Avoid cervical 'over-dilatation'.
- Minimize uterine trauma.
- Purge inflow tubing.
- Avoid multiple hysteroscope insertions/instrument changes.

Recognition

Symptoms include acute breathlessness (with or without chest pain), hypotension and hypoxia. It should also be suspected with changes in end tidal CO_2 (decrease), oxygen saturation (hypoxia), heart rate (tachycardia), respiratory rate (increased) and blood pressure (hypotension). A machine-like murmur may be heard over the precordium. Asystole may occur in severe cases.

Management

The procedure should be immediately abandoned, the hysteroscope removed, the vagina occluded (e.g. with a wet sponge) and the patient put into the recovery position (left side). The patient should be resuscitated on a bed (intravenous fluid, oxygen), a full blood count and electrolytes and arterial blood gases analysed, an electrocardiograph ± chest X-ray performed and an anaesthetic/cardiology opinion obtained. The acute episode usually resolves rapidly, although cardiopulmonary resuscitation and intensive care may be required if pulmonary oedema/adult respiratory disease syndrome (ARDS) occurs.

Evidence Box 4.1   Acceptability, feasibility and safety of outpatient hysteroscopy

- *Acceptability.* Small qualitative observational series have shown outpatient hysteroscopy to be an 'acceptable' procedure to women. This has mainly been judged in relation to acceptance of pain, but it should be borne in mind that women may not find such a procedure acceptable owing to other factors, such as perceived loss of dignity and embarrassment. Most women are 'satisfied' with the procedure, and prepared to recommend it or undergo the experience again if necessary. Further research is needed to identify the 3–5 per cent of women who, with hindsight, would have preferred the procedure under a general anaesthetic. The gynaecologist, when planning diagnostic work-up, should also bear in mind observations from the literature that women generally prefer ultrasound over hysteroscopy because it generates less discomfort and is a more discrete examination. Instrumentation and distension of the uterine cavity, whether using saline infusion sonography or hysteroscopy, is comparatively more painful than transvaginal ultrasound (TVS) but both procedures appear to be equally well tolerated. Proponents of ultrasound frequently purport hysteroscopy to be poorly tolerated in comparison to saline infusion sonography (SIS). This view may have been sustainable with older, larger diameter hysteroscopes, but there is scarce supporting evidence for such claims in relation to the modern miniaturized hysteroscopes used today. Abrasive, blind endometrial biopsy, although well tolerated, is more painful than standard outpatient hysteroscopy.

- *Feasibility.* The pooled failure rate derived from 26 000 diagnostic hysteroscopies was 3.5 per cent. The rate in the outpatient setting was marginally higher than that in the inpatient setting (4 versus 3 per cent respectively). We can therefore conclude that diagnostic outpatient hysteroscopy is a highly successful procedure. The reason for failure was most commonly technical difficulty owing to anatomical factors, including cervical stenosis followed by inadequate visualization and finally patient intolerance. It is important to note that inadequate visualization (e.g. obscured by bleeding, debris) was more common in the traditional inpatient setting as a reason for failure The failure rate of TVS is negligible, but that of SIS is generally reported to be higher when compared to outpatient hysteroscopy using endoscopes <5 mm in outer diameter. Although common factors contribute to failure of operative outpatient hysteroscopy, it is generally procedure dependent.

- *Safety.* Outpatient diagnostic hysteroscopy appears to be a very safe procedure. In an analysis of over 25 000 diagnostic outpatient hysteroscopies, only two serious potentially life-threatening complications were reported: one angina attack and one hypocalcaemic crisis. There were five uterine perforations although reporting bias may have underestimated the complication rate to some degree. The low rate of direct procedure-related complications may reflect improved image quality and miniaturization of hysteroscopes, obviating the need for blind cervical dilatation, which risks visceral perforation and haemorrhage. Operative hysteroscopy is associated with a higher adverse event rate, but large data sets pertaining to the outpatient setting are unavailable, reflecting its relative infancy.

KEY POINTS

- Outpatient hysteroscopy is feasible and well tolerated in over 95 per cent of women if a competent operator employs good basic technique.

- Outpatient hysteroscopy is safe with few absolute contraindications. Complications are limited to the procedure, as those occurring from distension media and anaesthesia are all but obviated in an outpatient setting.

- Problems such as pain and anxiety, occurrence of vasovagal attacks, cervical stenosis, non-visualization of cervical canal or uterine landmarks and inadequate uterine distension and cavity visualization can be easily resolved in the majority of cases if the operator has a knowledge of the simple strategies required to avoid/overcome them.

- Indications for hysteroscopy and diagnostic findings should be recorded and overall service performance audited.

FURTHER READING

Cicinelli E, Parisi C, Galantino P, Pinto V, Barba B, Schonauer S. Reliability, feasibility, and safety of minihysteroscopy with a vaginoscopic approach: experience with 6,000 cases. *Fertil Steril* 2003;**80**:199–202.

Clark TJ, Voit D, Song F, Hyde C, Gupta JK, Khan KS. Accuracy of hysteroscopy in the diagnosis of endometrial cancer and disease: A systematic review. *JAMA* 2002;**288**:1610–21.

Gimpelson RJ, Rappold HO. A comparative study between panoramic hysteroscopy with directed biopsies and dilatation and curettage. A review of 276 cases. *Am J Obstet Gynecol* 1988;**158**:489–92.

Kremer C, Duffy S, Moroney M. Patient satisfaction with outpatient hysteroscopy versus day case hysteroscopy: randomised controlled trial. *BMJ* 2000;**320**:279–82.

Tahir MM, Bigrigg MA, Browning JJ, Brookes ST, Smith PA. A randomised controlled trial comparing transvaginal ultrasound, outpatient hysteroscopy and endometrial biopsy with inpatient hysteroscopy and curettage. *Br J Obstet Gynaecol* 1999;**106**:1259–64.

5

Diagnostic hysteroscopy

Successful hysteroscopy depends upon good surgical technique, an understanding of the limitations of the technology and incorporation of information obtained from earlier in the clinical process (history and examination). Hysteroscopy should be avoided during menses because the view is likely to be compromised. Although normal endometrial appearances during the secretory phase could potentially be misinterpreted (e.g. as polyps or hyperplastic endometrium), with experience the likelihood of this is small and so timing of the procedure to coincide with the proliferative phase of the menstrual cycle is not necessary nor indeed practical.

Studies investigating the accuracy of hysteroscopy in diagnosing endometrial disease rarely define their diagnostic criteria. Where morphological descriptions of features suggestive of, say, endometrial hyperplasia or cancer are reported, they are often vague and conflicting or employ arbitrary scoring systems. Consequently, there are no agreed standardized criteria for hysteroscopic diagnosis. The difficulty in establishing such criteria stems from the fact that there is considerable overlap between hysteroscopic features of functional and pathological endometrium. More importantly, the limitations of hysteroscopic diagnosis have not been appreciated, i.e. macroscopic inspection of the uterine cavity cannot directly make more subtle, histological diagnoses. Within the practical clinical context therefore, hysteroscopic diagnoses incorporating these morphological features would be better classified as normal, abnormal (thickened), abnormal (suspicious) or abnormal (cancerous), consistent with the capability of the technology (see pages 86–87). In contrast to the difficulties with endometrial evaluation, hysteroscopy is the gold standard for detecting intrauterine structural pathology.

To formulate a hysteroscopic diagnosis requires an assessment of the endometrium and the uterocervical cavity. An appreciation of normality is fundamental to this assessment. The endometrial parameters and uterocervical features that need to be assessed are summarized in Information Box 5.1, and a description of normal and abnormal findings detailed in Tables 5.1 and 5.2. Thus, a normal examination requires a normal uterine cavity, with a normal-looking endometrium and an absence of any focal lesions.

Information Box 5.1 Uterine assessment

ENDOMETRIAL PARAMETERS (TABLE 5.1)

- Endometrial thickness
- Endometrial surface
- Endometrial colour
- Vasculature
- (Glandular openings – only appropriate if using high magnification)

UTEROCERVICAL CAVITY FEATURES (TABLE 5.2)

- Endocervical canal
- Uterine fluid
- Uterine axis
- Uterine shape
- Uterine size
- Uterine focal lesions or foreign bodies

TRADITIONAL 'HISTOLOGICAL' CLASSIFICATION OF HYSTEROSCOPIC ENDOMETRIAL APPEARANCE

Normal endometrium

Normal functional endometrium has a generally smooth, homogeneous and non-vascular appearance. The phases of the menstrual cycle can be differentiated with experience:

- *Menstrual.* The endometrium may be thin if menstruation is nearly completed, or have a patchy reddened 'shaggy' appearance caused by irregular endometrial sloughing. Blood and menstrual debris frequently obscure visualization.

- *Proliferative endometrium.* The endometrium is thin and yellow-white or pale pink with little vascularization (Plate 8).

- *Secretory.* The endometrium is globally thickened, 'fluffy' and more difficult to interpret, especially if it has a polypoid appearance. The delicate superficial vascular network is more prominent, resulting in an increasingly red-pink endometrial appearance (Plate 9).

Atrophic (postmenopausal) or inactive endometrium

The endometrium is thin, white and smooth. The lack of surface irregularities gives an overall featureless appearance. However, the exposed, thin underlying stroma may impart a trabeculated appearance (caused by revealed myometrial fibres) and fragile, but regular vasculature is visible (Plate 10).

Table 5.1 *Endometrial parameters to be assessed at diagnostic hysteroscopy*

Endometrial parameters*	Normal	Abnormal
Endometrial thickness	Thin (proliferative), uniform thickening (secretory), and thin or absent (inactive)	Focal or diffuse increase in endometrial thickness
Endometrial surface	Smooth and regular (proliferative), smooth, gently undulating, 'fluffy' or polypoid appearance (secretory) and smooth or trabeculated appearance caused by exposed, thin underlying stroma (inactive)	Focal or diffuse surface, irregularity of varying appearance (polypoid, papillary, cystic, necrotic, friable [haemorrhagic], etc.)
Endometrial colour	Yellow-white (proliferative), increasingly red (secretory) and white (inactive)	Grey-white, red (haemorrhagic)
Vasculature	Minimal (proliferative), uniform superficial network of blood vessels (secretory) and minimal (inactive)	Ranges from marked, but regular superficial vascular injection (hyperaemia) to a highly irregular vascular network containing frankly atypical vessels (large and bizarre, often free-running single vessels). In these circumstances, the endometrium is intensely haemorrhagic (friable). Areas of tissue necrosis and bleeding may be present
Glandular openings (density, size, colour)[†]	Regularly spaced and non-crowded arrangement of non-dilated glandular openings of the same colour as the surrounding endometrium (proliferative), more visible and pronounced (proliferative), non-visible (inactive)	Concentrated, thickened and irregular arrangement of dilated yellow glandular openings (up to 2–3 mm in diameter). Glandular cystic changes usually seen in association with a thickened endometrium

* All parameters dependent upon hormonal status. Note that appearances of all parameters vary in women on hormone replacement therapy. Generally those on a continuous combined preparation will have appearances akin to the atrophic (inactive) postmenopausal woman and those on sequential preparations will have appearances between active (functional) and inactive endometrium
[†] Assumes inspection under higher magnification ($\times$ 20–150)

Table 5.2 *Uterocervical parameters to be assessed at diagnostic hysteroscopy*

Uterocervical parameters	Normal	Abnormal
Endocervical canal	Easy passage of the hysteroscope through a regular, 2–4 cm cylindrical canal. The mucosa of the endocervix is folded (cervical crypts) and glandular (premenopausally) and may be polypoidal. It may also have a trabeculated appearance in the lower part because of the underlying fibrous connective tissue, which is more pronounced postmenopausally. Nulliparous women have a pin-point external cervical os, which may require dilatation to traverse	The most common anomaly is cervical stenosis resulting from a hypo-oestrogenic state or acquired following cervical cone biopsy (a deficient ectocervix, flush with the vaginal vault, can be found in association that may present further difficulties inserting the hysteroscope). The dark circle representing the cervical canal can be hard to locate especially after previous uterine surgery or instrumentation, where false passages may have been created. Polyps are commonly seen and the stalk should be located to define their origin – ecto- or endocervical or prolapsed from the endometrial cavity
Uterine fluid	Small amounts of clear or turbid (containing debris) intracavity fluid are normal findings especially in the presence of outflow obstruction (cervical stenosis). Brown/blood-stained fluid can be found in premenopausal women	Brown/blood-stained intracavity fluid or fluid of any description in the presence of postmenopausal endometrial thickening. Purulent fluid suggests infection or underlying malignancy and is an abnormal finding in any age group
Uterine axis	Most women (approximately 70 per cent) will have an anteverted uterus (long axis tilting forward in relation to the vaginal axis). The remainder will have axial of retroverted uteri	There is no 'abnormal' uterine axis although acute degrees of ante/retroflexion (flexion at the level of the isthmus) and ante/retroversion can present difficulties in inserting the hysteroscope and obtaining panoramic views. An immobile retro-verted uterus may suggest pelvic pathology

Uterine shape	The uterine contour should be regular with a saddle-shaped fundus, containing two cornual recesses (<1 cm from deepest median point of the fundus) in which are found the tubal ostia. An arcuate uterus is a normal variant (more pronounced 'saddle')	Congenital uterine malformations (Müllerian developmental defects) can lead to a variety of abnormal uterine shapes and sizes. The most common are bicornuate and septate uteri. Acquired structural anomalies (e.g. fibroids, adhesions) can also distort the cavity
Uterine size	The average uterocervical cavity measurement in women of reproductive age is around 7 cm and the uterine body:cervical length ratio is approximately 2–3:1 as compared to a 1:1 ratio before puberty and after the menopause. Parous women have larger uteri than nulliparous women	Uteri >10 cm absorb more light and so panoramic hysteroscopic views can be compromised. Uterine enlargement is most probably due to benign causes (e.g. fibroids, adenomyosis or diffuse myometrial hypertrophy), although uterine malignancy should always be considered in association with other clinical and hysteroscopic features. Hypoplastic uteri have a long cervical canal in association with a small, narrow cavity
Uterine focal lesions or foreign bodies	No focal lesions (e.g. polyps, submucous fibroids or adhesions) should be present. Correctly placed known intrauterine contraceptive devices (IUCDs) within the uterine cavity are considered normal	Presence of any focal lesion or incorrectly sited IUCD (twisted, non-fundal). Endometrial assessment should be completed prior to removing an IUCD to prevent bleeding or artefacts compromising diagnostic interpretation

Inflammatory endometrium

The endometrium can be of varying thickness, usually without surface irregularities, but will appear uniformly red as a result of globally increased vascularization. The endometrium is touch sensitive and bleeds easily. Such features in association with a suggestive history may indicate endometritis.

Hyperplastic endometrium

Endometrial hyperplasia is characterized by focal or diffuse, greyish-white endometrial thickening resulting in an irregular endometrial surface. Projections arising from the endometrium have been variously described as polypoid, mamillated, button-like, finger-like or cystic clusters morphologically. The endometrium is often hypervascular containing large superficial blood vessels, which may be irregular and frankly atypical. Bleeding may occur from friable endometrium, and tissue necrosis may be evident. With higher magnification, an increased and irregular arrangement of dilated glandular openings may be seen. A differential diagnosis between the grades of hyperplasia is not possible by hysteroscopy. It is important to realize that hyperplasia and adenocarcinoma exist along a continuum. The more pronounced these features, the more the likelihood of atypical hyperplasia or frank carcinoma being confirmed histologically is increased.

Cancerous endometrium

The endometrium is focally or more globally thickened and irregular surface lesions are visible, which most often have a papillary appearance. These exophytic lesions are characteristically friable, partly or extensively necrotic, and haemorrhagic as a result of abnormal vascularization. Profuse intrauterine bleeding triggered by uterine distension or contact commonly results, compromising visualization. The extent of the malignancy (i.e. cervical involvement) may be assessed, although such 'staging' is often unreliable (Plate 11).

SUGGESTED 'PRACTICAL' CLASSIFICATION OF HYSTEROSCOPIC ENDOMETRIAL APPEARANCE

Normal (functional or inactive)

The appearance of normality will depend upon the woman's hormonal status. Thus, premenopausal women or those receiving exogenous hormones should have a generally smooth and homogeneous endometrium, which is relatively non-vascular. In postmenopausal women, the endometrium is much thinner or absent, giving the cavity a featureless white smooth or trabeculated (caused by exposed, thin underlying stroma), usually avascular, appearance (Plates 8–10).

Abnormal (thickened)

The endometrium is focally or diffusely thickened, but does not display prominent surface irregularity or vascular abnormality.

Abnormal (suspicious)

The endometrium is focally or diffusely thickened containing surface irregularities usually in association with prominent or abnormal vascularization and/or areas of necrosis or haemorrhage (Plate 11).

Abnormal (cancerous)

The endometrium is focally or diffusely thickened and irregular surface excrescencies are visible, which most often have a papillary appearance. The exophytic growths are friable and extensively necrotic and haemorrhagic as a result of abnormal vascularization. Profuse intrauterine bleeding triggered by uterine distension or contact commonly results, compromising visualization.

STRUCTURAL ABNORMALITIES

Intrauterine polyps

An intrauterine polyp appears as a discrete outgrowth of endometrium, attached by a pedicle, which moves with the flow of the distension medium. The intracavity formation is usually soft (glandular), but may be firm and fibrous making it difficult to distinguish from a submucous fibroid. Polyps can be broad based or pedunculated mucosal projections, single or multiple, and of varying size and vascularity. The covering endometrium may be thin (appearing translucent and revealing a delicate vascular network) or thick (obliterating surface vascularity) and should be carefully assessed to exclude features suggestive of hyperplasia.

Submucous (intracavity) fibroids

Submucous fibroids appear as a firm, smooth and irregular sessile or pedunculated, intracavity formation, covered by a thin, pale and transparent layer of endometrium revealing superficially large blood vessels, distorting the regular contour of an otherwise normal endometrial cavity. Some operators attempt to estimate the intramural extension of sessile tumours hysteroscopically, by observing the angle of the fibroid in relation to the myometrium at the attachment with the uterine wall (classification of European Hysteroscopic Society: 0, no intramural extension; 1, ≤50 per cent intramural extension; 2, >50 per cent intramural extension). In the absence of a discrete submucous projection, multiple intramural fibroids within the uterus can be suspected as they often impart a gently undulating appearance to the cavity.

Uterine adhesions (synechiae)

Adhesions appear hysteroscopically as isolated or extensive band(s) of filmy or firm, white or grey tissue, which lead to varying degrees of uterine cavity distortion. The uterine walls may be coapted without discrete tissue bands visible. The uterine fundus and cornual recesses may be partially or completely occluded. In true Asherman's syndrome, the endometrium is denuded and the cavity is extensively scarred with coaptation of the uterine walls (similar to the appearance following endometrial ablation). Note that an iatrogenic lesion (false passage) should be excluded. A common hysteroscopic finding following previous uterine instrumentation (e.g. dilatation and curettage (D&Cs)) or past infection (e.g. endometritis) is the presence of fibrosis (fibrotic cords of tissue) at the fundus, imparting a somewhat rigid look to the fundus, cornual recesses and tubal ostia, which appear less distinct as a result.

Classifications systems based on hysteroscopic appearances have been produced, although none has been universally accepted. These include classifications of adhesions based primarily upon tissue type (endometrial, myofibrous, connective), extent (minimal, moderate or severe), location (central, marginal) or according to some combination of features.

Congenital malformations (Müllerian duct anomalies)

Hysteroscopy can be usefully employed for the evaluation of congenital uterine anomalies arising from abnormal development or fusion of the Müllerian ducts during embryonic development. The most common of such anomalies encountered are arcuate- and bicornuate-shaped uteri or the presence of a uterine septum, which may be complete (septate) or incomplete (subseptate). A hypoplastic uterus may also be encountered.

ARCUATE

The fundus appears to gently bulge into the uterine cavity, so that the cornual recesses are more pronounced (i.e. producing a space (<1 cm) between the tubal ostia and the deepest median point of the fundus). This is a physiological normal variant.

BICORNUATE UTERUS

A two-chambered uterus is discovered. The diagnosis should be suspected when only one tubal ostia or cornual recess is seen in a narrow, cylindrically shaped uterus. This appearance could represent a unicornuate or hypoplastic uterus, but a careful exploration for an additional entrance into another uterine horn must be carried out. A bicornuate uterus cannot be distinguished hysteroscopically from a completely septate uterus, without additional investigation.

UTERINE SEPTUM

An incomplete uterine septum (*subseptate uterus*) partially separates the uterine cavity into two chambers. The septum is covered with endometrial mucosa and the other uterine chamber can be easily overlooked, the more the septum projects into the uterine cavity. The septum is usually thin proximally, becoming wider towards the fundus. A complete uterine septum (*septate uterus*) separates the uterine cavity completely so that only one tubal ostia/cornual recess is seen. Careful withdrawal of the hysteroscope and exploration for an entrance into another cavity is necessary in order to bypass any intervening tissue.

UTERINE HYPOPLASIA

A small, cylindrical uterine cavity (typically uterine length <6 cm) is detected. The contracted uterus frequently takes on a 'T-shape', with well-formed cornual recesses, but a tubular uterine body, making the ostia difficult to access.

OTHER FINDINGS

Adenomyosis

This condition cannot be reliably diagnosed by hysteroscopy, as it is a histological diagnosis of ectopic endometrium within the myometrium. Hysteroscopy cannot inspect the myometrium, although some authors suspect adenomyosis when the endometrium has a punctate appearance caused by the presence of raised blue-brown spots (small channels of endometrium penetrating into the myometrium).

Pregnancy-related lesions

Retained products of conception and placental polyps appear as irregular endometrial outgrowths, and trophoblastic disease may be more diffuse. The appearance and degree of vascularity or necrosis will depend upon the natural history. Hysteroscopy is not the principal investigative tool and such findings are often incidental, but can be suspected with an appropriate history. Postpregnancy endometritis and subsequent synechiae appear as previously described.

Information Box 5.2 summarizes our suggested practical approach to hysteroscopic diagnosis.

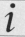

Information Box 5.2 Diagnostic criteria to be assessed and recorded at hysteroscopy

ENDOMETRIUM

- Normal
- Abnormal (thickened, suspicious, cancerous)

CAVITY

- Normal
- Abnormal (polyps, fibroids, adhesions, congenital malformations)

Evidence Box 5.1 Accuracy of outpatient hysteroscopy in diagnosis of uterine disease in women with abnormal uterine bleeding (see relevant chapters)

Diagnostic accuracy refers to the change in our ability to predict whether a particular pathology is present or absent. It should be remembered that this discriminative ability depends not only upon the performance of hysteroscopy, which is summarized below, but also upon other factors. These include the disease prevalence, the disease spectrum and the clinical context (i.e. information provided by preceding components of the clinical process – history, examination and complementary tests).

- *Endometrial cancer.* A systematic review and meta-analysis has demonstrated that hysteroscopy has high overall accuracy in diagnosing endometrial cancer. A positive test (disease detection) is more accurate than a negative test (disease exclusion) (Chapter 6).

- *Endometrial hyperplasia.* A systematic review and meta-analysis has demonstrated that hysteroscopy has moderate overall accuracy in diagnosing endometrial hyperplasia and so adjuvant endometrial sampling should be used. Accuracy is higher in the presence of cytological atypia (Chapter 7).
- *Endometrial polyps.* Hysteroscopy is generally considered to be the gold standard for diagnosis of intracavity structural pathology such as polyps and fibroids. However, accuracy data are scarce for endometrial polyps and, where available, are often not presented separately from other endometrial pathology. The prevalence of cancerous or hyperplastic polyps is estimated to be 1 per cent and 10–20 per cent respectively. It is reassuring to note that overall accuracy of hysteroscopy in diagnosing endometrial cancer or hyperplasia is not influenced by the presence of endometrial polyps (Chapter 15).
- *Submucous fibroids.* As for endometrial polyps. A systematic review of symptomatic premenopausal women has shown accuracy to be high and comparable between saline infusion sonography and hysteroscopy (Chapter 16).
- *Intrauterine adhesions.* Data are scarce. Accuracy is high if hysteroscopy is feasible (i.e. entry into the cavity possible) (Chapter 18).
- *Congenital malformations.* Data are scarce. The most common 'dual-chamber' anomalies, bicornuate and septate uteri, cannot be differentiated without ultrasound or laparoscopic inspection of the serosal surface (Chapter 18).

ULTRASOUND

This book describes the role of modern outpatient hysteroscopy, highlighting its potential and pointing the way for future gynaecological practice based on an outpatient hysteroscopic clinic set-up. There often appears to be an apparent conflict between enthusiasts of hysteroscopy and enthusiasts of transvaginal ultrasound (TVS). Yet in reality there should be no conflict. Both modalities offer the gynaecologist and the women they care for many benefits. The decision about the roles of ultrasound and hysteroscopy should be based primarily upon the available evidence regarding feasibility (Table 5.3), accuracy (see Further reading and subsequent chapters) and cost-effectiveness.

In the absence of decisive evidence in specific circumstances (e.g. postmenopausal bleeding [PMB] and endometrial cancer – see Chapter 6), clinicians rightly remain pragmatic. Local factors will dictate how hysteroscopy and ultrasound are deployed. Those hysteroscopists working in units with external sources of high-quality ultrasound are likely to practise differently from those reliant upon their own ability with TVS (Table 5.4). The suboptimal scenario where outpatient hysteroscopy is not available is thankfully becoming rarer in modern gynaecological practice. Such a situation should be rectified.

Place of pelvic ultrasound

In our opinion, the availability of TVS within an outpatient hysteroscopy clinic is a prerequisite for optimal practice. Although much of what is described in this book is not reliant upon access to TVS, the ideal situation requires the hysteroscopist to both have access to, and be proficient in, TVS. This is because TVS is safe, acceptable to women, practical, versatile and

Table 5.3   *Ultrasound and hysteroscopy: test characteristics*

Features	Transvaginal ultrasound	Saline infusion sonography	Outpatient hysteroscopy	Evidence and prevailing clinical opinion
Safety	333	333	333	All safe, with very low rates of adverse effects reported
Acceptability	333	33	33	All acceptable, ultrasound least painful and invasive. Instrumentation and distension of the uterine cavity is more painful
Feasibility	333	33	33	Typical failure rates higher in procedures requiring uterine instrumentation – saline infusion sonography (7 per cent) higher than hysteroscopy (4 per cent)
Other	Provides extracavity/pelvic information	Facilitates diagnosis of intracavity lesions/provides extracavity information	Directed endometrial biopsies and removal of focal pathology possible	Advances in the technology and application of ultrasound (three-dimensional, colour Doppler) techniques gives this modality the greatest future potential in diagnosis. Hysteroscopy has therapeutic potential

Table 5.4 *Ultrasound or hysteroscopy? Factors influencing practice*

Context	Consequent practice
Access to outpatient hysteroscopy clinic (*contemporary* practice)	
Non-expertise in TVS Non-enthusiast of TVS Availability of external (third party) TVS	*Hysteroscopy predominant diagnostic tool* Hysteroscopy used to confirm presence of structural cavity pathology following TVS. Simultaneous outpatient treatment unless assessed to be non-feasible or failed surgery
Expertise in TVS Enthusiast of TVS No availability of external (third party) TVS	*USS predominant diagnostic tool* SIS used to confirm presence of structural cavity pathology following TVS Scheduling of outpatient/inpatient hysteroscopic surgery

(*Continued*)

Table 5.4 (*Continued*)

Context	Consequent practice
No access to outpatient hysteroscopy clinic (anachronistic practice)	
Non-expertise in TVS Non-enthusiast of TVS Availability of external (third party) TVS	*USS predominant diagnostic tool (by default)* Scheduling of inpatient hysteroscopic surgery
Expertise in TVS Enthusiast of TVS No availability of external (third party) TVS	*USS predominant diagnostic tool* SIS used to confirm presence of structural cavity pathology following TVS Scheduling of inpatient hysteroscopic surgery

Abbreviations: SIS, saline infusion sonography; TVS, transvaginal ultrasound; USS, ultrasound

cheap. The modality generally provides far more information than a clinical pelvic examination and is less invasive. The findings from TVS, when used properly, direct subsequent management (discharge, follow-up, testing and treatment) in a rational manner. TVS is thus a hugely important part of gynaecology today and is recognized by many as the gynaecologists, 'stethoscope'. It would thus be remiss not to emphasize the role of TVS. To this end, the place of pelvic ultrasound (and endometrial biopsy) in relation to outpatient hysteroscopy in the diagnosis of specific gynaecological complaints is discussed throughout this handbook.

KEY POINTS

- Outpatient hysteroscopy is easy to perform and acceptable to women. Supervised training and practice will improve the operator's expertise.

- The technique allows direct visualization of the uterine cavity and cervical canal in a convenient outpatient setting.

- The limitations of visual inspection of the uterine cavity need to be appreciated when interpreting findings so that clinical management is optimized and alternative tests used appropriately.

- Accuracy is high for serious endometrial disease (endometrial cancer and atypical endometrial hyperplasia) and common structural pathology (polyps and submucous fibroids), enhancing the utility of hysteroscopy as a testing modality.

- High-resolution, transvaginal ultrasound is safe, acceptable to women and relatively easily learnt.

- Pelvic ultrasound can provide valuable information to aid management of many common gynaecological complaints.

- Although ultrasound or hysteroscopy may be preferred in particular clinical circumstances, they should generally be considered complementary outpatient tests.

FURTHER READING

Bachmann LM, ter Riet G, Clark TJ, Gupta JK, Khan KS. Probability analysis for diagnosis of endometrial hyperplasia and cancer in postmenopausal bleeding: an approach for a rational diagnostic workup. *Acta Obstet Gynecol Scand* 2003;**82**:564–69.

Clark TJ, Voit D, Gupta JK, Hyde C, Song F, Khan KS. Accuracy of hysteroscopy in the diagnosis of endometrial cancer and hyperplasia: a systematic quantitative review. *JAMA* 2002;**288**:1610–21.

Farquhar C, Ekeroma A, Furness S, Arroll B. A systematic review of transvaginal ultrasonography, sonohysterography and hysteroscopy for the investigation of abnormal uterine bleeding in premenopausal women. *Acta Obstet Gynecol Scand* 2003;**82**:493–504.

Gupta JK, Chien PF, Voit D, Clark TJ, Khan KS. Ultrasonographic endometrial thickness for diagnosing endometrial pathology in women with postmenopausal bleeding: a meta-analysis. *Acta Obstet Gynecol Scand* 2002;**81**:799–816.

Smith-Bindman R, Kerlikowske K, Feldstein VA *et al.* Endovaginal ultrasound to exclude endometrial cancer and other endometrial abnormalities. *JAMA* 1998;**280**:1510–17.

Part 2

Common Presentations in Outpatient Hysteroscopy

6

Postmenopausal bleeding

AETIOLOGY AND EPIDEMIOLOGY OF POSTMENOPAUSAL BLEEDING

Postmenopausal bleeding (PMB) is a common clinical problem in both general practice and secondary care, hospital settings. Women are most likely to present with PMB in the sixth decade of life, where consultation rates in primary care are 14.3/1000 population. Similarly, in the hospital setting, abnormal patterns of uterine bleeding account for more than 50 per cent of all gynaecological consultations in the peri- and postmenopausal years. The majority of women with PMB have benign endometrial pathology (Table 6.1). However, rapid referral for endometrial assessment is mandatory because 5–10 per cent of women with PMB will have endometrial cancer and 10–25 per cent will have endometrial hyperplasia, both conditions that may impact adversely on patient prognosis.

INVESTIGATION AND SERVICE PROVISION

Published recommendations state that women should be seen within 2–6 weeks of referral. The endometrial assessment service has to be efficient in order to meet such targets and optimize patient prognosis (Fig. 6.1). Traditional investigation of women with postmenopausal bleeding using inpatient blind dilatation of the cervix and curettage of the endometrium (D&C) is now considered outdated practice and has been replaced by initial outpatient endometrial evaluation. These new diagnostic modalities include miniature endometrial biopsy (EB) devices (Plate 12), transvaginal ultrasound scan (TVS – Fig. 6.2) and outpatient hysteroscopy (OPH). However, despite the widely accepted advantages of outpatient investigation, there is uncertainty regarding the individual value of these tests and the best sequence or combination in which to use them. Consequently practice varies throughout Europe and North America, largely dependent upon prejudice (of individual clinicians) and pragmatism (resources available to them).

Table 6.1 *Causes of postmenopausal bleeding*

Causes of postmenopausal bleeding	Mechanism
Malignant/premalignant	
Endometrial cancer	Abnormal endometrium
Endometrial hyperplasia (cytological atypia)	Abnormal endometrium
Benign	
Endometrial hyperplasia (no cytological atypia)	Abnormal endometrium
Submucous fibroids	Fragile overlying vasculature
Endometrial polyps	Friable vascular network. May contain foci of hyperplasia or cancer
Chronic endometritis	Inflamed, fragile endometrium associated with IUCD use, pelvic inflammatory disease and retained products of conception
Atrophic endometrium	Fragile vascular support provided by thin underlying stroma resulting in superficial petechial haemorrhages and mucosal ulceration
Hormone replacement therapy	Unstable endometrium (inadequate progestogenic support). Consider poor compliance, variable gastrointestinal absorption and drug interactions. Increased prevalence of polyps
Coagulation defects/anticoagulation (e.g. warfarin)	Propensity to bleeding from endometrial vessels

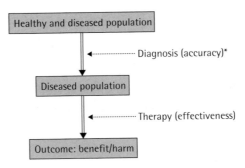

* The incidence of endometrial cancer has increased during the last decade and unlike other malignancies affecting women, endometrial cancer often presents at an early stage (80 per cent FIGO stage 1) with the possibility of curative treatment by hysterectomy. Prognosis is increasingly bleak the more advanced the disease. As there have been no recent advances in the treatment of endometrial cancer that can be expected to increase survival, the importance of accurate and timely diagnosis of endometrial cancer is paramount in order to reduce mortality further.

Figure 6.1 *Clinical process.*

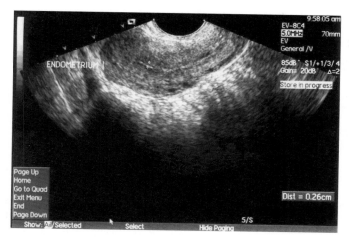

Figure 6.2 *Endometrial thickness measured by transvaginal ultrasound scan. Normal, thin (atrophic) postmenopausal endometrium (3 mm thickness).*

EVIDENCE-BASED APPROACH

A diagnostic test is useful if it changes our ability to predict whether a patient has a particular condition or not. Ideal tests that detect or exclude disease with 100 per cent certainty do not exist. However, the closer diagnostic test results are to such levels of certainty, the more useful they are likely to be. Traditional concepts of diagnostic accuracy using measures such as sensitivity and specificity are confusing and not clinically intuitive or indeed useful. This is because the patient and her doctor do not know whether disease (in this case endometrial cancer) is present or not. They base management decisions primarily on probabilities of disease, although other factors (e.g. disease prognosis if left untreated, and effectiveness and morbidity of treatment) are also relevant. A measure of accuracy, called the likelihood ratio, incorporates both sensitivity and specificity and more importantly allows clinically relevant post-test probabilities to be generated.

The accuracy of OPH, EB and TVS in diagnosing endometrial cancer in women with PMB has been estimated by performing systematic reviews of the world literature. Accuracy estimates (likelihood ratios) have been quantified through meta-analysis. This appraisal of the evidence has shown that OPH and EB are useful tests in ruling in endometrial cancer, whereas ultrasound is highly accurate in excluding it. These results and the concepts for determining accuracy and utility of tests outlined above are presented graphically in Fig. 6.3.

How should we investigate PMB?

Tests are not generally performed in isolation. They are normally employed later in the clinical process after clinical assessment by history-taking and examination. During investigation of PMB, the available outpatient tests may be used in sequence or combination, and how best to do this has generated considerable debate and controversy. The following section tries to introduce some clarity to the debate, applying principles of evidence-based medicine.

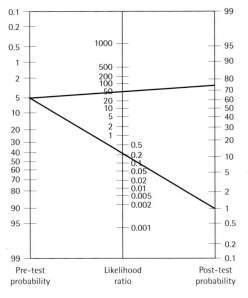

(a) Outpatient hysteroscopy. For a postmenopausal woman with vaginal bleeding and a 5 per cent pre-test probability of endometrial cancer, her probability of cancer is increased to approximately 80 per cent following a positive hysteroscopy, which is above most clinical thresholds for recommending advanced management (i.e. therapeutic intervention).

Her corresponding probability of cancer is 1 per cent following a negative hysteroscopy. Many may consider this a significant risk, as untreated endometrial cancer is invariably fatal and so additional testing is likely to be requested. A negative hysteroscopy result is thus less clinically useful than a positive one.

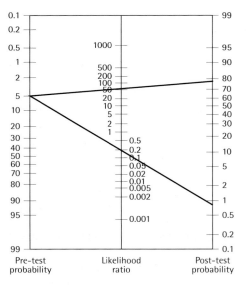

(b) Endometrial biopsy. The accuracy of endometrial biopsy is similar to that of hysteroscopy. A positive test is associated with a significant increase in the likelihood of endometrial cancer, which will be valuable in influencing clinical decision-making.

The patient's probability of cancer is < 1 per cent following a negative test result. Endometrial biopsy thus performs better than hysteroscopy for excluding cancer.

Figure 6.3 *Accuracy of outpatient endometrial tests in the diagnosis of endometrial cancer. (Nomogram adapted with permission. Fagan TJ. Nomogram for Baye's Theorem. NEJM 1975; 293:257. © 1975, Massachusetts Medical Society. All rights reserved.)*

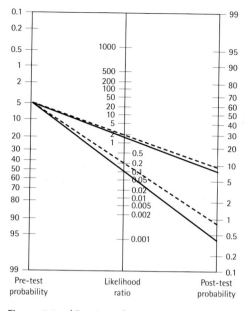

(c) Ultrasound. The accuracy of endome-trial thickness measurement by transvagi-nal ultrasound using both ≤4 mm (line) and ≤5 mm (broken line) to define abnor-mality is shown.

A positive test using either threshold is not useful for diagnosing endometrial cancer as the pre-test probability of cancer (5 per cent) is changed little following an abnormal result. In contrast a negative (normal) ultrasound result reduces the likelihood of endometrial cancer to <1 per cent (5 mm cut-off) and <0.5 per cent (4 mm cut-off) respectively. Ultrasound is thus useful in excluding endometrial cancer, negating the need for additional testing.

Figure 6.3 (*Continued*).

ENDOMETRIAL CANCER AND ATYPICAL HYPERPLASIA

The main purpose of undertaking investigation of women with PMB is to exclude serious endometrial pathology, namely cancer and hyperplasia. An economic model (decision analysis) employing evidence from systematic reviews, has shown that diagnostic work-up based on EB or TVS are the most cost-effective strategies. The analysis demonstrated that in most circumstances, where high-quality ultrasound services are available, women with PMB should undergo initial evaluation with pelvic ultrasound. Women with a normal ultrasound (negative test) should be discharged (assuming a normal clinical examination). Those with an abnormal ultrasound (positive test) should undergo endometrial biopsy followed by advanced management (usually hysterectomy) if cancer is confirmed histologically. There are insufficient data to determine which threshold (4 mm or 5 mm) should be used to define abnormal results, although costs are generally lower if a 5 mm threshold is chosen (see Further reading). A practical, evidence-based algorithm is set out in Fig. 6.4. This approach will ensure best practice and facilitate compliance with recommended (and increasingly compulsory) waiting time targets.

The surgical and medical treatments of benign causes of PMB are discussed in the pro-ceeding chapters. Management of endometrial cancer falls outside the remit of this book. A specialist in gynaecological oncology should undertake advanced management.

BENIGN DISEASE

It has long been argued that blind endometrial biopsy is inaccurate because it does not rep-resentatively sample the endometrial cavity and misses focal pathology. As demonstrated above, such opinions are not borne out in the diagnosis of endometrial cancer. However, these limitations are more apparent where benign pathologies are the underlying causes of PMB. These pathologies include endometrial hyperplasia without atypia, endometrial polyps and submucous fibroids. Observational series report that, together, these diagnoses account for between 25 and 75 per cent of women with PMB according to population spectrum (characteristics, referral patterns, etc.). Although such diagnoses are of less significance in terms of survival, persistent PMB can impact adversely on quality of life, because of continued abnormal bleeding resulting in anxiety and inconvenience. Accurate diagnosis is important to reassure the patient and tailor treatments to produce optimal outcomes.

Modern miniature office hysteroscopy is the gold standard for diagnosing structural pathology within the uterus (polyps, fibroids – see Chapters 15 and 16) and may also reveal focal endometrial anomalies (e.g. hyperplasia, petechial haemorrhages), which may account for bleeding symptoms. In contrast to endometrial cancer, evidence regarding diagnostic effectiveness (i.e. best resulting clinical outcomes) is lacking for PMB caused by benign disease. In the absence of this, three approaches should be considered (Fig. 6.5). All are based on screening with ultrasound because this modality is the most cost-effective in excluding any malignant disease that may be present (see above).

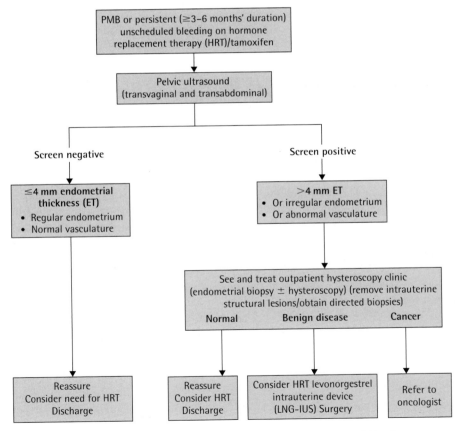

Figure 6.4 *Suggested algorithm for the investigation of postmenopausal bleeding.*

The strategies differ in their use of outpatient hysteroscopy. Adoption of strategy 1 will avoid unnecessary hysteroscopy. Furthermore, although benign pathology may be more prevalent in symptomatic postmenopausal women, this association does not necessarily imply causation (i.e. treatment may not be necessary). However, many believe that such pathology is important and requires investigation and treatment, in which case strategy 2 should be adopted. Access to adequate outpatient hysteroscopy facilities is essential if this approach is taken, because identifiable benign pathology (hyperplasia, fibroids and polyps) will be

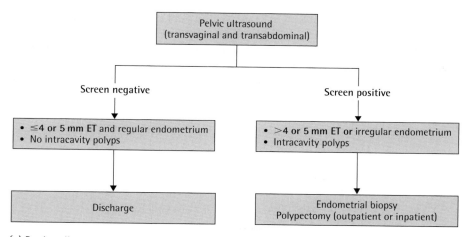

(a) Benign disease: strategy 1: ultrasound ± biopsy.

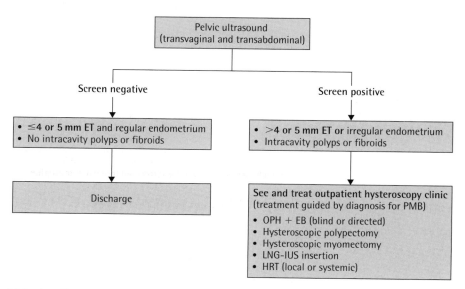

(b) Benign disease: strategy 2: ultrasound ± outpatient hysteroscopy.

Figure 6.5 *Investigation of postmenopausal bleeding.*

present in over 50 per cent who screen positive on ultrasound. Immediate treatment can then be instituted in keeping with the 'see and treat' philosophy. Furthermore, the finding of a normal atrophic cavity may be reassuring. Strategy 3 is an amalgam of strategies 1 and 2. This strategy may be appropriate where 'see and treat' outpatient hysteroscopy services are available, but would be overwhelmed without a further tier of patient selection (Fig. 6.5).

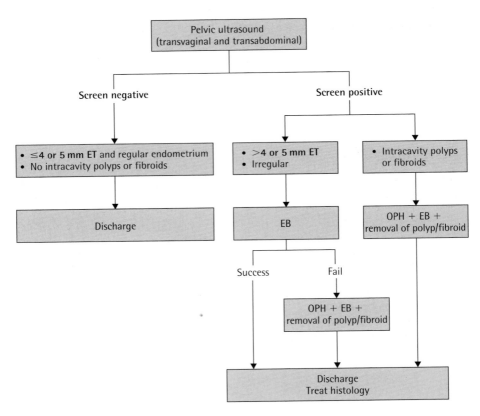

(c) Benign disease: strategy 3: ultrasound ± biopsy ± outpatient hysteroscopy.

Figure 6.5 (*Continued*).

KEY POINTS

- The incidence of endometrial cancer is between 5 and 15 per cent in women presenting with postmenopausal vaginal bleeding.

- Initial evaluation with transvaginal ultrasound represents the most cost-effective strategy for excluding *endometrial cancer* using a threshold of 4 mm or 5 mm double layer endometrial thickness to define abnormal results on pelvic ultrasound.

- Outpatient hysteroscopy and endometrial biopsy are useful tests for detecting, rather than excluding endometrial cancer.

- Outpatient hysteroscopy provides clarification when the endometrium is thickened on transvaginal ultrasound but a non-diagnostic endometrial biopsy sample has been obtained.

- Outpatient hysteroscopy facilitates global and directed biopsy of the endometrium and removal of focal pathology.

FURTHER READING

Clark TJ, Barton PM, Gupta JK, Khan KS. Ambulatory diagnosis of endometrial cancer in women with postmenopausal bleeding. West Midlands Health Technology Assessment Collaboration Report 2003. University of Birmingham (in press, but will be available at www.publichealth.bham.ac.uk).

Clark TJ, Mann CH, Shah N, Song F, Khan KS, Gupta JK. Accuracy of outpatient endometrial biopsy in the diagnosis of endometrial cancer: A systematic review. *Br J Obstet Gynecol* 2002;**109**:313–21.

Clark TJ, Voit D, Gupta JK, Hyde C, Song FS, Khan KS. Accuracy of hysteroscopy in the diagnosis of endometrial cancer and hyperplasia: a systematic quantitative review. *JAMA* 2002;**288**:1610–22.

Gupta JK, Chien PF, Voit D, Clark TJ, Khan KS. Ultrasonographic endometrial thickness for diagnosing endometrial pathology in women with postmenopausal bleeding: a meta-analysis. *Acta Obstet Gynecol Scand* 2002;**81**:799–816.

Smith-Bindman R, Kerlikowske K, Feldstein VA *et al*. Endovaginal ultrasound to exclude endometrial cancer and other endometrial abnormalities. *JAMA* 1998;**280**:1510–17.

7

Endometrial hyperplasia

DEFINITION OF ENDOMETRIAL HYPERPLASIA

Hyperplasia refers to an increase in cell numbers. The term endometrial hyperplasia comprises a spectrum of proliferative disorders and epithelial alterations (architectural and cytological changes to glands and stroma) ranging between normal proliferative endometrium and well-differentiated adenocarcinoma.

EPIDEMIOLOGY AND SIGNIFICANCE

Endometrial hyperplasia is more prevalent than endometrial cancer and affects both pre- and postmenopausal women. The probability of endometrial hyperplasia in women presenting with postmenopausal bleeding (with or without hormone replacement therapy (HRT)) is between 10 and 25 per cent. The risk factors for developing hyperplastic endometrium are the same as for endometrial cancer and thus relate mainly to unopposed oestrogen exposure. This can result from endogenous (anovulatory cycles, ovarian tumour and extra-ovarian oestrogen production – adipose, adrenal, etc.) or exogenous (administration of unopposed oestrogens and combined HRT) production of oestrogen. Endometrial hyperplasia is categorized histologically by the degree of architectural disruption (simple or complex hyperplasia) and by the presence of abnormal cytology (atypia).

The importance of endometrial hyperplasia relates not only to the symptoms of genital tract bleeding it can cause, but to its oncogenic potential. The natural history of endometrial hyperplasia is not fully understood. What is known is that a proportion of simple and complex hyperplastic processes will regress without treatment, although the time scale over which such regression may occur is unclear. However, a small proportion (estimated to be between 1 and 3 per cent) will progress to frank endometrial cancer. The main prognostic factor is the presence of atypical cells. Malignant progression has been reported to occur in 30 per cent of atypical endometrial hyperplasias if left untreated. Atypical hyperplasia can arise *de novo*, without oestrogenic stimulation from otherwise atrophic or inactive endometrium.

DIAGNOSIS AND ROLE OF HYSTEROSCOPY

Hysteroscopy used in isolation has modest accuracy in identifying and excluding hyperplastic endometrium (Fig. 7.1). Confirmation of diagnosis is histological and requires endometrial sampling. Endometrial hyperplasia without cytological atypia results from an oestrogen-dominant milieu and the resulting disease is normally global. Hysteroscopy is particularly useful in detecting focal endometrial disease (atypical hyperplasia) or hyperplastic endometrial polyps (10–25 per cent of polyps).

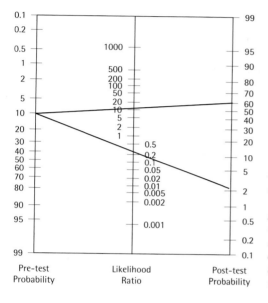

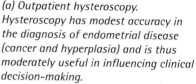

(a) Outpatient hysteroscopy. Hysteroscopy has modest accuracy in the diagnosis of endometrial disease (cancer and hyperplasia) and is thus moderately useful in influencing clinical decision-making.

For a postmenopausal woman with vaginal bleeding and a 10 per cent pre-test probability of endometrial disease, her probability of disease is increased to approximately 60 per cent following a positive hysteroscopy and reduced to 3 per cent following a negative hysteroscopy. Some gynaecologists may be prepared to initiate or withhold treatment based on these post-test probabilities, whereas the majority will request additional testing (e.g. endometrial biopsy, transvaginal ultrasound) on which to base management.

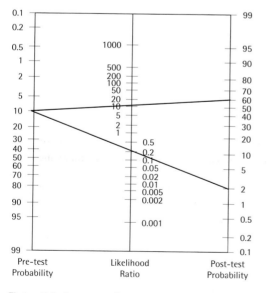

(b) Endometrial biopsy. The accuracy of endometrial biopsy in endometrial hyperplasia is shown. This is similar to that of hysteroscopy in diagnosing endometrial disease (cancer plus hyperplasia). The predictive ability of endometrial biopsy increases with more severe disease, i.e. atypical hyperplasia and cancer.

Figure 7.1 *Accuracy of outpatient endometrial tests in the diagnosis of serious endometrial disease (cancer and hyperplasia). (Nomogram adapted with permission, Fagan TJ. Nomogram for Baye's Theorem. NEJM 1975; 293:257. © 1975, Massachusetts Medical Society. All rights reserved.)*

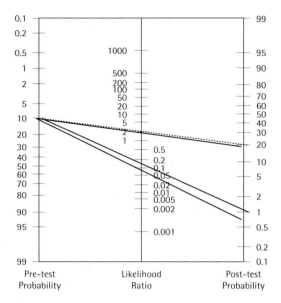

(c) Ultrasound. The accuracy of endometrial thickness measurement by transvaginal ultrasound using both ≤4 mm (line) and ≤5 mm (broken line) to define abnormality is shown.

A positive test using either threshold is not useful for diagnosing endometrial disease as the pre-test probability of cancer (10 per cent) is changed little following an abnormal result (20 per cent).

In contrast a negative (normal) ultrasound result reduces the likelihood of endometrial disease to <2 per cent (5 mm cut-off) and <1 per cent (4 mm cut-off) respectively. Ultrasound is thus useful in excluding endometrial disease, negating the need for additional testing.

Figure 7.1 (*Continued*).

MANAGEMENT

Management options are listed in Information Box 7.1. Choice of treatment depends upon presence of cytological atypia (oncogenic potential), the woman's age, fertility considerations, menopausal status and symptoms (bleeding, climacteric, etc.). Conservative treatment of endometrial hyperplasia is based on administration of agents with either anti-oestrogenic action and/or direct antiproliferative effects on the endometrium. Hysterectomy represents definitive treatment and allows complete endometrial sampling. However, the malignant potential of endometrial hyperplasia without cytological atypia has been overplayed in the past and so conservative treatments should be considered first-line therapy.

CYTOLOGICAL ATYPIA

It is important to note that the qualitative difference between atypical hyperplasia and a well-differentiated endometrioid adenocarcinoma is small and a matter of judgement.

Information Box 7.1 Management of endometrial hyperplasia

EXPECTANT

Endometrial hyperplasia without atypia can be managed without the need for treatment as the condition may regress spontaneously, but regular endometrial assessment is required to exclude disease progression if this approach is taken.

MEDICAL (HORMONAL)*

- *Systemic progestogen.* This can be administered via the oral, transdermal or parenteral route. Compliance is limited by side effects of high-dose progestins, which include weight gain, oedema, headaches and mood disturbance. Disease regression does not appear to be dependent upon type of progestin (e.g. norethisterone, medroxyprogesterone (MDP), etc.). Suggested regimens range from low dose, cyclical regimens (e.g. 10–20 mg MDP × 14 days/month) to high dose, continuous ones (e.g. MDP 40–100 mg daily) for between 3 and 6 months.
- *Local progestogen.* Local (intrauterine) progestogens to reverse the oestrogen dominant milieu directly. Local delivery is advantageous because compliance is 100 per cent, constant drug concentrations are better achieved, liver breakdown is avoided and systemic side effects are minimized. Useful as an adjunct to HRT or tamoxifen. Vaginally administered natural micronized progesterone (3 months) has also been reported to induce disease regression in a small series.
- *Combined oral contraceptive pill.* This can be given cyclically or continuously for at least 6 months. Useful in younger women with anovulatory cycles.
- *Hormone replacement therapy (HRT).* Continuous combined HRT preparations (daily progestogen) have been shown to reverse non-atypical endometrial hyperplasias found in association with sequential regimes.
- *Gonadotrophin-releasing analogues.* These induce disease regression in non-atypical hyperplasia (with fewer dysfunctional uterine bleeding episodes compared with systemic progestins). Duration of use is limited by menopausal side effects and risk of osteoporosis. Regression rates of 80 per cent have been reported in atypical hyperplasias when they are given for 6 months in conjunction with systemic progestins.
- *Other.* Danazol and clomiphene citrate have been used in the past to good effect. Use is limited because of side effects.

SURGICAL

- *Endometrial resection/ablation.* Useful if hyperplasia is confined within a focal lesion (e.g. polyp). However, this approach is not recommended for two main reasons. First, endometrial hyperplasia is usually global in response to a relatively hyperoestrogenic state. Corrective hormonal therapy or hysterectomy is thus required to ensure complete treatment/eradication of disease. Second, endometrial assessment following conservative surgical therapy is compromised such that endometrial cancers have been missed.
- *Hysterectomy.* Traditional treatment is with hysterectomy. In the presence of atypical cells, hysterectomy is usually recommended in view of the potential for malignant transformation. Should be reserved in non-atypical hyperplasias for those cases that are refractory to medical treatment from a histological or symptomatic perspective.

* Follow-up at 6-monthly intervals is recommended using endometrial biopsy with or without endometrial imaging (hysteroscopy or ultrasound).

In view of this, the poor response to hormonal therapy and a substantial oncogenic potential, hysterectomy is recommended unless fertility considerations (desire to retain their reproductive potential) or other medical factors (high risk for surgery) come into play.

HORMONAL STATUS

Anovulatory cycles are common in perimenopausal women and so endometrial hyperplasia is increasingly likely at this stage of reproductive life, especially in association with abnormal bleeding patterns. Similarly oestrogenic stimulation of the endometrium can occur in post/perimenopausal women taking HRT or tamoxifen. However, further investigation is required where endometrial hyperplasia (without atypia) is diagnosed in postmenopausal women not taking exogenous hormones, in order to look for a source of oestrogen. An ultrasound assessment of the ovaries is recommended to exclude tumour. Endometrial cancer and hyperplasia with cytological atypia are thought to be able to arise *de novo* without oestrogen as a cofactor.

Progestogens

Progestogens exert a direct antiproliferative effect on the endometrium and indirect anti-oestrogenic effect, through decrease of endometrial oestrogen receptors and conversion of 17-β-estradiol to less potent estrone. Endometrial hyperplasia without atypia will regress in the majority of women (> 90 per cent) treated with progestogens. Regression rates are much lower (20 per cent) when cytological atypia is present. What is unclear is the duration of therapy required to ensure complete resolution or regression of the hyperplastic process. Traditionally systemic progestogens have been administered for a 3–6-month period. However, there have been no long-term follow-up studies to evaluate the prognosis or recurrence of disease following cessation of therapy.

Levonorgestrel intrauterine system (LNG–IUS – Mirena)

The hysteroscopy clinic is an ideal environment to fit a LNG-IUS. Endometrial hyperplasia and coexisting bleeding symptoms can be successfully treated with local intrauterine progestogen, although the product is not licensed for this indication (see Information Box 7.2). The LNG-IUS is typically fitted for 5 years' use thereby affording longer term treatment. Rates of complete regression approaching 100 per cent have been reported, although these uncontrolled series are small, with short-term follow-up to date. Close follow-up utilizing endometrial biopsy ± hysteroscopy is required at 6-monthly intervals for at least 2 years. Surveillance can be stopped at this time as long as the woman remains asymptomatic from a bleeding perspective and histology is consistently negative. Alternatively, transvaginal ultrasound (TVS) can be performed annually for 5 years with further hysteroscopy and biopsy reserved if the endometrial thickness exceeds 5 mm or is irregular. The LNG-IUS can be removed, but we would recommend leaving it in place for 5 years if well tolerated. The LNG-IUS is also useful in treating hyperplasia in women on HRT, providing adequate endometrial protection with minimal side effects (see above).

A summary of our current treatment algorithm, based on the use of local progestogens, is given in Fig. 7.2. A longer-term observational study is being conducted to assess the longer-term effects of local progestogens delivered via the LNG-IUS on the natural history of endometrial hyperplasia.

Information Box 7.2 Unlicensed preparations

The LNG-IUS (levonorgestrel intrauterine system) is licensed for use as a contraceptive and for the treatment of menorrhagia. Prescription for other unlicensed indications is legal as long as personal professional responsibility is taken. Named patient prescribing involves ensuring that the doctor:

- is adopting a practice that would be endorsed by a responsible body of professional opinion;
- has explained to the woman that this is an unlicensed prescription;
- has clearly explained the perceived risks and benefits, so that informed consent can be obtained and recorded;
- keeps a record of the woman's details and the prescription;
- ensures that all practices regarding the product are acceptable to those responsible for the doctor's professional indemnity.

(From Sturridge and Guillebaud, 1997.)

Evidence Box 7.1 Diagnosis and natural history of endometrial hyperplasia

Endometrial biopsy is required to diagnose endometrial hyperplasia. Hysteroscopy is highly accurate for diagnosing atypical hyperplasia and polyps, but its accuracy is only modest in diagnosing lesser degrees of disease without the aid of biopsy. The natural history of endometrial hyperplasia has been elucidated from published cohort studies. Cytological atypia is the main predictor of malignant transformation, which occurs in 30 per cent (20–80 per cent) of cases within 10 years if left untreated. Hysterectomy is thus indicated in most instances. This view is reinforced by the finding that up to one-third of women with atypical hyperplasia are found subsequently to have well-differentiated adenocarcinoma at hysterectomy. Spontaneous regression frequently occurs in simple, and to a lesser degree, complex hyperplasia without cytological atypia. However, persistence and progression of disease (and symptoms) is common. Small, uncontrolled series have demonstrated that regression occurs in the majority of patients treated with systemic or local progestogens. A larger series has shown the incidence of complex endometrial hyperplasia to be 5 per cent and atypical hyperplasia 0.7 per cent in women receiving sequential hormone replacement therapy (HRT) regimens (median duration 2.5 years). All cases of complex hyperplasia regressed in response to 9 months of continuous combined HRT.

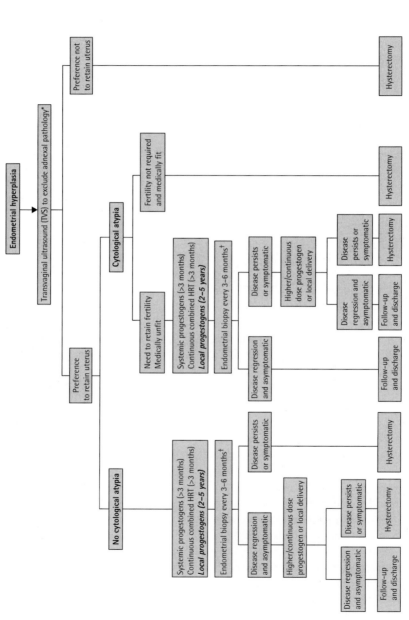

* Especially if source of oestrogen stimulation not identified (e.g. ovarian, exogenous hormones, etc.).

[+] Follow up endometrial biopsy ± outpatient hysteroscopy at 6-monthly intervals for minimum of 1 year. *Systemic treatment:* annual TVS after first year, with biopsy reserved if TVS abnormal (>5 mm, irregular); *local progestogen:* endometrial evaluation by TVS compromised with an intrauterine system (LNG-IUS). The LNG-IUS is unlicensed for treatment of endometrial hyperplasia; therefore close follow-up is compulsory with biopsy ± outpatient hysteroscopy every 6 months for a minimum of 2 years.

KEY POINTS

- Endometrial hyperplasia is a common cause of abnormal uterine bleeding in women of reproductive and non-reproductive age and is frequently encountered in the outpatient hysteroscopy clinic.

- Endometrial hyperplasia can progress to cancer if undiagnosed or inappropriately managed.

- The diagnostic potential of outpatient hysteroscopy in endometrial hyperplasia is optimized if risk factors for disease and characteristic visual appearances are appreciated, as well as an understanding of diagnostic limitations.

- The outpatient hysteroscopy clinic is a useful setting for initiating treatment and maintaining endometrial surveillance.

- The LNG-IUS shows promise in affording an effective long-term (5 years) therapy for endometrial hyperplasia with 100 per cent patient compliance. It can also provide endometrial protection as part of a hormone replacement regimen.

FURTHER READING

Clark TJ, Mann CH, Shah N, Song F, Khan KS, Gupta JK. Accuracy of outpatient endometrial biopsy in the diagnosis of endometrial hyperplasia: A systematic review. *Acta Obstet Gynecol Scand* 2001;**80**:784–93.

Clark TJ, Voit D, Gupta JK, Hyde C, Song FS, Khan KS. Accuracy of hysteroscopy in the diagnosis of endometrial cancer and hyperplasia: a systematic quantitative review. *JAMA* 2002;**288**:1610–22.

Kurman RJ, Kaminski PF, Norris HJ. The behaviour of endometrial hyperplasia: A long-term study of 'untreated' hyperplasia in 170 patients. *Cancer* 1985;**56**:403–12.

Sturridge F, Guillebaud J. Gynaecological aspects of the levonorgestrel-releasing intrauterine system. *Br J Obstet Gynaecol* 1997;**104**:285–9.

Wells M, Sturdee DW, Barlow DH *et al.* Effect on endometrium of long term treatment with continuous combined oestrogen-progestogen replacement therapy: follow-up study. *BMJ* 2002;**325**:239.

Hormone replacement therapy

Recent evidence has shaken the status quo regarding universal prescription of opposed hormone replacement therapy (HRT – oestrogen plus progestogen). However, prescription of HRT will still be necessary for treatment of menopausal symptoms, and abnormal bleeding on HRT will still be a common complaint and indication for outpatient hysteroscopy. The prevalence of endometrial cancer in postmenopausal women with bleeding on HRT is lower (2–5 per cent) than for those not taking exogenous hormones (5–15 per cent). However, vigilance is important because endometrial disease in the form of hyperplasia, and structural anomalies in the form of endometrial polyps and submucous fibroids may be more prevalent, although data are conflicting. Interpretation of endometrial thickness by transvaginal ultrasound is more difficult when exogenous hormones are being taken, and so direct hysteroscopic visualization of the uterine cavity is often useful.

INVESTIGATION AND INDICATIONS FOR HYSTEROSCOPY

Women with persistent unscheduled bleeding on HRT are candidates for diagnostic hysteroscopy in order to exclude uterine pathology. However, an appreciation of other possible causes of bleeding is required to avoid unnecessary investigation (Information Box 8.1). The prime purpose of investigating women with uterine bleeding associated with HRT is to exclude the relatively small risk of endometrial cancer. Secondary reasons for investigation include diagnosis and eradication of underlying causes of bleeding (Information Box 8.2) thereby providing symptom relief, improving compliance and allaying anxiety. Abnormal bleeding patterns are highly prevalent in the first few months of commencing therapy and this should be appreciated in order to avoid overinvestigation. The decision to investigate women with abnormal uterine bleeding associated with HRT use will depend upon several factors including the amount, timing and duration of symptoms, time since HRT commenced (>6 months if light bleeding), previous amenorrhoea, woman's age and other risk factors for endometrial cancer, and the degree of patient anxiety.

A careful history and clinical examination is required to avoid missing vulval, vaginal and cervical causes for bleeding (Chapter 11). Transvaginal ultrasound is a useful preliminary test to exclude endometrial cancer and adnexal disease (see Chapter 6). Endometrial

Information Box 8.1   Causes of abnormal bleeding on Hormone Replacement Therapy (HRT)*

- *Poor compliance.* Risk of endometrial disease increased if progestogen component alone omitted (sequential preparation).
- *Malabsorption.* Avoid oral preparations if gastrointestinal disease.
- *Endogenous ovarian activity.* Endogenous ovarian activity often unpredictable if perimenopausal dysfunctional uterine bleeding. Coincide exogenous administration of progestogen with endogenous production to minimize erratic bleeding.
- *Ovarian pathology.* Oestrogen-secreting neoplasms.
- *Endometrial pathology.* Polyps, submucous fibroids, endometrial hyperplasia, endometritis, cancer.
- *Cervical pathology.* Ectopy, polyps, cancer.
- *Vaginal/vulval pathology.* Atrophic vaginitis, vaginal intraepithelial neoplasia, cancer.
- *Previous implant therapy.* Continued release of estradiol (up to 4 years) can result in bleeding. Progestogenic endometrial protection should be maintained whilst withdrawal bleeding occurs.
- *Drug interactions.* Check prescribed medications for known interactions with HRT.
- *Coagulation defects.* Endometrial disease should still be excluded in women on anti-coagulant therapy or coagulopathies.
- *'Unstable' atrophic endometrium.* Typical features (Chapter 5) of an atrophic cavity with a fragile vascular network, can be seen in women receiving continuous progestogen.

* *Adapted from Spencer CP et al., 1997.*

Information Box 8.2   Treatment of abnormal bleeding on hormone replacement therapy (HRT)

NO PATHOLOGY

Sequential preparations

- *Scheduled (heavy or prolonged).* Alter type/delivery route of progestogen and/or oestrogen (e.g. change sequential HRT preparation or convert to continuous combined preparation/levonorgestrel intrauterine system (LNG-IUS). Mefanamic or tranexamic acid administered during the withdrawal bleed may help.
- *Unscheduled*
  - *Too early in progestogen phase.* Increasing the progestogen dosage (progesterone only pill, LNG-IUS, change of preparation e.g. micronized progesterone) or type/delivery route (change sequential HRT preparation, LNG-IUS), especially if endometrial biopsy fails to show secretory change.
  - *No pattern.* Exclude causes in Information Box 8.1. Alter type/delivery route of progestogen and/or oestrogen (e.g. change sequential HRT preparation, LNG-IUS).
  - *Perimenopausal.* If <1 year amenorrhoea prior to onset of HRT, then residual intermittent and unpredictable ovarian function likely (follicular activity seen on

transvaginal ultrasound), which may interfere with externally administered oestrogen. Options include review need for HRT, reassurance as self-limiting problem, prescribe combined oral contraceptive if no contraindications or fit LNG-IUS.

Continuous combined preparations

* *Unscheduled ('unstable' atrophic endometrium).* Increase the oestrogen or progestogen dose ± type, consider LNG-IUS, or revert to sequential therapy.

PATHOLOGY

* *Atrophic vaginitis.* Local oestrogen (ring, pessary, topical creams).
* *Polyps.* Hysteroscopic removal indicated.
* *Submucous fibroids.* Hysteroscopic removal indicated especially if bleeding is unpredictable, persistent and there is evidence of enlargement. Use the lowest effective oestrogen dosage.
* *Endometrial hyperplasia without atypia.* Increase progestogen (e.g. continuous combined HRT, or use systemic or local progestogens ± temporarily stop oestrogen). If symptoms persist or no disease regression then hysterectomy indicated.
* *Endometrial cancer or atypical hyperplasia.* Hysterectomy. Referral to oncology.

thickness ≤5 mm negates the need for hysteroscopy unless symptoms persist. Outpatient endometrial biopsy is mandatory if endometrial thickness is >5 mm and as an adjunct to hysteroscopic diagnosis. Evidence does not support hysteroscopic uterine screening of asymptomatic women prior to commencing HRT, but incidental findings of endometrial ultrasound abnormalities should be investigated.

HYSTEROSCOPIC DIAGNOSIS AND HRT

From a practical viewpoint, failure rates of hysteroscopy are lower in postmenopausal women taking exogenous oestrogen, because the need for local anaesthesia and cervical dilatation is reduced. Compared with symptomatic postmenopausal women not receiving exogenous hormones, the prevalence of endometrial hyperplasia is similar (but is dependent on compliance with progestogen), but the incidence of endometrial cancer and atypical hyperplasia is lower (typically <5 per cent). 'Functional' endometrium is generally encountered with sequential HRT regimens, but atrophy is common if the endometrium has been subject to suppression from continuous progestogen. Structural lesions such as submucous fibroids may be more common as they are oestrogen dependent, but endometrial polyps appear with a comparable frequency in most studies.

TREATMENT OF UNSCHEDULED BLEEDING ON HRT

Uterine bleeding problems and progestogenic side effects are the prime reasons for high non-compliance and drop-out rates associated with opposed HRT. Approaches to managing women with abnormal genital tract bleeding on HRT are summarized in Information Box 8.2.

Hysteroscopic

Polyps and vascular submucous fibroids should be hysteroscopically treated as outlined in Chapters 15 and 16. Bleeding is usually unpredictable (as with endometrial cancer), being unrelated to opposed or unopposed phases of therapy in the case of sequential preparations. Focal endometrial lesions should be biopsied under direct vision and a global endometrial biopsy taken in all women to provide histological diagnosis (primarily to exclude endometrial cancer and hyperplasia). A levonorgestrel intrauterine system (LNG-IUS) may be fitted if indicated (see page 118).

Medical

It is important to determine the pattern of abnormal bleeding on HRT. The cause (Information Box 8.1) and type of preparation guide treatment of heavy or unscheduled bleeding on HRT. In the absence of organic pathology, the continued need for HRT should be reviewed in terms of risk and benefits and consideration of non-hormonal therapy (e.g. clonidine for hot flushes, testosterone for improving sexual enjoyment and libido) considered (Information Box 8.3). If HRT remains indicated, then hormonal manipulation is often the solution.

 Information Box 8.3 Indications for prescribing hormone replacement therapy (HRT)

TREATMENT (SEQUENTIAL)

- *Menopausal symptoms.* This is the prime indication for HRT. Very effective in treating symptoms of oestrogen deficiency – vasomotor symptoms (hot flushes, night sweats-insomnia) and symptoms of urogenital atrophy (dyspareunia, urinary frequency and urgency – add local oestrogen/lubricants/bioadhesive moisturizers if solely for this purpose). Quality of life is improved in all domains (sexuality, sleep, physical functioning etc.).
- *Perimenopausal dysfunctional uterine bleeding (DUB).* A trial of HRT can sometimes regulate anovular DUB in this age group, but frequently the interaction between exogenous and endogenous oestrogen can lead to more refractory bleeding patterns. Levonorgestrel intrauterine system (LNG-IUS), combined oral contraceptive or systemic progestogens represent better options unless significant vasomotor symptoms are present.
- *Premature menopause.* Women <40 years should take hormone replacement (combined oral contraceptive, HRT) in order to treat symptoms and maintain bone mass (benefits outweigh risks, clinical trial data not transferable to this population).
- *Chemically induced menopause.* Suppression of ovarian function for >3–6 months (e.g. gonadotrophin-releasing hormone analogues), for the treatment of chronic gynaecological conditions (e.g. endometriosis, premenstrual syndrome) necessitates HRT in order to maintain bone mass.

PREVENTION (SEQUENTIAL/CONTINUOUS)

- *Predisposition for osteoporosis.* Advice regarding diet and lifestyle ± use of biphosphonates should be first line. Consider selective oestrogen receptor modulators if not tolerated, or HRT if there are menopausal symptoms.

HRT PRESCRIBING IN THE HYSTEROSCOPY CLINIC

The one-stop hysteroscopy clinic is an excellent setting to discuss issues relating to HRT. As well as excluding or treating endometrial disease, the need to commence, continue or change HRT can be assessed. The evidence section at the end of this chapter summarizes data from epidemiological studies (i.e. studies of health and related interventions as applied to populations). As clinicians we treat individuals with varying background risks for diseases, varying opinions regarding the weights applied to these risks and varying attitudes to the menopause, accompanying symptoms and their treatment. Individualized prescribing of HRT is thus required. A detailed discussion about HRT prescribing is beyond the scope of this book, but can be found in the references given under Further reading. Indications for prescribing HRT in light of the current evidence are given in Information Box 8.3. The lowest effective doses should be given for the shortest duration consistent with treatment goals and in relation to risk–benefit balance. Consideration should be given to lower than standard doses (e.g. 0.25–0.5 mg β-estradiol tablet or 0.025 mg patch, which may relieve vasomotor/vulvovaginal symptoms while still preserving bone density). Long-term prescription of HRT as a preventative measure is no longer justified in the vast majority of women. Healthy lifestyle changes and non-hormonal evidence-based interventions are preferred (e.g. exercise, perhaps calcium/vitamin D, biphosphonates, calcitonin and selective oestrogen receptor modulators (SERMs) for osteoporosis, and diet, smoking cessation, exercise, blood pressure control, aspirin, statins for cardiovascular health).

In the short term, the benefits of HRT in the treatment of symptomatic menopausal women appear to outweigh risks, but the risk–benefit ratio is likely to become less favourable with increasing duration of use. Annual medical review is necessary. Once the decision to stop HRT has been made, sudden cessation or gradual withdrawal of HRT (reducing daily dose, e.g. cutting matrix patches – 'dose tapering'; alternate day dosing – 'day tapering', etc.) can achieve this. It is unclear whether one approach confers more benefit in terms of minimizing recurrence of symptoms and maintaining abstinence.

ALTERNATIVES TO STANDARD HRT

In view of clinical and research developments in menopausal health, the hysteroscopist will increasingly be faced with symptomatic postmenopausal women on 'alternative' hormone therapies. It is important, despite pressure from the pharmaceutical industry, not to assume that these alternative agents are safer or more effective than standard HRT, which has been more rigorously investigated. Practical considerations are outlined below.

Levonorgestrel-releasing intrauterine system (Mirena)

This system is not licensed for this use in the UK (see Chapter 7), but there is some evidence for its effectiveness in providing adequate endometrial protection (see Further reading). However, unscheduled bleeding after the initial 3–6 months should be promptly investigated by hysteroscopy and endometrial biopsy. There is hope that local delivery of progestogen will avoid the demonstrated adverse effects of systemic progestogens on the breast and cardiovascular system (NB: There was no increase in breast cancer or cardiovascular disease in the oestrogen-alone arm of the Women's Health Initiative (WHI) study), as well as increased compliance. Further research is needed.

Tibolone

Tibolone is a synthetic steroid that acts on oestrogen, progesterone and androgen receptors. It is effective in relieving menopausal symptoms, improving vaginal lubrication and libido and increasing bone density compared (data demonstrating fracture prevention is lacking) with placebo. Most women taking tibolone with uterine bleeding are found to have a normal atrophic cavity. The incidence of endometrial pathology (polyps, submucous fibroids and hyperplasia) is comparable to women with spontaneous postmenopausal bleeding (PMB). Its effect on the breast and cardiovascular function is unclear and requires further study.

Selective oestrogen receptor modulators (SERMs)

Depending upon the target tissue, SERMs can act as oestrogen agonists or antagonists. Tamoxifen is the best known SERM and its oestrogen antagonist action is used in the treatment of breast cancer, but its oestrogen agonistic function on the endometrium increases the risk of endometrial cancer (see Chapter 9).

Raloxifene has been developed to competitively inhibit oestrogen activity in the breast and endometrium (the frequency of postmenopausal vaginal bleeding is no higher than in a non-treated population), while maintaining an agonistic action on bone and lipid metabolism. Raloxifene has been shown to lower the frequency of breast cancer and increase bone density, reducing the risk of vertebral, although not non-vertebral, fractures (see Further reading). Raloxifene has no effect on vasomotor symptoms and so its use is limited to treatment/ prevention of osteoporosis. Further research is awaited to ascertain the balance of effects on the cardiovascular system.

Phyto-oestrogens

Experimental data for effectiveness of natural plant oestrogens (e.g. soya supplements, isoflavone, yams) in reducing vasomotor symptoms are conflicting and absent for other outcomes such as urogenital/psychological effects and impact on quality of life. The hysteroscopist should be aware that substantial dietary intake via supplements of unopposed phyto-oestrogens can lead to endometrial proliferation, PMB and even hyperplasia.

 Evidence Box 8.1 Benefit and harm of combined hormone replacement therapy (HRT)

Although the clinical evidence base for HRT is large, most is based on less reliable and often conflicting observational data. The recent publication of more valid experimental data in the form of large randomized controlled trials has helped clarify the benefits and harms associated with widespread use of HRT. The results from recent clinical trials of HRT versus placebo are given in Fig. 8.1 and the clinical inferences described in this chapter. For a more detailed analysis see Further reading.

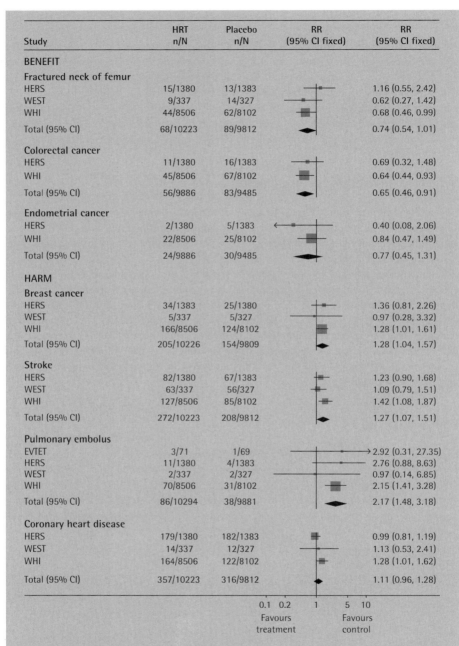

Study	HRT n/N	Placebo n/N	RR (95% CI fixed)	RR (95% CI fixed)
BENEFIT				
Fractured neck of femur				
HERS	15/1380	13/1383		1.16 (0.55, 2.42)
WEST	9/337	14/327		0.62 (0.27, 1.42)
WHI	44/8506	62/8102		0.68 (0.46, 0.99)
Total (95% CI)	68/10223	89/9812		0.74 (0.54, 1.01)
Colorectal cancer				
HERS	11/1380	16/1383		0.69 (0.32, 1.48)
WHI	45/8506	67/8102		0.64 (0.44, 0.93)
Total (95% CI)	56/9886	83/9485		0.65 (0.46, 0.91)
Endometrial cancer				
HERS	2/1380	5/1383		0.40 (0.08, 2.06)
WHI	22/8506	25/8102		0.84 (0.47, 1.49)
Total (95% CI)	24/9886	30/9485		0.77 (0.45, 1.31)
HARM				
Breast cancer				
HERS	34/1383	25/1380		1.36 (0.81, 2.26)
WEST	5/337	5/327		0.97 (0.28, 3.32)
WHI	166/8506	124/8102		1.28 (1.01, 1.61)
Total (95% CI)	205/10226	154/9809		1.28 (1.04, 1.57)
Stroke				
HERS	82/1380	67/1383		1.23 (0.90, 1.68)
WEST	63/337	56/327		1.09 (0.79, 1.51)
WHI	127/8506	85/8102		1.42 (1.08, 1.87)
Total (95% CI)	272/10223	208/9812		1.27 (1.07, 1.51)
Pulmonary embolus				
EVTET	3/71	1/69		2.92 (0.31, 27.35)
HERS	11/1380	4/1383		2.76 (0.88, 8.63)
WEST	2/337	2/327		0.97 (0.14, 6.85)
WHI	70/8506	31/8102		2.15 (1.41, 3.28)
Total (95% CI)	86/10294	38/9881		2.17 (1.48, 3.18)
Coronary heart disease				
HERS	179/1380	182/1383		0.99 (0.81, 1.19)
WEST	14/337	12/327		1.13 (0.53, 2.41)
WHI	164/8506	122/8102		1.28 (1.01, 1.62)
Total (95% CI)	357/10223	316/9812		1.11 (0.96, 1.28)

0.1   0.2   1   5   10

Favours   Favours
treatment   control

Figure 8.1 *Summary of results from randomized trials of HRT versus placebo: risks and benefits of serious disease. (Adapted from Beral et al., 2002.)*

Abbreviations: CI: confidence interval; EVTET: Estrogen in Venous ThromboEmbolism Trial; HERS: Heart and Estrogen/Progestogen Replacement Study; RR: relative risk; WHI: Women's Health Initiative; WEST: Women's Estrogen for Stroke Trial.

INFERENCES

- *Confirmed.* Objective trial data have confirmed previous observations for cancer of the breast and colon, pulmonary embolism and fractured neck of femur so that the findings are true effects of HRT and not due to bias or confounding.
- *Rejected.* There is consistent evidence from all trials of little or no benefit for a substantial protective effect of HRT against coronary heart disease. Observational heart data must be regarded as severely biased and should now be discounted. HRT *per se* does not improve quality of life unless taken to reduce significant vasomotor menopausal symptoms (hot flushes, night sweats, urogenital atrophy). There is no evidence to support cognitive benefits arising from use of HRT in women with or without dementia (Alzheimer's disease).
- *Conflicting* (more evidence required). Observational data regarding cerebrovascular accidents (CVAs) is conflicting. The increased risk of all types of CVA combined from randomized controlled trials (RCTs) is a new finding, but this aggregated measure is crude, and further investigation is warranted for the role of HRT on subtypes of stroke. There is little evidence to support a favourable impact on altering the course of mood disturbance.

VALIDITY

Concerns have been raised regarding the validity of data arising from these RCTs. Methodological shortcomings highlighted include biased population selection (e.g. inappropriate old age where reversal of trends towards disease is required rather than 'maintenance of protection'), confounding arising from population surveillance, choice of HRT preparations studied (dose, route, compliance), and non-examination of case fatalities, amongst others. In contrast, identified benefits, but more importantly harms, may have been underestimated from non-adherence to allocated treatment, i.e. relatively high rates of HRT non-compliance compared with non-allocated HRT in placebo arms (intention-to-treat analyses). Subgroup analyses by age show consistent results, suggesting that this is not a confounding factor. Clearly, more and better science is required to answer outstanding questions and controversies about the role of HRT. However, to most objective observers, the clinical bottom lines from the results of adequate RCTs are clear (see above and current indications for prescribing HRT).

TRANSFERABILITY

The likelihood of qualitatively different (i.e. beneficial) results being obtained with other preparations (e.g. non-oral delivery routes, varying doses of HRT) are unknown. The magnitude of effects may vary (and perhaps affect certain risk–benefit ratios), but overall directional change is unlikely. In the absence of reliable supportive data, one cannot assume that these alternative agents are safe or effective.

LESSONS

- Biological theory cannot reliably predict the effects of hormones on cancer and cardiovascular disease.

- Observational findings of putative benefits (therapeutic or preventative) of HRT need to be validated in large RCTs with adequate follow-up before recommending mass prescribing.
- Judicious analysis and interpretation of available evidence (especially where there is uncertainty) is required to optimize treatment decisions and care for women.
- Conflicts of interest should be made explicit so that the degree of scientific independence of opinions given by experts and industry can be more reliably ascertained.

KEY POINTS

- Hysteroscopy is indicated to diagnose endometrial pathology when there is unscheduled uterine bleeding in menopausal women receiving hormone replacement therapy (HRT).
- An appreciation of the organic and non-organic causes of abnormal bleeding on HRT will help dictate investigation and management.
- The outpatient hysteroscopy clinic is an ideal setting to manage HRT problems and advocate menopausal health.
- Unbiased counselling and rational prescribing of HRT requires a comprehensive understanding of the current best evidence regarding risks and benefits.

FURTHER READING

Beral V, Banks E, Reeves G. Evidence from randomised trials on the long-term effects of hormone replacement therapy. *Lancet* 2002;**360**:942–4.

Hays J, Ockene JK, Brunner RL *et al.* Women's Health Initiative Investigators. Effects of estrogen plus progestin on health-related quality of life. *N Engl J Med* 2003;**348**:1839–54.

Nagele F, O'Connor H, Baskett TF, Davies A, Mohammed H, Magos AL. Hysteroscopy in women with abnormal uterine bleeding on hormone replacement therapy: a comparison with postmenopausal bleeding. *Fertil Steril* 1996;**65**:1145–50.

Rossouw JE, Anderson GL, Prentice RL *et al.* Writing Group for the Women's Health Initiative Investigators. Risks and benefits of estrogen plus progestin in healthy postmenopausal women: principal results From the Women's Health Initiative randomized controlled trial. *JAMA* 2002;**288**:321–33.

Spencer CP, Cooper AJ, Whitehead MI. Management of abnormal bleeding in women receiving hormone replacement therapy. *BMJ* 1997;**315**:37–42.

Tamoxifen

Tamoxifen is an effective and widely used adjuvant therapy for women with breast cancer because it reduces recurrence rates and prolongs disease-free survival. In future it may also be employed in a preventative capacity in women at high risk for breast cancer. It is a non-steroidal, partial oestrogen agonist; it exhibits anti-oestrogenic activity in the breast, but has a stimulatory effect on the endometrium. This hormonal activity results in a higher incidence of postmenopausal vaginal bleeding and endometrial pathology such as endometrial polyps, hyperplasia and cancer. However, the benefits of tamoxifen in terms of reducing contralateral breast cancers, outweigh these unwanted effects.

Genital tract bleeding in women on tamoxifen therapy is a common reason for referral to an outpatient hysteroscopy clinic. Endometrial evaluation is indicated in this situation, primarily to exclude serious endometrial disease, but also to detect and treat endometrial polyps, which appear with an increased frequency (30–80 per cent). Some gynaecologists advocate endometrial screening in asymptomatic women on tamoxifen therapy. These contentious issues along with role of hysteroscopy and ultrasound are discussed.

DIAGNOSIS AND SCREENING: TRANSVAGINAL ULTRASOUND (TVS), HYSTEROSCOPY OR BIOPSY?

In the absence of reliable data to guide practice, the simple answer to this question is probably initial TVS followed (if positive >5 mm) by hysteroscopy and outpatient endometrial biopsy. Hysteroscopy has a major role to play in view of the high endometrial disease prevalence and the limitations of TVS (high false positive rate) and biopsy (non-diagnostic samples). These considerations are detailed below.

Ultrasonography

Several studies have examined the usefulness of endometrial thickness measurement using TVS in asymptomatic women on tamoxifen therapy, as they, along with symptomatic women,

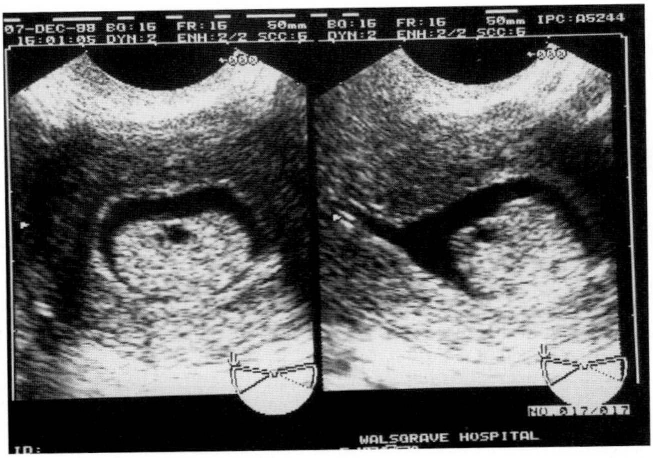

Figure 9.1 *Ultrasound: tamoxifen-induced endometrial changes as seen on ultrasound (saline contrast). The endometrium contrains a tamoxifen-induced polyp. This appears as a focal area of cystic thickening. (Image courtesy of Mr K Cietak.)*

are at increased risk of significant endometrial disease. These studies have consistently shown the accuracy of TVS, with the use of traditional endometrial thickness cut-offs, to be poor, especially in detecting endometrial disease, and thereby of limited value as a screening test. This is because tamoxifen can induce specific morphological endometrial changes, particularly subendometrial cysts, and such appearances can make characterization and measurement of the endometrium difficult (Fig. 9.1). A normal TVS (normal endometrial morphology and thickness ≤5 mm) may negate the need for further testing, but a positive test result is of little value, further testing being required (see below). Only a few studies have assessed the accuracy of TVS in symptomatic women taking tamoxifen (i.e. those with postmenopausal bleeding), and these women have represented small subgroups of larger asymptomatic populations. The role of TVS in the diagnosis of endometrial pathology in symptomatic women taking tamoxifen is thus less clearly defined.

Hysteroscopy

Tamoxifen stimulation of atrophic, postmenopausal endometrium can cause proliferative, hyperplastic or cancerous changes. Typical glandulocystic endometrial polyps are found in up to 50 per cent of women and these are often large and multiple. A wide range of hysteroscopic appearances is thus encountered, although a typical 'tamoxifen-induced' endometrial appearance is described (Plate 13). This consists of an atrophic-looking endometrium (smooth and white), but with increased vascularity. Stromal fibrosis with dilated endometrial glands may be seen through this overlying thin endometrial mucosa resulting in an undulating patchy 'cystic' or 'oedematous' appearance (so called 'glandulocystic' atrophic endometrium). Direct cavity visualization via hysteroscopy is a reliable diagnostic method in combination with endometrial biopsy. Furthermore, hysteroscopically guided biopsies of focal endometrial lesions (e.g. patches of atypical hyperplasia), and excision biopsy of endometrial polyps are facilitated. Such lesions appear with increased frequency, especially in thickened endometria (>5 mm), so that an outpatient hysteroscopic 'see and treat' approach is not only convenient and reassuring, but also cost-efficient (see below).

Endometrial biopsy

The subendometrial changes induced by tamoxifen affect the clinical usefulness of blind endometrial biopsy. This is because an insufficient, non-diagnostic sample is often reported in an apparently thickened endometrium. In view of the increased incidence of endometrial cancer and hyperplasia, it is unwise to attribute this to benign tamoxifen-induced subendometrial changes without direct visualization by hysteroscopy or perhaps saline infusion sonography (SIS).

ASYMPTOMATIC WOMEN ON TAMOXIFEN: SCREENING OR PROPHYLAXIS?

In view of the increased incidence of benign and malignant endometrial pathology associated with tamoxifen use, various management strategies have been recommended. These include screening and prophylactic administration of intrauterine progestogens (levonorgestrel intrauterine system).

Screening

Despite being slightly more invasive, hysteroscopy has advantages over ultrasound. Tamoxifen-induced changes to endometrial morphology (epithelial and subepithelial) explain the poor predictive ability of ultrasound (with or without colour Doppler flow measurement) and, although accuracy is improved with saline contrast, failure rates are high because of atrophic induced cervical changes. The only value of ultrasound is a normal result. Hysteroscopy on the other hand is more discriminatory and facilitates directed or global endometrial biopsy and polypectomy. Furthermore, the frequent inability to obtain endometrial tissue samples from women taking tamoxifen can be explained by the presence of directly visualized inactive endometrium at hysteroscopy. Although the incidence of endometrial cancer is 2–3 times greater in tamoxifen users compared with baseline (0.4 per cent versus 1.2 per cent), the absolute risk remains low in an asymptomatic population. Furthermore, over 95 per cent of endometrial cancers present with vaginal bleeding. Endometrial assessment using ultrasound, hysteroscopy and endometrial biopsy should therefore be reserved for women with abnormal uterine bleeding, and the costs and morbidity associated with screening protocols are not justified. A baseline hysteroscopy may be justified prior to commencing tamoxifen therapy in women at high risk of developing endometrial lesions (e.g. late menopause, chronic anovulation, history of endometrial polyps and hyperplasia, HRT use, diabetes and obesity).

Local progestogens

Local administration of progestogen may render the endometrium incapable of responding to the tamoxifen-induced oestrogenic stimulation. However, the preventative role of LNG-IUS needs further, longer-term investigation to enable a more thorough assessment of any net benefits. Rates of unscheduled bleeding are >50 per cent at 1 year, and endometrial assessment may be compromised. However, such disadvantages may be offset if the incidence of significant pathology necessitating treatment (i.e. polyps, fibroids, hyperplasia and cancer) can be reduced.

TREATMENT

Hysteroscopic approach to unscheduled vaginal bleeding on tamoxifen

The incidence of unscheduled bleeding on tamoxifen is around 20 per cent over a 1-year period. As tamoxifen use is recommended for at least 5 years, many women are likely to be referred for hysteroscopic investigation. The most common causes for unscheduled bleeding are polyps or an unstable endometrium that has been subject to weak oestrogenic stimulation. Submucous fibroids may grow in response to tamoxifen stimulation, and endometrial cancer and hyperplasia are also more prevalent. Investigation with hysteroscopy and endometrial biopsy is indicated. Polyps and fibroids should be removed under direct hysteroscopic vision, directed biopsies taken from focal, cystic lesions, and a global biopsy performed. Hyperplastic endometrium should be treated with progestogens, preferably administered locally using a LNG-IUS (avoiding potential compromise of tamoxifen efficacy on the breast), and such women should be kept under hysteroscopic surveillance.

Selective oestrogen receptor modulators (SERMs)

The pure anti-oestrogens (e.g. anastrazole) and the new generation of selective oestrogen receptor modulators (e.g. raloxifene) have less stimulatory effect on the endometrium. Their use may become more widespread if they can be shown to be as protective against breast cancer as tamoxifen.

 Evidence Box 9.1

Women on tamoxifen for >2 years have a 2–3 times greater risk of endometrial cancer than non-users. Screening asymptomatic women on tamoxifen in order to lower mortality resulting from endometrial cancer has not been demonstrated to be cost-effective. Investigation of abnormal vaginal bleeding is necessary because the likelihood of significant endometrial disease (polyps, hyperplasia and cancer) is high (30–80 per cent). Future research should be aimed at improving diagnostic testing and establishing the role, if any, of LNG-IUS and SERMs.

KEY POINTS

- Both malignant (endometrial cancer, atypical hyperplasia) and benign (hyperplasia, polyps) endometrial pathology are more common in symptomatic women taking tamoxifen.

- Tamoxifen-induced changes to endometrial morphology can make endometrial evaluation problematic.

- Outpatient hysteroscopy has a major role to play in characterizing tamoxifen-affected endometrium, thereby aiding interpretation of complementary tests, as well as diagnosing serious endometrial disease.

- Outpatient hysteroscopic surgery is frequently indicated to remove endometrial polyps, which are detected in at least one-third of women with abnormal uterine bleeding.

- The role of screening, preventative therapies and the impact of newer, 'endometrial friendly' chemotherapeutic agents requires further evaluation.

FURTHER READING

Bergman L, Beelen ML, Gallee MP, Hollema H, Benraadt J, van Leeuwen FE. Risk and prognosis of endometrial cancer after tamoxifen for breast cancer. Comprehensive Cancer Centres' ALERT Group. Assessment of liver and endometrial cancer risk following tamoxifen. *Lancet* 2000; **356**:881–7.

Fung MF, Reid A, Faught W *et al.* Prospective longitudinal study of ultrasound screening for endometrial abnormalities in women with breast cancer receiving tamoxifen. *Gynecol Oncol* 2003;**91**:154–9.

Gardner FJ, Konje JC, Abrams KR *et al.* Endometrial protection from tamoxifen-stimulated changes by a levonorgestrel-releasing intrauterine system: a randomised controlled trial. *Lancet* 2000;**356**:1711–17.

Neven P, Vergote I. Should tamoxifen users be screened for endometrial lesions? *Lancet* 1998;**351**:155–7.

Timmerman D, Deprest J, Bourne T, Van den Berghe I, Collins WP, Vergote I. A randomized trial on the use of ultrasonography or office hysteroscopy for endometrial assessment in postmenopausal patients with breast cancer who were treated with tamoxifen. *Am J Obstet Gynecol* 1998;**79**:62–70.

10

Excessive menstrual bleeding

Menorrhagia or excessive menstrual bleeding is a common problem in both gynaecological and general practice. One in five women undergo hysterectomy by the age of 60 years, the majority have menorrhagia with no detectable pelvic pathology. This, along with the high cost associated with medical management, means that menorrhagia places a huge financial burden on the health service. Diagnosis and treatment within an outpatient hysteroscopy clinic setting has great potential in optimizing management of this common complaint and reducing the need for major surgery.

DIAGNOSIS OF EXCESSIVE MENSTRUAL BLEEDING

Periods become problematic to women when they impact adversely upon important aspects of their life (e.g. social and family relationships, professional commitments, etc.). This typically occurs when menstrual bleeding is heavy, prolonged, frequent, unpredictable or painful. Although menorrhagia is objectively defined as blood loss of $\geq$80 ml per period, the woman's subjective perception of menstrual blood loss and how it affects her overall quality of life is should be considered more important.

Selection of diagnostic tests

The diagnostic process involves taking a careful history, performing a thorough clinical examination and employing appropriate tests. The selection of suitable tests requires an appreciation of the potential causes underlying excessive menstrual blood loss (Table 10.1).

General approach: initial investigation

A comprehensive history and clinical examination should be undertaken. A cervical smear should be performed during the pelvic examination if it is due. A full blood count should be performed so that oral iron therapy can be instituted if anaemia is diagnosed. The prevalence of anaemia in women complaining of menorrhagia varies depending upon definition and population factors, but is thought to be between 3 and 20 per cent.

Table 10.1 *Potential causes of excessive menstrual bleeding*

Common	Less common	Rare
Dysfunctional uterine bleeding • Ovular • Anovular (endometrial hyperplasia) Fibroids • Submucous • Intramural	Gynaecological disease • Endometriosis • Adenomyosis • Diffuse myometrial hypertrophy • Pelvic inflammatory disease • Intrauterine polyps Pregnancy-related • Retained products of conception Iatrogenic • Intrauterine contraceptive devices • Exogenous sex hormones • Anticoagulants	Gynaecological cancer • Uterus • Ovary (theca and granulosa cell tumours) Endocrine • Thyroid dysfunction Haematological • von Willebrand's disease • Idiopathic thrombocytopenia

Further investigation: is it necessary?

The choice for further endometrial assessment is between hysteroscopy, ultrasound and endometrial biopsy. However, remember that unnecessary investigation can be associated with patient morbidity (e.g. anxiety and side effects of tests) and wastage of limited resources. The decision whether to simply reassure, institute treatment or recommend further testing will depend upon the likelihood of disease, as elicited from the preceding history and examination, as well as the performance of available tests (feasibility, accuracy and morbidity). Severe or sudden change in the pattern or amount of menstrual blood loss, particularly when associated with other symptoms such as pain, may point to the presence of local or systemic pathology (Table 10.1). Further testing may then be indicated. Organic pathology necessitating additional investigation should also be considered where risk factors for serious endometrial disease exist or when examination findings are abnormal.

Outpatient hysteroscopy: when is it indicated?

Although some enthusiasts argue for non-selective outpatient hysteroscopy in women with menorrhagia of all ages, we believe such a policy to be inappropriate and extremely resource heavy. This is because most women will have no detectable uterine pathology (dysfunctional uterine bleeding – DUB), and so diagnostic yield will be low. Indeed, a randomized study (see Further reading) has demonstrated that the non-selective use of hysteroscopy does not influence subsequent management compared with a policy of endometrial biopsy alone. Furthermore, if uterine imaging is deemed necessary, then transvaginal ultrasound (TVS) may be more appropriate as it is marginally less invasive, will diagnose the most common

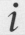

Information Box 10.1   Risk factors for uterine pathology

- Menstrual dysfunction refractory to appropriate, evidence-based medical treatments (Information Box 10.2)
- Persistent intermenstrual bleeding (±postcoital bleeding)
- Risk factors for serious endometrial disease – hyperplasia and cancer (e.g. age >40 years, obesity, polycystic ovaries)
- Focal pathology suspected on transvaginal ultrasound or saline infusion sonography
- Local (or systemic) pathology suspected clinically (severe/sudden change in the pattern/ amount of menstrual blood loss, excessive pain, abnormal examination)

pathology with a high level of accuracy (i.e. uterine fibroids) and, in addition, provide useful extracavity information.

Outpatient hysteroscopy should be performed on a selective basis so that the consequences of unnecessary intervention are avoided. In general, hysteroscopy should be reserved for women with menstrual dysfunction thought to be due to focal intracavity pathology (polyps, fibroids and endometrial disease). Such pathology is more likely in the clinical situations shown in Information Box 10.1.

If such an approach is adhered to then the vast majority of women undergoing outpatient hysteroscopy for menstrual dysfunction will be over 40 years old. This is a reflection of the increased incidence of menstrual dysfunction, organic pathology and detrimental effects on health-related quality of life in parous women and those approaching the end of reproductive life. Clinics with markedly younger demographics should review the indications for hysteroscopy in menorrhagia, and the impact it has on directing further management.

Other outpatient tests and menorrhagia

These tests are often complementary rather than competing testing modalities. However, one should always consider carefully the additional information afforded by additional or alternative tests.

ULTRASOUND

Pelvic ultrasound is widely practised, safe and acceptable to women. The advent of TVS has allowed high-resolution imaging of the uterus and surrounding pelvic structures. The most likely positive finding will be uterine fibroids as they are found in at least 25 per cent of the general adult female population and are estimated to be associated with menorrhagia in 30–50 per cent of cases. Ultrasound can detect, measure and localize fibroids with a high degree of accuracy.

Endometrial thickness measurement using transvaginal ultrasound is of limited usefulness in premenopausal women (Fig. 10.1). This is because specific cut-off levels do not accurately define the presence or absence of endometrial hyperplasia or cancer, as is the case in postmenopausal women. Moreover, the prevalence of serious endometrial disease is much lower in the reproductive group, further limiting its impact on clinical decision-making.

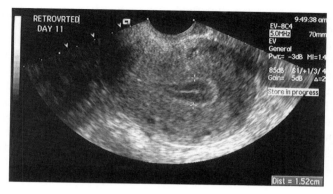

Figure 10.1 *Measurement of endometrial thickness by transvaginal ultrasound in a premenopausal woman. The endometrium is regular, thickened and hyperechoic, characteristic of the late proliferative phase of the menstrual cycle.*

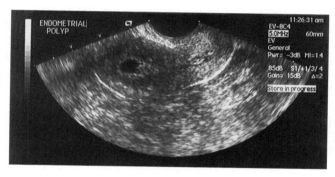

Figure 10.2 *Transvaginal ultrasound showing an endometrial polyp. The polyp appears as a smooth-margined, homogeneous, echogenic mass arising from the endometrium. Fluid is also seen within the endometrial cavity.*

Intrauterine polyps are present in up to 25 per cent of women with menstrual dysfunction, and may be indirectly suggested by a thickened endometrium. However, benign intracavity pathology, such as polyps and submucous fibroids, are more specifically detected in the presence of characteristic ultrasound features (Fig. 10.2). Intrauterine injection of saline contrast markedly increases the diagnostic performance of TVS in diagnosing intracavity pathology. This is a simple procedure, but is more invasive, has an increased failure rate and prolongs the examination. Saline infusion sonography should therefore only be considered when the ultrasound scan is suggestive of focal pathology.

One of the main advantages of ultrasound over other methods of endometrial assessment is that it is not restricted to visualization of the uterine cavity, but also allows the myometrium and ovaries to be imaged. In addition to intramural fibroids, other potential causes of excessive menstrual blood loss may be looked for (e.g. adenomyosis, endometriomas or other ovarian pathology).

Despite the advantages of TVS, its routine use as a first-step procedure in women with excessive menstrual blood loss is not recommended for two main reasons. First, a specific gynaecological cause of bleeding is identified in less than 50 per cent of affected women. Second, most published accuracy data of transvaginal ultrasound for detecting or excluding intracavity uterine pathology (submucous fibroids, polyps and hyperplasia) in premenopausal women are not high enough to be clinically useful in an unselected population. It remains to be seen whether emerging technology such as three-dimensional ultrasound improves accuracy sufficiently to play an important future role in the diagnosis of gynaecological pathology.

ENDOMETRIAL SAMPLING

Initial investigation of menstrual dysfunction using dilatation of the cervix and curettage of the endometrium (D&C) under general anaesthetic is outdated and has been replaced by less invasive outpatient biopsy devices. The technique is safe and simple, requiring less training than ultrasound or hysteroscopy. Outpatient biopsy is highly accurate for diagnosing endometrial cancer and to a lesser extent endometrial hyperplasia. The diagnosis of these potentially serious conditions can only be made histologically, and so endometrial biopsy is mandatory when they are suspected (age over 40 years, historical risk factors, failed medical treatment). As the technique is blind and the amount of endometrium sampled restricted, there are concerns that focal pathology (e.g. polyps) may be missed unless it is used in conjunction with ultrasound or hysteroscopy.

Additional laboratory tests

HAEMATOLOGICAL

Coagulation disorders, mainly von Willebrand's disease and idiopathic thrombocytopenia, are present in 17 per cent of women with objectively defined menorrhagia. Coagulation studies (including activated partial thromboplastin time, factor VIII activity, von Willebrand factor antigen and activity) in addition to a routine full blood count should be ordered when hereditary bleeding disorders are suspected from the history. Suggestive historical features include a severe, long history of menorrhagia since menarche, a history of bleeding postoperatively or after parturition, and continued heavy bleeding after gonadotrophin-releasing hormone (GnRH) suppression or use of the levonorgestrel intrauterine system (LNG-IUS). They should also be considered in severe adolescent menorrhagia where 10–20 per cent of affected girls referred to hospital are found to have a coagulopathy.

ENDOCRINE

Thyroid function tests should be restricted to women with symptoms of thyroid dysfunction, as the prevalence of thyroid disease is low in women with menorrhagia. Recent studies suggest that the incidence of menstrual disturbance in women with proven thyroid dysfunction is around 20 per cent, which is much lower than previously reported. Furthermore, most affected women complain of infrequent or lack of periods rather than excessive menstrual loss. It is not necessary to measure other hormones of the hypothalamus–pituitary–ovarian axis unless fertility is an issue.

TREATMENT

Treatments for menorrhagia are shown in Information Box 10.2. Those for abnormal menstrual bleeding that are relevant to an outpatient hysteroscopy clinic (i.e. polypectomy, myomectomy, LNG-IUS insertion, and endometrial ablation) are described in detail in the following chapters. A general, evidence-based strategy is shown in Fig. 10.3 for the treatment of DUB (i.e. no organic pathology identified). Treatment should be tailored to specific pathologies where identified (Table 10.1, page 129). However, the treatments outlined for

---

i **Information Box 10.2 Evidence-based medical treatments for menorrhagia (based on Royal College of Obstetricians and Gynaecologists (RCOG) guidance – see Further reading)**

- Mefanamic acid 500 mg t.d.s. (prostaglandin synthetase inhibitor)
- Tranexamic acid 1 g t.d.s. (antifibrinolytic agent)
- Combined oral contraceptive pill
- Levonorgestrel intrauterine system

NB: Low dose oral progestogen therapy is not effective in ovulatory cycles.

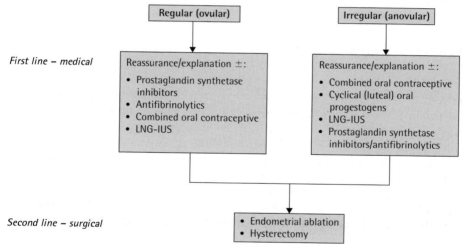

Figure 10.3 *Treatment of dysfunctional uterine bleeding. Some treatments may be used in combination, e.g. prostaglandin synthetase inhibitors in addition to antifibrinolytics where dysmenorrhoea is substantial. The haemostatic agent etamsylate and cyclical oral progestogens have not been demonstrated to be effective in reducing menstrual blood loss in women with regular menstrual cycles. The use of danazol and long-term oral progestogens are limited by their side effect profiles. The use of depot or implanted progestogenic contraceptives (e.g. depot medoxyprogesterone acetate) and hormone replacement therapy may be used in appropriate circumstances (i.e. where fertility control or treatment of vasomotor symptoms is also required). However, iatrogenic dysfunctional bleeding can result, and such an approach should not be considered as a first-line treatment.*

DUB in Fig. 10.3 may also be appropriate under certain circumstances where specific pathologies have been identified (e.g. microwave endometrial ablation for small submucous fibroids, LNG-IUS following polyp resection, etc.).

CONCLUSION

An outpatient hysteroscopy-based menorrhagia clinic is a potentially cost-effective way of delivering high-quality, patient-centred services for a common condition. To increase diagnostic yield and be influential in directing further management, whether this be simultaneous 'see and treat' interventions or scheduling subsequent treatment, a rational basis for selecting patients is required. This will necessitate the use of explicit referral criteria and the use of additional outpatient tests, namely ultrasound and endometrial sampling.

 Evidence Box 10.1 Investigation of excessive menstrual bleeding

Excessive menstrual bleeding is infrequently associated with recognizable organic pathology and if so, it is generally of a benign origin. Most women do not therefore require any investigation apart from a full blood count. The need for further investigation will be directed from information acquired earlier in the clinical process or when empirical treatment fails.

Specific evidence-based diagnostic strategies for use in women with excessive menstrual blood loss cannot be formulated because of the lack of relevant, high-quality diagnostic research and cost-effectiveness studies. A single decision analysis has examined the cost-effectiveness of transvaginal ultrasound (TVS), saline infusion sonography (SIS) and hysteroscopy in the management of menorrhagia. It showed that, although a strategy based on evaluation with outpatient hysteroscopy resulted in the best clinical outcomes (most effective for 'cure' of menorrhagia), the most cost-effective strategy was one based on SIS, followed by a combination strategy of TVS and SIS. However, study weaknesses limit the internal and external validity of these findings.

As pelvic ultrasound is the most versatile, acceptable and cheapest imaging modality currently available, and has high accuracy for diagnosing the most common organic pathology associated with menstrual dysfunction (uterine fibroids), it should be considered a first-line test when further investigation is deemed necessary. Selective use of hysteroscopy will increase diagnostic yield and facilitate efficient use of a 'see and treat' outpatient service. Economic evaluations are required to support further development of an outpatient hysteroscopy-based menorrhagia service.

 ## KEY POINTS

- Menstrual bleeding is deemed excessive (menorrhagia) if blood loss is quanitified at 80 ml per period. However, the threshold for managing menorrhagia is determined by patients' expectation, not by measurement of blood loss during a period.

- The overall aim of management of chronic, benign conditions such as menorrhagia is to reduce the adverse impact of the condition, thereby improving the sufferer's 'quality of life'.

- Pelvic ultrasound is the most versatile, acceptable and cheap imaging modality currently available, has high accuracy for diagnosing the most common organic pathology associated with menstrual dysfunction (uterine fibroids) and should be considered a first-line test when further investigation is deemed necessary.
- Outpatient hysteroscopy is indicated when focal intrauterine pathology or significant endometrial disease is suspected.
- Outpatient hysteroscopic surgery facilitates directed biopsy of focal lesions, insertion of LNG-IUS and hysteroscopic surgery for polyps and fibroids and endometrial ablative techniques.

FURTHER READING

Bain C, Parkin DE, Cooper KG. Is outpatient diagnostic hysteroscopy more useful than endometrial biopsy alone for the investigation of abnormal uterine bleeding in unselected premenopausal women? A randomised comparison. *Br J Obstet Gynaecol* 2002;**109**:805–11.

Coulter A, Kelland A, Long AEA. The management of menorrhagia. *Eff Health Care Bull* 1995;**9**.

Dijkhuizen FP, Mol BW, Bongers MY, Brolmann HA, Heintz A. Cost-effectiveness of transvaginal sonography and saline infused sonography in the evaluation of menorrhagia. *Int J Gynecol Obstet* 2003;**83**:45–52.

Royal College of Obstetricians and Gynaecologists. *The Initial Management of Menorrhagia*. Evidence-Based Clinical Guideline No.4. London: RCOG Press, 1999.

Royal College of Obstetricians and Gynaecologists. *The Management of Menorrhagia in Secondary Care*. Evidence-Based Clinical Guideline No.5. London: RCOG Press, 1999.

11

Intermenstrual and postcoital bleeding, abnormal cervical smears and vulvovaginal disorders

Abnormal vaginal bleeding that is unrelated to the menstrual periods is a common symptom. Such bleeding is usually classed as intermenstrual (IMB) or postcoital (PCB) and can be related to any part of the lower genital tract or uterus. Although the vast majority of women with unscheduled bleeding do not have any significant underlying pathology, such symptoms tend to provoke a disproportionate amount of anxiety to patients and their doctors. The decision to refer or perform further investigation will be dependent upon the perceived probability of significant disease and the impact the symptoms are having on her quality of life. This will become apparent from information obtained via the history and examination. Indications for referral/testing are given in Information Box 11.1 and potential causes for IMB and PCB given in Information Box 11.2.

INVESTIGATION

Over a 6-month period, 7–10 per cent of women will experience IMB and 2–4 per cent PCB. Most cases are benign and self-limiting. Repeated episodes in women of reproductive age, require initial diagnostic work-up, which should include a cervical smear and genital tract swabs (including testing for chlamydia). Contraception should be reviewed and changed as appropriate. If unexplained bleeding persists then further cervical and endometrial assessment is required. In general, hysteroscopy should be the primary imaging procedure in women with persistent IMB, as endometrial pathology is most likely, while colposcopy should be the primary procedure with persistent PCB or if a suspicious lesion is present on the cervix. Both investigations may be required.

Endometrial pathology is increasingly prevalent in women >40 years and so a lower threshold to perform hysteroscopy should be applied. All postmenopausal women with PCB warrant hysteroscopic and histological assessment of the endometrium unless a local cause can be identified with confidence (e.g. atrophic vaginitis) and symptoms abate following treatment.

Information Box 11.1 Intermenstrual and postcoital bleeding: indications for referral/further investigation

NORMAL PELVIC EXAMINATION

- Recurrent and persistent symptoms especially if hormonal contraceptives or the IUCD not being used
- Pelvic pain or dyspareunia

ABNORMAL PELVIC EXAMINATION

- Suspect appearance or lesions on vulva, vagina and cervix
- Friable cervix/contact bleeding*
- Pelvic mass not thought to be fibroids

ABNORMAL CERVICAL SMEAR

- Squamous or glandular dyskaryosis
- BNA, HPV, mild atypia on repeated testing*

* In association with persistent symptoms.

NB: Duration, volume and frequency of bleeding need to be taken into account in determining whether symptoms are persistent.

NB: Postmenopausal bleeding of any sort warrants urgent referral to exclude endometrial cancer. Unscheduled bleeding on HRT is dealt with in Chapter 8.

Abbreviations: BNA, borderline nuclear abnormalities; HPV, human papilloma virus; IUCD, intrauterine contraceptive device.

Information Box 11. 2 Intermenstrual and postcoital bleeding: potential causes

PHYSIOLOGICAL

- Mid-cycle – periovulatory hormonal fluctuations (occurs in 1–2 per cent of normal cycles)
- Luteal phase defect – inadequate progestogenic endometrial support

TRAUMA

- Laceration and abrasion may occur during intercourse (e.g. from a fingernail) and with inadequate vaginal lubrication (e.g. oestrogen deficiency, psychosexual dysfunction)

CONTRACEPTION

- Hormonal contraception (COC, POP, progesterone depot injections or implants, LNG-IUS). Break-through bleeding is common with all preparations especially

in the first few cycles of treatment, and is usually self-limiting. Poor compliance, drug interactions (e.g. from anticonvulsants) or malabsorption should be considered
- IUCD (premenstrual spotting is common)

GENITAL TRACT INFECTION (CERVICITIS/ENDOMETRITIS)
- *Chlamydia trachomatis* (IMB or PCB reported in 18 per cent)
- *Candida* spp. (cause vulvovaginitis; usually found in association with a creamy white discharge)

CERVIX
- Benign lesions – ectopy (exposed columnar cells), polyps (endometrial dysregulation), cervicitis (inflammation)
- Dyskaryosis (up to 17 per cent of women with PCB will have CIN)
- Cancer (uncommon; <1 per cent of PCB in women with a normal looking cervix and smear)

ENDOMETRIUM
- Benign lesions – polyps (common finding in IMB), submucous fibroids (generally cause menorrhagia)
- Hyperplasia and cancer (uncommon, generally present with menorrhagia or PMB)

Abbreviations: BTB, breakthrough bleeding; CIN, cervical intraepithelial neoplasia; COC, combined oral contraceptive; IMB, intermenstrual bleeding; IUCD, intrauterine contraceptive device; LNG-IUS, levonorgestrel intrauterine system; PCB, postcoital bleeding; PMB, postmenopausal bleeding; POP, progesterone-only pill.

TREATMENT

This is dependent upon the suspected cause. Prominent cervical ectopies may be excised or ablated using a variety of outpatient methods, and cervical intraepithelial neoplasia (CIN) should be treated by large loop excision of the transformation zone (LLETZ). It should be noted, however, that, although a modest association between presence of cervical ectopy and vaginal discharge has been shown, no such association has been found with PCB or IMB. In PCB associated with urogenital atrophy, local oestrogen or lubricants can help maintain natural secretions and improve coital comfort. Polyps and intracavity fibroids should be hysteroscopically excised or ablated. Endometrial hyperplasia should be treated and followed up (see Chapter 7). Genital tract malignancy should be managed by a specialist with appropriate expertise.

ABNORMAL CERVICAL SMEARS

Hysteroscopic assessment of the endometrial cavity may be indicated when cervical smears report the presence of cytological abnormalities of glandular cells.

The majority of abnormal Papanicolaou cervical smears relate to squamous cell lesions and they report various degrees of cytological nuclear change suggestive of CIN (dyskaryosis). Cytological abnormalities of glandular cells can also be detected and they account for 1 per cent of referrals for colposcopy. Although glandular cell neoplasia is less common, its evaluation is more problematic. This is because glandular abnormalities are not confined to the accessible reaches of the cervix, but can originate from high in the endocervical canal and the endometrium.

Glandular abnormalities

The diagnosis of atypical glandular cells is made on less than 1 per cent of smears. Atypical cells refer to cells that display greater cellular abnormalities than those attributable to reactive or reparative changes. They are not considered diagnostic of dyskaryosis or frankly invasive cancer unless actually specified as such. The international community favours this term (Bethesda 2001 classification), whereas the British Society of Cervical Cytology (BSCC) report such findings within the broader term of borderline nuclear abnormalities.

Atypical glandular cells can be further subclassified by origin (e.g. endocervical, endometrial, not specified) and likely neoplastic potential. Where neoplasia is suspected these are categorized as 'favouring neoplasia' or adenocarcinoma (Bethesda 2001) or query glandular abnormality, query invasive (BSCC).

CLINICAL SIGNIFICANCE

Atypical glandular cells on cervical smears are associated with a wide spectrum of lesions, the epithelial origin of which may be either squamous or glandular, and the location can be cervical, uterine or extrauterine. Possible diagnoses range from benign glandular conditions (e.g. reactive atypia and endometrial polyps) to preinvasive (squamous cell dyskaryosis, endocervical adenocarcinoma *in situ*, endometrial hyperplasia) and frankly malignant conditions of the endocervix, endometrium and, rarely, ovary. Underlying lesions are usually restricted to the cervix in younger women (<40 years), whereas lesions (e.g. cancer, hyperplasia and polyps) are increasingly likely to be found within the endometrium in older and postmenopausal women. The overall prevalence of endometrial pathology is approximately 20 per cent. Descriptive cytological criteria appear unable to reliably predict the nature, origin and location of the lesion.

MANAGEMENT

Smears showing neoplastic glandular abnormalities or possible invasive cancer are considered as suspicious as cancer and warrant urgent referral. Diagnostic work-up should include colposcopic and endometrial evaluation. The colposcopic management of atypical glandular cytology is contentious and beyond the scope of this book. Appropriate clinical evaluation of the endometrium includes taking an endometrial biopsy and/or undertaking hysteroscopic assessment, especially in older women (>40 years), menopausal women and those with abnormal uterine bleeding where the likelihood of significant endometrial pathology (cancer, hyperplasia, polyps) is highest. The identification of polyps and other focal endometrial lesions requires hysteroscopic polypectomy or directed biopsy respectively. An ultrasound to exclude ovarian pathology should be considered, especially if cervical and endometrial assessment are negative.

Benign endometrial cells

Although most investigators agree on the significance of finding atypical glandular cells or atypical/malignant endometrial cells on cervical smears, the significance of benign glandular or endometrial cells, especially from asymptomatic women, is the subject of some debate. Shed endometrial cells may be detected on smears obtained during the first 14 days of the menstrual cycle, in women with abnormal uterine bleeding, submucous fibroids or intrauterine devices, and in association with withdrawal bleeding on hormone replacement therapy.

CLINICAL SIGNIFICANCE AND MANAGEMENT

The chances of finding significant endometrial pathology (cancer or hyperplasia) among women with endometrial cells on cervical cytology increases with increased patient's age, postmenopausal status and abnormal uterine bleeding. The majority of postmenopausal women with endometrial disease are symptomatic and consequently there is little evidence to indicate that the presence of benign endometrial cells results in additional diagnoses of otherwise clinically unsuspected endometrial disease. Hysteroscopy and endometrial biopsy is only indicated if there is abnormal uterine bleeding.

VULVA AND VAGINA

Although hysteroscopy is primarily involved with uterine assessment, the lithotomy position provides excellent exposure of the lower genital tract. A complete visual assessment of the perineum, vulva and vagina is essential in order to avoid missing both incidental pathology and pathology relevant to symptoms. *Postmenopausal bleeding and discharge is often explained by disorders in the lower genital tract.*

VULVA AND PERINEUM

Common findings are atrophy and inflammation arising from urinary leakage or candidal vulvitis. Vulval biopsies are indicated when lesions suggestive of vulval dermatoses, non-neoplastic epithelial disorders (e.g. lichen sclerosis and squamous hyperplasia) and vulval intraepithelial neoplasia or malignancy (nodules, ulceration and fissures) are found. Persistent pruritis vulvae, especially in association with vulvoperineal lesions, should be referred for vulvoscopy.

VAGINA

Atrophic vaginitis (urogenital atrophy)

Postmenopausal oestrogen deficiency results in atrophic changes to the lower genital tract with thinning and shrinkage of the skin, retraction and fusion of the labia and contraction of the introitus. Resulting symptoms of vaginal atrophy are common (10–40 per cent of postmenopausal women) and include vaginal dryness, pruritis, dyspareunia, superimposed infection (yellow malodorous discharge) and bleeding. Urinary tract symptoms are also common. Atrophic vaginitis should be diagnosed if such symptoms are found in association with pronounced atrophic changes in the vagina epithelium, which appears thin, smooth, shiny, inflamed and sometimes ulcerated. The epithelium is easily traumatized, especially at the posterior fourchette, and petechial haemorrhages are common and bleeding easily triggered. Treatment should be with local (creams, pessaries, vaginal ring) or systemic oestrogen replacement to restore normal acidic vaginal pH levels and thicken and revascularize the epithelium. Antibiotics should be prescribed for any superimposed infection.

Vaginal discharge

Lactobacilli spp. (Doderlein's bacillus) is a normal commensal organism which suppresses the growth of pathogens and obligate anaerobes so that a mildly acidic pH is maintained through the production of lactic acid from breakdown of glycogen contained within the thick, oestrogenized, vaginal epithelium. Troublesome vaginal discharge arises when this normal vaginal microbiological environment is disturbed leading to infection from overgrowth of commensal organisms (e.g. *Candida albicans, Streptococci* spp., *Staphylococci* spp., *Gardnerella vaginalis* and coliforms) or 'foreign' pathological organisms (e.g. *Chlamydia trachomatis, Neisseria gonorrhoea*). Sexually transmitted infections (STIs) or STI-related conditions are common in both symptomatic and asymptomatic sexually active young women. Bacterial vaginosis, vulvovaginal candidiasis, chlamydial infection and trichomoniasis are the commonest infective conditions in that order of prevalence. Common infections leading to troublesome vaginal discharge are given in Table 11.1.

An appreciation and understanding of vaginal discharge is valuable when hysteroscopy is performed. Women frequently complain of such symptoms and appropriate advice and/or treatment needs to be given. The presence of acute cervicitis or purulent vaginal discharge requires hysteroscopy to be deferred until results of genital tract swabs are available. Antibiotic cover should be administered (e.g. oral azithromycin 1 g) with a history of recurrent pelvic infection. IMB and PCB, particularly in association with an inflamed, friable cervix and vaginal discharge may be related to chlamydial infection. Postmenopausal women with blood-stained or brown vaginal discharge are a frequent indication for hysteroscopy. Assessment here should exclude pyometra and endometrial malignancy, but if the endometrium appears normal, high vaginal swabs should again be taken. Foreign bodies may be encountered during assessment.

Table 11.1 *Common causes of vaginal discharge**

Condition/organism	Presentation	Management
Physiological	Copious or perceived 'offensive' discharge white-clear discharge	Still perform swabs to exclude infection, followed by reassurance and explanation. May be COC-related. Avoid excess vaginal douching/perfumes
Prominent cervical ectopy/polyps	Copious or perceived 'offensive' discharge white-clear discharge	As for physiological discharge. Avulse polyp. Consider local ablative therapy (e.g. cryocautery)
Bacterial vaginosis (high concentrations of anaerobic bacteria – *Gardnerella vaginalis*, *Mobiluncus* spp., *Mycoplasma hominis*, *Ureaplasma urealyticum*, *Bacteroides* spp.)	Malodorous (fishy), white discharge, worse after intercourse or during menstruation	Topical or oral metronidazole or clindamycin. Advise stopping smoking and removal of IUCD if refractory. Consider empirical treatment if persistent and suggestive history. There is no evidence that treating the partner provides benefit
Vulvovaginal candidiasis (*Candida albicans*, *C. tropicalis* and *C. glabrata*)	White 'cottage cheese' adherent discharge ± itching and burning. Vagina/vulva may be inflamed, oedematous and excoriated	Topical or oral antifungals (e.g. nystatin, clotrimazole and fluconazole). Consider prophylactic treatment if predisposed to recurrent episodes (e.g. antibiotic/steroid therapy, menstrual-related)
Chlamydial infection (*Chlamydia trachomatis*)	STI. Often asymptomatic. Copious discharge, urinary frequency, IMB, PCB ± pelvic pain and cervicitis	Doxycycline, erythromycin, azithromycin
Trichomoniasis (*Trichomonas vaginalis*)	STI. Often asymptomatic. Copious grey-green, offensive smelling mucopurulent discharge ± 'strawberry cervix'	Metronidazole
Foreign body (e.g. tampon, IUCD)	May be purulent or blood stained	Remove. IUCD may be associated with actinomyces-like organisms – treat with long-term penicillin
Tumour (vagina, cervix and uterus)	Blood-stained discharge plus characteristic lesions	Refer to oncologist when histological diagnosis made

*In all cases take genital tract swabs and give general health advice. Preventative measures include avoiding clothes that keep the genital area moist (e.g. natural fibres such as cotton are preferable to nylon) and thoroughly rinsing underwear. Daily washing the vulva, perineum and anal area may be helpful, but avoid vaginal douching (especially with perfumed soaps) as this practice is associated with a relative reduction in the numbers of protective bacteria. Irritant soaps, bubble baths and shampoos should be avoided, and advise using soft clean towels, and dab rather than rub or use a 'cold' hair dryer. Use soft toilet paper to wipe the anal area from front to back.
Abbreviations: COC, combined oral contraceptive; IMB, intermenstrual bleeding; IUCD, intrauterine contraceptive device; PCB, postcoital bleeding; STI, sexually transmitted infection.

KEY POINTS

- Examination of the lower genital tract forms part of the hysteroscopic procedure.
- Abnormal 'vaginal' bleeding and discharge may have cervical, vaginal or vulval rather than uterine origins.
- The hysteroscopist should be aware of possible disorders affecting the lower genital tract in order to arrive at the correct diagnosis and treatment.
- Outpatient hysteroscopy can be useful in women with intermenstrual/postcoital bleeding and glandular cervical smear abnormalities.

FURTHER READING

Mount SL, Wegner EK, Eltabbakh GH, Olmstead JI, Drejet AE. Significant increase of benign endometrial cells on Papanicolaou smears in women using hormone replacement therapy. *Obstet Gynecol* 2002;**100**:445–50.

Rosenthal AN, Panoskaltsis T, Smith T, Soutter WP. The frequency of significant pathology in women attending a general gynaecological service for postcoital bleeding. *Br J Obstet Gynaecol* 2001;**108**:103–6.

Zweizig S, Noller K, Reale F, Collis S, Resseguie L. Neoplasia associated with atypical glandular cells of undetermined significance on cervical cytology. *Gynecol Oncol* 1997;**65**:314–18.

Part 3

Operative Outpatient Hysteroscopy

12

Combating anxiety and pain

Successful implementation of an outpatient interventional service requires effective attenuation of anxiety and pain. This is achieved by an appreciation of the sources of anxiety, and implementation of strategies to combat potential distress. Optimal ambulatory analgesic and anaesthetic requirements must be delivered. This goal can only be accomplished if the operator appreciates relevant uterine neuroanatomy (described in Chapter 1), the psychological and physical factors underlying uterine pain, and the action and role of pharmacological agents.

ANXIETY AND PSYCHOLOGICAL FACTORS

Pain and compliance with surgery are closely related to the level of anxiety experienced. Women attending an interventional outpatient clinic, such as a colposcopy or hysteroscopy clinic, experience higher levels of anxiety compared with women attending a conventional gynaecology outpatient appointment. One-fifth of women admit to being very anxious, with levels of emotional distress comparable to those found in women awaiting major surgery. This increased anxiety may be attributable to the expectation of unpleasant procedures to come as well as the presenting complaint itself (e.g. postmenopausal bleeding and fear of cancer). Anxiety can only be successfully combated if the operator has insight into precipitating factors.

Suggested strategies shown to reduce anxiety include:

- comprehensive verbal and written (and/or multimedia productions) preprocedural information outlining the reason for the test/treatment, what the intervention entails and likely patient experience;
- adequate numbers of suitably trained staff and a clinic infrastructure able to create a private, caring and calm environment;
- expeditious and informative diagnosis and treatment delivered by a skilled operator;
- ensuring patient choice (the option of inpatient investigation and treatment under general anaesthetic should be offered).

The clinical advantages of outpatient diagnosis and treatment are potentially eroded if levels of anxiety are high and patient acceptability low. However, attention to attenuating anxiety and pain (see below) effectively will prevent this so that the patient experience is a positive one. Evidence for this lies in the high levels of patient satisfaction (>90 per cent) and willingness (>90 per cent) to choose the outpatient route in the future, reported from established centres offering a comprehensive 'see and treat' hysteroscopic service.

ANALGESIA

Analgesic drugs reduce sensibility to pain (Table 12.1). In ambulatory uterine surgery, analgesics can be administered pre-, peri- and postoperatively. In addition to effectiveness and safety, a number of other factors, including patient profiles, operator preference, type of procedure and cost, will determine the choice of analgesic(s) and type of regime. Although the perfect elixir does not exist, good pain control is achievable in most instances with some combination of paracetamol, non-steroidal anti-inflammatory drugs (NSAIDs) or opiate analgesic agents (Table 12.2).

Preoperative analgesia

The costs and any side effects associated with pre-emptive analgesics or cervical preparation (e.g. vaginal prostaglandin) are probably not justified for routine diagnostic mini-hysteroscopy if an atraumatic, low-pressure and efficient technique is followed. Some advocate a selective analgesic policy based on menopausal status. Although postmenopausal women are more likely to require cervical dilatation, rates are still well below 10 per cent and potential adverse effects, such as gastric irritation, are more likely with advancing age, so such

Table 12.1 *Definitions*

Technique	Definition	Side effects
Analgesia	The reduction of pain in the conscious patient	NSAIDs can cause indigestion and exacerbate asthma. Opiates can cause problems such as constipation as well as more serious sequelae such as depression of the central nervous and cardiovascular systems
Local anaesthesia	The eradication of pain (and other sensations) in a localized body area, by the topical application or injection of a drug	Intravascular injection or overdose can lead to depression of the central nervous and cardiovascular systems and subsequent cardiac arrest
Conscious sedation	The depression of the central nervous system that enables treatment to be carried out, but during which verbal contact is maintained throughout	Can cause disorientation and dysphoria. Can lead to loss of consciousness and impair respiration, circulation or both
General anaesthesia	The controlled induction and maintenance of depressed consciousness or unconsciousness accompanied by partial or complete loss of protective reflexes	Potential for serious cerebrovascular and cardiovascular morbidity

Table 12.2 *Analgesia in outpatient hysteroscopy*

Analgesic	Information	Examples
Paracetamol	Safe and effective for the treatment of mild–moderate pain. May be given as part of a compound opiate analgesic (e.g. co-codamol (codeine), co-dydramol (dihydrocodeine), co-proxamol (dextropropoxyphene)). Analgesic activity is equivalent to that of NSAIDs in single doses and may thus be preferred in the elderly	*Preoperative:** 0.5–1 g oral or rectal *Postoperative:* 0.5–1 g 4–6 hourly (max 4 g/24 hours) oral or rectal
Opioids	Relieve mild–moderate pain (codeine, dihydrocodeine) or moderate–severe pain (e.g. morphine, diamorphine, tramadol, fentanyl). Codeine causes constipation, but is otherwise well tolerated. Nausea and vomiting are generally more common with more potent opioids and so an anti-emetic should be administered simultaneously. Drowsiness may also occur and larger doses or sensitivity may induce respiratory depression and hypotension (care in the elderly)	*Preoperative:** Codeine phosphate 30–60 mg oral Tramadol hydrochloride 50–100 mg oral/i.m. *Perioperative:* Morphine 2.5–5 mg slow i.v. injection Fentanyl 25–50 mcg slow i.v. injection *Postoperative:* Codeine phosphate 30–60 mg 4–6 hourly (max 240 mg/24 hours) Morphine 10 mg oral/i.m. 4–6 hourly
NSAIDs	Non-steroidal anti-inflammatory drugs (NSAIDS) inhibit the biosynthesis of prostaglandins (prostaglandin synthetase inhibitors). These wide selections of agents have both an analgesic and anti-inflammatory effect. They are all effective in the treatment of dysmenorrhoea caused by prostaglandin-induced myometrial contraction and ischaemia. For this reason NSAIDs would appear to be the ideal analgesic for attenuating uterine pain. They can cause gastric irritation (give with food/milk to obviate this) and bronchospasm, and should thus be avoided in those with peptic ulceration and asthma.	*Preoperative:** Diclofenac sodium 100 mg rectal Mefenamic acid 500 mg Piroxicam 20 mg sublingual, oral or rectal *Postoperative:* Diclofenac sodium 50 mg 8 hourly/75 mg 12 hourly Mefenamic acid 500 mg 8 hourly after food

*Timing of preoperative analgesia depends upon the half life and chosen route of the agent. In general administration 1–2 hours prior to the procedure is sufficient time to obtain adequate drug plasma levels. A steadier state may be achieved by instructing the patient to self-medicate before arrival at hospital (e.g. mefenamic acid 8 hours prior to preoperative dose). Non-oral routes will avoid non-absorption as a result of vomiting.

an approach is equally contentious. However, if a 'see and treat' philosophy is adopted, then routine prescribing of preoperative analgesia may be supported, given that approximately one in three to four women in an unselected population will require some form of intervention (intrauterine device insertion, polypectomy, etc.). It needs to be emphasized, however, that there is no substitute for good technique (Chapter 4), which should be adopted from the outset to prevent a 'snowballing' effect of increasing sensitivity to pain and propensity to anxiety as the procedure continues.

Suggested regimens for specific procedures are described in the relevant chapters. Overall, in the absence of contraindications, premedication with NSAIDs is preferred. Convincing reduction in perioperative pain has not been demonstrated (which may reflect inadequate time for drugs to reach peak plasma concentrations), but postoperative discomfort is substantially reduced.

Perioperative analgesia

Intravenous administration of 'rescue' narcotic analgesics during ambulatory uterine procedures is infrequently required. Some use parenteral opiates as part of conscious sedation regimes (see below). Abdominal transcutaneous electrical nerve stimulation (TENS) has been shown to suppress pelvic pain induced by hysteroscopy, but is not widely employed.

Postoperative analgesia

Immediate postoperative pain control is most effectively achieved by administering preoperative analgesics. Immediate supplementary analgesics will be required in a minority of patients who experience unanticipated levels of discomfort, and such patients should be allowed to lie supine in a quiet environment and observed regularly. Increased postoperative pain may follow long or complicated procedures. Significant delayed uterine pain can be expected following destructive endometrial techniques (e.g. tissue necrosis and release of inflammatory mediators following endometrial ablation) and so strong opiate analgesia should be considered despite the initial absence of pain. Routine postoperative analgesics are not required following a well-tolerated diagnostic procedure or simple uterine intervention. Following more complex ambulatory intervention, instructions should be given to take regular simple analgesics for 24–48 hours and to contact the clinic if pain is not adequately controlled or persists. We adopt a policy of contacting the patient the following day by telephone following outpatient hysteroscopic surgery to check on progress and address any concerns. Women receiving potent opiate analgesics (or conscious sedation) should not be allowed to drive home and must be accompanied on discharge because of induced drowsiness. Alcohol should be avoided as effects may be enhanced. Morphine may confer a state of mental detachment and euphoria that may bias patient-centred research outcomes if this not taken into account.

ANTI-EMETICS

In addition to pain, the other main unpleasant symptoms following outpatient (and for that matter inpatient) gynaecological surgery are nausea and vomiting. In our experience, anti-emetics are not required routinely for outpatient hysteroscopic procedures apart from destructive procedures, namely endometrial ablation. However, consider prescribing anti-emetics to women prone to motion sickness, those receiving opiate analgesia and those with a previous history of postoperative nausea and vomiting.

LOCAL ANAESTHESIA

The aim is to provide reversible local nerve blockade thereby eliminating pain both during and immediately after the procedure. Pain from the cervix is transmitted via the pelvic splanchnic nerves. Pain from the upper cervix and uterine body is carried with the sympathetic nerves to the spinal cord at the T10–L1 level. Uterine anatomy and the nature of the nerve supply make complete abolition of pain impossible using appropriate office local anaesthetic techniques (as opposed to regional spinal blocks). Cramping and pain will still occur, especially at the fundus. However, in combination with preoperative analgesics and adequate psychological patient preparation, the patient can be maintained in a comfortable state, enabling completion of short procedures with high rates of postoperative acceptability.

As with any hollow viscus, pain in the uterus is triggered by distension (i.e. cervical dilatation and uterine expansion), although these structures are relatively insensitive to touching, cutting and diathermy, with the exception of the region around the tubal ostia. Local anaesthesia should therefore be used in all procedures requiring cervical dilatation, prolonged periods of uterine distension or operations in the vicinity of the tubal ostia.

Choice of local anaesthetic agent depends upon duration of action required and safety considerations. Local anaesthetics of use in office gynaecology are intermediate or longer-acting amides. Vasoconstrictor agents are commonly used in conjunction with the local anaesthetic to minimize blood loss and reduce rapid systemic absorption, thereby prolonging its local effect and reducing toxicity. Types of commonly available local anaesthetics are listed in Table 12.3. All agents can cause cardiovascular and central nervous system toxicity following rapid systemic absorption, usually as a result of overdose, especially in areas of high vascularity or following inadvertent intravascular injection. The operator should remain vigilant for danger symptoms signifying possible local anaesthetic toxicity. These are listed in Information Box 12.1. Maximum systemic concentrations develop within 10–25 minutes, so careful surveillance is recommended for at least 30 minutes after injection. For management of acute toxicity, see Information Box 12.2.

To help avoid serious side effects from excessive systemic absorption, standard protocols of anaesthetic dosage and administration should be implemented, with wide safety margins. However, the dosage may still need to be reduced in circumstances where increased systemic absorption (e.g. vascular region) or concentration (e.g. poor clinical condition, low body mass index) or reduced excretion of the agent (old age) is expected. Combinations of intermediate acting with longer-acting agents (bupivacaine, levobupivacaine) can be used to acquire fast onset of action and prolonged postoperative pain relief pain. Combination dosages should be altered accordingly so that the overall dose of local anaesthetic does not exceed safe limits (Table 12.3).

Techniques

Local anaesthesia can be delivered topically into the cervix and uterus or injected directly into and around the cervix.

Table 12.3 *Local anaesthetic agents used commonly in gynaecological intervention*

Local anaesthetic agent (duration)*	Vasoconstrictor	Suggested maximum dose[†]	Maximum dose by weight[†]	Availability	Comment
Intermediate duration (1–2 hours)					
Lidocaine (Xylocaine)	Adrenaline 1:200 000 (5 μ/ml)	20 ml of 1% (10 mg/ml) = 200 mg	7 mg/kg (total dose <500 mg)	2, 5, 10 & 20 ml ampoules	Immediate onset of action
Mepivacaine (Scandonest)	Adrenaline 1:100 000 (10 μ/ml)	7.2 ml of 2% (20 mg/ml) = 144 mg	7 mg/kg (total dose <180 mg)	1.8 ml cartridges	Immediate onset of action
Prilocaine (Citanest)	Felypressin 0.03 unit/ml	8 ml of 3% (30 mg/ml) = 240 mg	8 mg/kg (total dose <300 mg)	2 mL cartridges	Immediate onset of action and low toxicity
Long duration (4–6 hours)					
Bupivacaine (Marcain)	Adrenaline 1:200 000 (5 μg/ml)	20 ml of 0.25% (2.5 mg/ml) = 50 mg	2 mg/kg (total dose <150 mg)	10 ml ampoules	Up to 30 minutes for effect

* The duration of local anaesthesia is variable and the addition of a vasoconstrictor, e.g. adrenaline (1 in 200 000) will increase the quality and prolong the duration of anaesthesia.
[†] Dosages are based on concurrent use of a *vasoconstrictor agent*. Maximum dosages are presented per unit of weight, but maximum total dosages are presented where stated by manufacturers or recommended according to the *British National Formulary*. Maximum dosages will vary according to individual patient factors (see text) and should be viewed with caution.
(NB: A 1% solution = 10 mg/ml = 1:100 = 1 g in 100 ml).

Information Box 12.1 Toxicity* arising from local anaesthetic: Danger symptoms and signs

Central nervous system
- Dizziness, lightheadedness and feeling of inebriation
- Nausea and vomiting
- Circumoral anaesthesia and feeling of numbness
- Auditory disturbance (tinnitus)
- Visual disturbance (difficulty focusing, blurred vision)
- Tingling ('pins and needles')
- Disorientation and nervousness
- Drowsiness and loss of consciousness
- Shivering and twitching
- Fitting

Cardiovascular system
- Arrhythmias
- Bradycardia
- Hypotension
- Asystole (cardiac arrest)

* CNS depression normally precedes cardiac toxicity with the exception of bupivacaine.

Information Box 12.2 Management of acute toxicity

- Call resuscitation team.
- Maintain the airway and administer oxygen by facemask (artificial ventilation if respiratory arrest).
- Cardiopulmonary resuscitation in cases of cardiac arrest.
- Convulsions should be treated with anticonvulsant drugs (e.g. diazepam 10–20 mg i.v.) repeated as necessary.
- Profound hypotension and bradyarrhythmias should be treated with intravenous atropine (0.5–1.5 mg), and colloid or crystalloid infusions as plasma expanders may be necessary.
- Adrenaline may be required for severe hypotension or bradycardia.
- Cardioversion may be necessary for persistent arrhythmias (e.g. ventricular fibrillation).

SURFACE ANAESTHESIA

Topical approaches involve smearing one of the following:

- anaesthetic gels (e.g. Instillagel – lidocaine hydrochloride 2 per cent and chlorhexidine gluconate solution 0.25 per cent)
- creams (e.g. EMLA – lidocaine 2.5 per cent and prilocaine 2.5 per cent)
- sprays (e.g. Xylocaine – lidocaine 10 per cent)

onto the ectocervix, as well applying directly into the endocervical canal and uterus. Absorption through mucous membranes and skin may be slow and unreliable (onset of action is at least 5 minutes). Unless you allow sufficient time for action, any benefit derived probably relates to its lubricant properties, enhancing ease of uterine instrumentation. The approach is safe, but the creation of 'blobs' of intrauterine gel can however, partially obscure hysteroscopic views.

DIRECT CERVICAL INFILTRATION

Local anaesthetic is injected directly into the cervix ('intracervical' or 'direct' cervical block), with the patient in the dorsolithotomy position (Fig. 12.1). A standard 21-gauge (green) or 23-gauge (blue) venepuncture needle, 25/27-gauge spinal needle or a 27-gauge dental syringe is used to inject the local anaesthetic solution, which should be distributed equally to all cervical quadrants. This can be achieved by injecting at the 3, 6, 9 and 12 o'clock positions, although some operators may prefer to use alternate sites (e.g. 2, 4, 8 and 10 o'clock). The block may be supplemented at the 5 and 7 o'clock positions, representing the insertions of the uterosacral ligaments into the cervix. The posterior injection sites should be addressed first, followed by the superior sites, as blood tracking down from the cervix can otherwise obscure the view. Application of a tenaculum to the anterior lip of the cervix (after superficially anaesthetizing the lip – 'blanching') can be useful to help expose the lateral aspect of the ectocervix in women with lax vaginal walls.

The majority of local anaesthetic should be injected at the deepest possible point in each quadrant, approximating the level of the internal cervical os, and the remainder distributed evenly throughout the length of the cervix on withdrawal (a 35 mm-long, 27G dental syringe or a 40 mm-long 21-gauge venepuncture needle facilitates this). Inadvertent intravascular injection is less likely with direct cervical blocks than with paracervical blocks. However, slow injection following aspiration to detect inadvertent intravascular injection is still recommended.

The patient should be prewarned of any potentially noxious stimuli so that her trust and confidence are maintained. Prior to injection, the patient should be told to expect a sharp, stinging sensation. Another commonly used strategy involves requesting the patient to

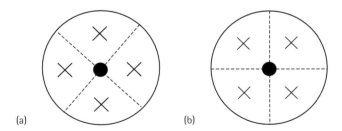

(a)   (b)

Figure 12.1 *Direct cervical infiltration. (a) The technique involves injection of local anaesthetic solution directly into the intravaginal cervix to provide nerve blockade in quadrants. In this example the 3, 6, 9 and 12 o'clock positions have been used. (b) The initial superficial injection blanches the surface, but the majority of local anaesthetic should be injected at the deepest possible point in each quadrant, approximating the level of the internal cervical os. The remainder is distributed evenly throughout the length of the cervix on withdrawal. In this example the 2, 4, 8 and 10 o'clock positions have been used.*

cough, when the needle tip is just over the site selected for insertion. The cervical epithelium is then breached with the woman's attention diverted. This block will allow cervical dilatation to be performed to Hegar 9 and may avoid vasovagal reactions. Some operators advocate administering a small 'test dose' in case of an allergic or idiosyncratic reaction. However, the benefit of such an approach is probably minimal, especially as such reactions are fortunately rare. However, an enquiry to identify a history of previous adverse responses to local anaesthetics should be routine, and administration of offending agents avoided.

PARACERVICAL INFILTRATION

Local anaesthetic is injected into the vaginal mucosa at the cervicovaginal junction ('paracervically'), with the patient in the lithotomy position (Fig. 12.2). Various techniques have been described, but in general a 21-gauge (green) to 23-gauge (blue) standard venepuncture needle or 25/27-gauge spinal needle is inserted just under the vaginal epithelium (<3 mm), and local anaesthetic (1–2 ml) is injected to produce swelling and blanching of the tissue around the cervix. Application of a tenaculum to the anterior lip of the cervix (after superficially injecting 1–2 ml of local anaesthetic into this region) facilitates slight traction and movement of the cervix. This may help identify the cervicovaginal junction and the attachment of the uterosacral ligaments ('tenting').

The needle is then advanced into the vaginal vault and anaesthetic delivered to a depth of 1–2.5 cm. There is some evidence to suggest that deeper injection (embedding the needle into the lower uterine segment at the paracervical nervous plexus) provides better pain reduction. Care should be taken to aspirate before injection to avoid inadvertent intravascular injection. The injection site may be 'tracked' by injecting as the needle progresses. The standard bilateral injection sites are the 4 and 8 o'clock positions (theoretically avoiding uterine vasculature), although 3 and 9 o'clock positions are often used. Additional anaesthetic is often injected between (6 o'clock) or into (5 and 7 o'clock) the uterosacral ligament attachments to the posterior cervix. Some operators also employ injection sites at the 2 and 10 o'clock positions.

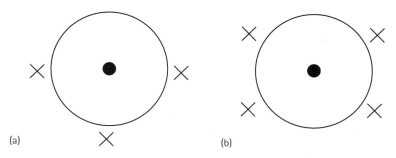

(a)   (b)

Figure 12.2 *Paracervical infiltration. The technique involves injection of local anaesthetic solution into the tissues adjacent to the cervix to provide regional anaesthesia to the cervix and uterus. Various injection sites have been described, but typical distributions are shown here. In addition to autonomic nerve blockade, a 'pressure' effect from nerve capsule distension may aid the local anaesthetic effect.*

The amount of anaesthetic solution used varies depending upon the agent and concentration used (see Table 12.3, page 152). If bupivacaine is used, sufficient time should be allowed to elapse (5–10 minutes) to take account of its slower onset of action. The proximity of the uterine blood vessels, within the broad ligaments, just deep to the lateral vaginal fornices, make bleeding (including parametrial haematoma) and intravascular injection the main risks associated with paracervical anaesthetic blocks.

CONSCIOUS SEDATION

Conscious sedation refers to an arousable, but drowsy state in which a patient can communicate and maintain an airway (Information Box 12.3). Sedation techniques aim to make potentially unpleasant gynaecological interventions more acceptable. However, any drug that depresses the central nervous system has the potential to impair respiration, circulation or both. Life-threatening complications can occur as a result. Any operator undertaking such techniques should be able to provide a level of care identical to that needed for general anaesthesia in the event of deep sedation and loss of verbal responsiveness. This means that the operator should have advanced training in airway management and anaesthesia or, more practically, have an anaesthetist present. In view of this, interventions requiring conscious sedation are frequently performed in day case theatres. Furthermore, it is arguable whether procedures necessitating this degree of complexity and additional manpower can still be classed as truly 'outpatient' or 'office' procedures. The cornerstones of safe sedation practice are given in Information Box 12.3.

Is sedation necessary?

None of the procedures described in this book requires routine use of sedation techniques. The outpatient hysteroscopist must appreciate that anxiety, discomfort and pain are interrelated. Such unpleasant feelings are invariably alleviated by a sympathetic attitude, an expert clinical approach and targeted use of appropriate analgesia and local anaesthesia. Recent reports and publications have confirmed the feasibility, effectiveness and patient satisfaction of gynaecological procedures (that conventionally were believed to require sedation or general anaesthesia) without the need for systemic medication. In all cases where conscious sedation is deemed necessary, the suitability of patients and the appropriateness of the setting should be carefully considered. Sedation should not be used for operator convenience, but as a supplement to behavioural management. Postoperative recovery is likely to be prolonged.

Which agent, which regimen?

Sedative drugs are administered by oral, intravenous or inhalational routes. Commonly used agents employed in conscious sedation are shown in Information Box 12.4. Various regimens have been published. The choice of regimen should be based on published recommendations from authoritative bodies, restricted maximum doses and in consultation with local anaesthetic departments. The key point is that safety will be optimized only if practitioners use defined methods of sedation for which they have received formal training. If a single sedative agent given in a restricted maximum dose via a traditional route is insufficient,

Information Box 12.3 Conscious sedation: Safety considerations (adapted from Royal College of Anaesthetists (RCA) 2001 guidelines – see Further reading)

- *Patient assessment.* Adequate preoperative patient assessment for potential risk factors (e.g. old age, obesity, cardiopulmonary and neurological disease etc.) should be undertaken.
- *Staffing and training.* There must be adequate levels of medical, nursing and support staff (ideally multidisciplinary teams). The 'operator-sedationist' should have received recognized training in sedation or have direct anaesthetic support. All staff should be able to locate resuscitation equipment and be familiar with use.
- *Set-up.* Published guidelines should be followed. Immediate access to adequate resuscitation equipment is mandatory. The operating table/trolley should be capable of being tipped head down. In addition to suitable monitoring devices, venous access must be secured, oxygen and facial delivery devices available and specific antagonist agents to hand.
- *Monitoring.* A designated, suitably trained person must take responsibility for monitoring patient safety. Continuous verbal contact must be maintained, and a pulse oximeter attached to measure oxygen saturation. Monitoring of blood pressure and ECG should be considered in specific cases.
- *Drug administration.* Drugs and techniques used should carry a margin of safety wide enough to render loss of consciousness unlikely (i.e. distance between 'conscious sedation' and 'deep sedation/anaesthesia'. Reversal agents should be available, e.g. naloxone (opiates) and flumazenil (benzodiazepines).
- *Recognition of potential dangers.* Patient response (sedative effect) to drug dosage can vary, but maximum doses should not be exceeded without anaesthetic input. Combinations of drugs, especially sedatives and narcotics, should be employed with particular caution (synergistic effect). The opioid should be given first and allowed time to become maximally effective before any sedative is added. Oxygen therapy is indicated if saturations drop below the resting figure.
- *Postoperative observation.* Clinical and instrumental (e.g. pulse oximetry) observation must be continued until discharge criteria are met. Aftercare instructions should be relayed to the accompanying person. These include not driving and avoidance of alcohol for 24 hours.

then anaesthetic advice should be sought. The operator should note that conventional doses of systemic sedatives and anxiolytics have no analgesic properties. Pain control requires administration of a specific analgesic agent or local anaesthetic block (see above).

FUTURE

The move towards more day case and ambulatory surgery in an attempt to increase health service capacity is going to place an increased emphasis on peri- and postoperative pain

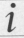

Information Box 12.4 Conscious sedation: commonly used agents

Anaesthetics

- *Ketamine, propofol, nitrous oxide.* Although drugs used primarily as intravenous anaesthetics have excellent properties for use in sedation, their administration requires specialized knowledge, skills and equipment, and is not recommended at present for use by the 'operator-sedationist'. Inhalational approaches using nitrous oxide mixed with oxygen are safe at analgesic non-sedative doses (i.e. 50 per cent fixed concentration).

Anxiolytics

- *Midazolam, diazepam.* Short-acting intravenous midazolam is the most commonly used anxiolytic agent. Benzodiazepines have a muscle-relaxing and amnesic as well as sedative effect. Oral and intramuscular administration is available.

Opioids

- *Fentanyl, alfentanil, morphine.* In addition to systemic analgesia, opioids produce a degree of sedation as well, but they have a respiratory depressant and other adverse effects (e.g. nausea and vomiting). In addition there may be potentially dangerous synergistic effects when they are used in combination with sedatives.

control. Technological advances and pioneering surgeons, pushing the limits of what is feasible in the conscious patient, will further compound the need for increasingly effective analgesia. There is likely to be an increase in the use of regional anaesthesia/analgesia (i.e. spinal and epidural anaesthesia) in an ambulatory setting, as well as the development of new techniques such as patient-maintained sedation and total intravenous anaesthesia. We are thus unlikely to dispense with the services of our anaesthetic colleagues just yet! Developments in pharmacology and patient-controlled anaesthesia should lead to improvements in postoperative pain control. There is also scope for reducing the prevalence of nausea and vomiting induced by anxiety, pain, hypotension and analgesics. In addition to individualized care and gentle surgery, attention to fluid hydration, use of newer anti-emetics and other pharmacological agents (e.g. steroids, ephedrine) are likely to play a role.

CONCLUSION

Outpatient surgery should be performed in the patient's best interest. No approach is infallible and consideration to the patient's level of comfort during a procedure should be a priority throughout. A minority of women will have a painful, nauseous, generally unpleasant experience of outpatient hysteroscopic surgery. However, in the vast majority of women, outpatient intervention is well tolerated, satisfaction rates are high and clinical outcomes excellent. Information Box 12.5 gives useful tips for optimizing success.

Information Box 12.5 Tips for optimizing feasibility of ambulatory hysteroscopic surgery

- Give an honest account to the patient of potential discomfort/other unpleasant symptoms that they may experience.
- Encourage joint decision-making between patient and doctor. Offer alternatives, e.g. inpatient procedure under general anaesthesia.
- Consider scheduling issues. Morning clinics are preferable to afternoon for more invasive procedures (e.g. endometrial ablation). This will allow adequate recovery time during daytime hours.
- A caring, efficient, but unrushed team approach (doctors, nurses *and* patient) is best.
- Combat pain with appropriate analgesic/local anaesthetic regimens.
- Combat nausea and vomiting (adequate pain control, oral/intravenous fluids, anti-emetics; consider other agents, e.g. dexamethasone, ephedrine for postural hypotension, and delay postoperative feeding).
- Make a gentle, efficient approach to minimize tissue damage.
- Achieve competence in performing the procedure under general anaesthesia first.
- Give attention to quality not quantity (limit *what* we do and *who* does it).
- Concentrate skills and experience in 'ambulatory diagnosis and treatment' centres.

Evidence Box 12.1 Attenuation of pain and anxiety

The complex nature of pain makes the assessment and interpretation of pain control interventions difficult. Large randomized trials are required to minimize the impact of confounding factors and selection bias (e.g. saline or carbon dioxide media, size of hysteroscope, rate of cervical dilatation and endometrial biopsy, parity, menopausal status, endometrial pathology, type of procedure, anxiety, patient choice, pre-emptive analgesia, etc.). Measures of effect often involve the use of visual analogue scales to record pain experience. However, statistically significant reductions in pain scores between interventions do not necessarily translate into clinically significant effects. The literature contains several small randomized trials evaluating different local anaesthetics in hysteroscopy, which include topical application (sprays, gels and creams for cervical and/or intrauterine use) and direct, paracervical and uterosacral infiltration. Interpretation is difficult because of the validity of outcome assessment and the conflicting estimates of effectiveness reported (pain relief, incidence of vasovagal reactions and procedure success).

Additional clinical messages include:

- Topical preparations appear beneficial for painless tenaculum placement only.
- Cervical infiltration allows cervical dilatation.
- Deep cervical injection may improve anaesthetic effect compared with superficial injection.
- Lower doses of lidocaine (50 mg versus 100 mg or 200 mg) appear to be as effective as higher doses.
- Satisfaction and feasibility of operative hysteroscopy using local anaesthetic or conscious sedation is the same.

- Higher operator experience, smaller diameter hysteroscopes and increased parity appear to be associated with less procedural pain.
- Overall local anaesthetic administration is safe, with a low incidence of complications and systemic toxicity.

In addition to randomized trials, qualitative research should be conducted aimed at identifying risk factors predictive of unacceptable anxiety or dissatisfaction with the experience in the outpatient setting and strategies to overcome this.

KEY POINTS

- 'See and treat' hysteroscopy clinics can provoke high levels of anxiety, and strategies to combat this should be employed.

- Successful implementation of an outpatient interventional service requires effective attenuation of pain.

- Rates of procedure feasibility and patient satisfaction are high following outpatient hysteroscopic intervention. Pharmacological and non-pharmacological factors are equally important in achieving this.

- Preoperative analgesics, especially non-steroidal anti-inflammatory drugs, are useful in reducing postoperative discomfort.

- Local anaesthetic infiltration is safe if a careful technique is used and safe maximum doses are observed.

- Conscious sedation, as an adjunct to good pain relief and sympathetic patient management, may improve patient tolerance and procedure feasibility in some instances. Attention to patient safety is paramount as life-threatening complications can occur unless the technique is performed in a controlled environment.

FURTHER READING

Campo R, Molinas CR, Rombauts L et al. Prospective multicentre randomized controlled trial to evaluate factors influencing the success rate of office diagnostic hysteroscopy. *Hum Reprod* 2005;**20**:258–63.

Guida M, Pellicano M, Zullo F *et al*. Outpatient operative hysteroscopy with bipolar electrode: a prospective multicentre randomized study between local anaesthesia and conscious sedation. *Hum Reprod* 2003;**18**:840–3.

Gupta JK, Clark TJ, More S, Pattison H. Patient anxiety and experiences associated with an outpatient 'one-stop' 'see and treat' hysteroscopy clinic. *Surg Endosc* 2004;**18**:1099–104.

Lau WC, Lo WK, Tam WH, Yuen PM. Paracervical anaesthesia in outpatient hysteroscopy: a randomised double-blind placebo-controlled trial. *Br J Obstet Gynaecol* 1999;**106**:356–9.

Nagele F, Lockwood G, Magos AL. Randomised placebo controlled trial of mefenamic acid for premedication at outpatient hysteroscopy: a pilot study. *Br J Obstet Gynaecol* 1997;**104**:842–4.

United Kingdom Academy of Medical Royal Colleges and their Faculties. *Implementing and Ensuring Safe Sedation Practice for Healthcare Procedures in Adults 2001*. pp.1–21. [Available at www.rcoa. ac.uk/docs/safesedationpractice.pdf, accessibility verified 6 May 2004.]

13

Mirena (levonorgestrel intrauterine system)

The Mirena (levonorgestrel intrauterine system – LNG-IUS) is a hormonally medicated intrauterine device. It consists of a 32-mm long T-shaped polyethylene frame holding a polydimethylsiloxane capsule, which contains the progestogenic hormone levonorgestrel. This 'intrauterine system' allows levonorgestrel to be released at a steady rate of 20 μg/day into the uterine cavity. The system is effective for 5 years. Two fine threads are attached to the bottom of the frame to check that the LNG-IUS is correctly placed and to allow easy removal (Plate 14).

OUTPATIENT HYSTEROSCOPY CLINIC AND MIRENA

A variety of common gynaecological complaints encountered in a typical outpatient hysteroscopy clinic are amenable to treatment with the LNG-IUS (Information Box 13.1). Moreover, the hysteroscopy clinic is an ideal environment for swift and painless fitting intrauterine devices such as the LNG-IUS. Careful patient positioning facilitates access and local anaesthetic infiltration to the cervix to allow cervical dilatation in 10 per cent of women who require it. Although not essential, it is likely that a pelvic ultrasound will have been performed to exclude uterine pathology in women with menorrhagia. A preceding hysteroscopic examination alerts the physician to potential problems such as stenosis, deviation of the cervical canal or uterine fibroids, as well as providing some dilatation of the canal, which aids LNG-IUS insertion. An endometrial biopsy should be taken when indicated (Chapter 10).

USES OF THE LNG-IUS

Local release of levonorgestrel within the uterine cavity renders the endometrium insensitive to oestrogen, causing endometrial atrophy. Histological features include stromal decidualization and glandular atrophy. There is minimal systemic absorption of the hormone thereby minimizing systemic side effects and increasing the likelihood of compliance with treatment. The LNG-IUS was developed initially as a reversible form of contraceptive (Chapter 19), but

Information Box 13.1 Levonorgestrel-releasing intrauterine system: therapeutic uses

ESTABLISHED USES

- *Contraception* (licensed in the UK in 1995 – see Chapter 19).
- *Menorrhagia* (licensed in the UK in 2001 – see below).

POTENTIAL USES

- *Endometrial hyperplasia.* Reverses hyperplastic process (endometrial suppression). May be useful in preventing formation of hyperplastic endometrium in women taking tamoxifen as part of breast cancer treatment (see Chapter 9).
- *Endometrial polyps.* May prevent recurrence polyp formation as a result of endometrial suppression (see Chapter 15).
- *Hormone replacement therapy.* Provides endometrial protection from exogeneous oestrogen with minimal systemic symptoms, hence increasing compliance (see Chapter 8).
- *Chronic pelvic pain, endometriosis and dysmenorrhoea.* Relieves menstrual pain whether congestive or in association with endometriosis. Reduces recurrence of dysmenorrhoea following surgical treatment of endometriosis.
- *Premenstrual syndrome.* Reduces progestogenic side effects when used in combination with oestrogen.

its potential versatility has been recognized and it has thus been employed for treating a variety of gynaecological conditions.

Idiopathic menorrhagia

The LNG-IUS is licensed for use in idiopathic menorrhagia (i.e. dysfunctional uterine bleeding (DUB)). This implies that organic causes of menorrhagia have been excluded (Chapter 10). In the absence of risk factors for endometrial hyperplasia (irregular cycles, obesity, age >40 years) and given a normal clinical examination (no uterine enlargement or pelvic tenderness), the LNG-IUS can be fitted without further testing. Additional testing will include some combination of transvaginal ultrasound, hysteroscopy and endometrial biopsy, in accordance with the clinical situation (see Chapter 10). Contraindications and side effects of the LNG-IUS are given in Information Box 13.2. There are additional relative contraindications relating to systemic absorption of progestogen (e.g. cardiovascular disease and diabetes; for a full list see manufacturer's information). However, alternative management is also likely to present potential disadvantages in chronic medical disorders and so suitability should be assessed on a individual basis.

Special circumstances – fibroids and adenomyosis

The LNG-IUS is licensed for use in idiopathic menorrhagia (i.e. DUB). The process of named patient prescribing is required if the LNG-IUS is used outside of this licensed indication (i.e.

Information Box 13.2 LNG-IUS: contraindications and adverse effects

CONTRAINDICATIONS

- Pregnancy
- Current genital tract infection/pelvic inflammatory disease
- Undiagnosed genital tract bleeding
- Congenital or acquired intrauterine abnormality giving rise to significant uterine cavity distortion
- Hypersensitivity to preparation constituents

SIDE EFFECTS

- Uterine insertion problems (expulsion and perforation [rare])
- Unscheduled bleeding (spotting, intermenstrual bleeding, vaginal discharge)
- Hormonal (mastalgia, acne, greasy skin, hirsutism, mood disturbance, headache, functional ovarian cysts)

full explanation to patient, general acceptance of practice, patient record kept – for a fuller explanation see Chapter 7).

The LNG-IUS is likely to be less effective in treating menorrhagia arising from recognizable organic pathology such as fibroids (especially submucous), adenomyosis and diffuse myometrial hypertrophy (resulting in a large cavity). However, some women with these conditions may benefit from treatment. These are normally women requiring future fertility, but with poor health-related quality of life because of menorrhagia refractory to standard medical treatments.

There is some empirical evidence, from uncontrolled observational series, supporting the use of the LNG-IUS in adenomyosis or fibroid-related menorrhagia. However, most high-quality (experimental) evidence has come from studies excluding submucous fibroids and enlarged uteri. We recommend that hysteroscopic myomectomy should be performed when submucous fibroids over 2 cm in diameter are encountered, to restore uterine anatomy prior to fitting a LNG-IUS.

INSERTION TECHNIQUE

A bimanual examination should be performed to establish the size and position of the uterus. An aseptic technique is used throughout. After introducing a vaginal speculum, the cervix is cleaned with saline or a non-foaming antiseptic. Rates of induced pelvic infection (PID) are lower in this population (idiopathic menorrhagia) than in younger women requiring contraception. Genital swabs and antibiotics are therefore not routinely required, although they should be considered with a past history of PID or presence of vaginal discharge.

Information Box 13.3 Fitting the LNG–IUS

LOADING DELIVERY SYSTEM

- Align the device horizontally, collapse and withdraw the device within the delivery sheath by pulling on the threads and then fix the threads tightly in the cleft at the end of the handle.
- Set the uppermost part of the flange to the appropriate sound measurement.

UTERINE PLACEMENT

- Introduce the delivery sheath into the cervical canal and uterine cavity whilst holding the slider firmly in the uppermost position (otherwise the device will be prematurely released). Stop further forward insertion once the flange is 2 cm from the cervix so that there is sufficient room for the arms of the device to open within the cavity.
- Release the device arms by retracting the slider to the mark.
- Introduce the delivery catheter further until the flange is in contact with the cervix. At this point the device should be in a fundal position.
- Retract the slider fully whilst holding the delivery catheter firmly in position. This releases the LNG–IUS.

REMOVAL OF DELIVERY SYSTEM

- The delivery catheter is then gently withdrawn and removed leaving the threads trailing into the vagina.
- Cut the threads about 2 cm below the cervix.

A urinary pregnancy test should be performed if there is a history of recent unprotected intercourse or a missed period.

A tenaculum applied to the anterior lip of the cervix is usually required to stabilize a mobile cervix, straighten the cervical canal and provide counter-traction whilst the LNG–IUS is being fitted. The use of local anaesthetic to the anterior lip is optional, as the injection itself may induce as much discomfort as application of the tenaculum. It is important, however, to prewarn the patient of a nipping sensation prior to gentle application of the tenaculum (use the first ratchet).

In general, blind uterine instrumentation ('sounding') should be avoided in modern gynaecology. However, gentle introduction of a metal sound or graded miniature biopsy catheter (if a preceding endometrial sample is indicated) allows the size and direction of the uterine cavity to be determined. The device is fitted (see Information Box 13.3) while gentle counter-traction is applied on the cervix. Remove all ancillary instruments and remove any collected blood from the vagina. Gentle pressure on the cervix is occasionally required to stem any bleeding from cervical puncture by the tenaculum. Simple analgesics are recommended for any postinsertion abdominal pain. Information Box 13.4 gives additional tips for fitting success.

> ### *i* Information Box 13.4 Tips for successful fitting of an intrauterine device
>
> - Counsel the patient beforehand and consider giving non-steroidal anti-inflammatory drugs (NSAIDs) prior to insertion.
> - Timing is not essential, but negotiating the cervical canal is easier towards the end of a period.
> - Anticipate difficult insertion (e.g. in nulliparous women and in those who have had cervical biopsies). Cervical dilatation is more likely to be required.
> - Have all equipment prepared and available.
> - Do not open the sterile packaging until the cavity has been successfully instrumented.
> - Recheck sound measurement if cavity <6 cm.
> - Recheck the uterine axis and resort to cervical dilatation early rather than repeatedly persevering to overcome cervical resistance while applying increasing forward pressure and counter-traction.
> - Dilate the cervix if significant resistance is encountered during passage of the uterine sound and/or perform a hysteroscopy.
> - Remove the device or perform an ultrasound if incorrect placement is suspected.

REMOVAL

This procedure can usually be completed by gentle, steady traction exerted on the string (see Chapter 19).

EXPULSION

The likelihood of expulsion of the LNG-IUS is minimized by careful patient selection and correct insertion technique. However, up to 5 per cent of LNG-IUS fitted may be spontaneously expelled when used for treating menorrhagia. This is more likely within the first 3 months, especially if there is heavy menstrual loss or uterine cavity fibroids. Women should be given a patient information booklet and be aware of the appearance of the LNG-IUS so it will be recognized if expelled. The woman should be advised how to check the threads, especially if the LNG-IUS is being used for contraceptive purposes (see Chapter 19). Later partial or complete expulsion may be suspected if menorrhagia or pain returns.

COUNSELLING

The following information, reinforced by more detailed written information, should be given to the patient to help them make a decision about their treatment and to optimize compliance:

- *LNG-IUS.* As many women may have heard from a third party or had personal experience of problems tolerating a traditional contraceptive 'copper' coil, it is important to make a clear distinction between copper devices and the LNG-IUS. Explain that the therapeutic 'ingredient' is the hormone (a derivative of a naturally occurring female sex hormone) and, in order to hold it in place within the womb (where its effect is needed), it requires attachment to a plastic frame.

- *Insertion.* Fitting the LNG-IUS is a short procedure that involves insertion of the device into the womb. Mild 'period-like' pain may be experienced during and for a short time after fitting, which is invariably relieved by simple analgesia. In some cases local anaesthetic and cervical dilatation may be required. Complications such as uterine perforation are rare.

- *Follow-up.* If the woman is comfortable with checking device strings herself, then this should be done on a monthly basis to exclude expulsion, which may occur in between 1 and 5 per cent of cases. Alternatively, they should be vigilant for expulsion around the time of a heavy period and attend their general practitioner/primary care physician for a 6-week re-examination to confirm strings visible, followed by a 6-month or yearly check. Continuing or recurrence of menorrhagia may suggest expulsion. The LNG-IUS should be changed every 5 years.

- *Unscheduled bleeding.* Light vaginal discharge or blood spotting (staining of the under-wear without the necessity for sanitary protection) occurs in 40 per cent of women at 6 months and 20 per cent at 1 year. Unscheduled bleeding or discharge is most common in the first 3–6 months after which time it normally resolves, so the LNG-IUS should be kept in place for at least 6 months to assess treatment efficacy and prior to any decision for removal. Amenorrhoea (absence of menses) occurs in approximately 50 per cent of women after a year of use. This amenorrhoea rate rises with increasing duration of use.

- *Hormonal side effects.* Although the system releases progestogen locally, some is absorbed into the blood circulation and up to 50 per cent of users may experience side effects such as breast tenderness, skin changes, mood change, nausea and headache, although these are usually mild and self-limiting.

- *Effectiveness.* The amount of menstrual blood loss will be significantly reduced in over 90 per cent of women, although the number of bleeding days may or may not. After 1 year of use, 70 per cent of women treated are satisfied, experience improvement in quality of life and will continue to use the LNG-IUS. After 5 years, at least 50 per cent of women will continue to use and benefit from the LNG-IUS.

 ## Evidence Box 13.1 Effectiveness of LNG-IUS in the treatment of dysfunctional uterine bleeding

There are no data available from randomized controlled trials comparing progesterone-releasing intrauterine systems with either placebo or other commonly used medical therapies for heavy menstrual bleeding. Although the LNG-IUS results in a smaller mean reduction in menstrual blood loss than transcervical resection of the endometrium, there is no difference in the rate of satisfaction with treatment and no difference in patients' perceived quality of life. The cost-effectiveness of Mirena has been established in a recent randomized controlled trial of Mirena versus hysterectomy for the treatment of menorrhagia scheduled for hysterectomy. The trial showed that hysterectomy can be avoided in 60 per cent of women (5 years' follow-up) and in this group of successfully treated women, quality of life indicators are comparable with women randomized to hysterectomy. The evidence for contraceptive and other uses of the LNG-IUS are addressed in the relevant Chapters.

KEY POINTS

- The LNG-IUS is a safe, well-tolerated and effective treatment for dysfunctional uterine bleeding. It also provides reliable contraception if required.
- Women should be counselled about the likelihood of troublesome unscheduled bleeding in the first 3–6 months following LNG-IUS placement.
- The outpatient hysteroscopy clinic setting is an ideal environment for fitting the LNG-IUS device. Successful uterine placement is achieved in 99 per cent of cases as access is improved, and local cervical anaesthetic can be administered with or without dilatation of the endocervical canal if this is narrowed or instrumentation is painful.
- The LNG-IUS should be considered following outpatient hysteroscopic resection of focal lesions in women with menorrhagia.

FURTHER READING

Hurskainen R, Teperi J, Rissanen P et al. Quality of life and cost-effectiveness of levonorgestrel-releasing intrauterine system versus hysterectomy for treatment of menorrhagia: a randomised trial. *Lancet* 2001;**357**:273–7.

Hurskainen R, Teperi J, Rissanen P A et al. Clinical outcomes and costs with the levonorgestrel-releasing intrauterine system or hysterectomy for treatment of menorrhagia: randomized trial 5-year follow up. *JAMA* 2004;**291**:1456–63.

Lethaby AE, Cooke I, Rees M. Progesterone/progestogen releasing intrauterine systems for heavy menstrual bleeding (Cochrane Review). In: *The Cochrane Library*, Issue 2, 2004. Chichester, UK: John Wiley & Sons, Ltd.

Marjoribanks J, Lethaby A, Farquhar C. Surgery versus medical therapy for heavy menstrual bleeding (Cochrane Review). In: *The Cochrane Library*, Issue 2, 2004. Chichester, UK: John Wiley & Sons, Ltd.

Stewart A, Cummins C, Gold L, Jordan R, Phillips W. The effectiveness of the levonorgestrel-releasing intrauterine system in menorrhagia: a systematic review. *Br J Obstet Gynaecol* 2001;**108**:74–86.

Bipolar intrauterine electrosurgery

The miniaturization of endoscopes combined with improvements in optical technology has revolutionized diagnostic hysteroscopy and facilitated outpatient practice. Further technological developments have made therapeutic outpatient hysteroscopic surgery possible. No other hysteroscopic advance has had a greater impact than the production of a diminutive bipolar electrodiathermy system for use in normal saline (Versapoint Bipolar Electrosurgical System, Gynecare, Ethicon Inc., Menlo Park, CA, USA).

THE BIPOLAR INTRAUTERINE SYSTEM

The bipolar intrauterine system (Versapoint) is shown in Plate 15. It consists of a dedicated bipolar generator, a reusable hand piece and connector cable to which is attached one of a choice of three single use, disposable coaxial electrodes, with differing distal geometric configurations – twizzle, spring and ball tips (Plate 16). Once connected, these electronic 'smart electrodes' automatically adjust the generated power to preprogrammed default (ideal) settings facilitating rapid set-up and electrode exchanges if required. The generator is programmed so that the electroluminescent screen displays quick-reference prompts to guide the operator through the simple set-up procedure. The operator controls activation of energy via a yellow and blue two-pedal foot switch (cut and desiccate).

There are six modes of operation (electrical waveforms) available so that tissue effects are tailored to the surgeon's requirements (cut, ablate and coagulate). These are VapourCut (VC) 1, 2 and 3, Blend (BL) 1 and 2 (yellow pedal) and a Desiccate setting (blue pedal). Operative procedures are performed in a conductive medium (0.9 per cent normal saline) using a continuous flow hysteroscope with a 2 mm (5 Fr) working channel (see below).

BIPOLAR ELECTROSURGICAL TECHNOLOGY

The principles of electrosurgery are summarized in Information Box 14.1 and a diagrammatic schema of how the bipolar technology works in saline is illustrated in Fig. 14.1.

Information Box 14.1 Principles of electrosurgery

A typical electrical circuit comprises an electrosurgical generator, which is the source of high-frequency alternating current (electron flow) and voltage (force pushing electrons) connected to an active electrode and return electrode. The intervening target tissue produces resistance (impedance) to current and this generates heat and desired tissue effects.

MONOPOLAR VERSUS BIPOLAR

In bipolar electrosurgery, both the active and return electrode functions occur at the site of surgery, whereas with monopolar diathermy, the current flows through the patient to a more distant return electrode. Bipolar circuits are inherently safer because the current path is confined to the intervening tissue, reducing the risk of stray current and alternate site burns.

ELECTRICAL WAVEFORMS AND TISSUE EFFECTS

Electrosurgical generators can produce a variety of electrical waveforms. A constant waveform produces a rapid and intense temperature rise (>200°C), which vaporizes and easily cuts through tissue (pure cut). If the duty cycle generated is interrupted (an intermittent or modulated waveform), less heat is produced resulting in different tissue effects. As the duty cycle is progressively reduced, cutting (vaporization) properties wane and desiccation (coagulation providing haemostasis) becomes the dominant tissue effect produced (80–100°C). The tissue effect is also influenced by other factors, e.g. more heat is generated the smaller the electrode (higher current density), with 'sparking' in close proximity to rather than direct contact with tissue and longer activation times.

ELECTROSURGICAL WAVEFORMS

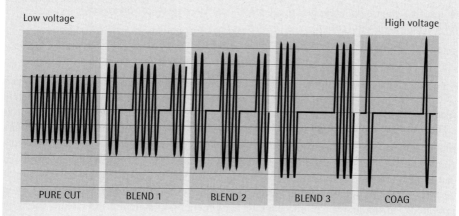

Note that lower voltage is used during coagulation than cutting with Versapoint, in contrast to conventional electrosurgery (shown here).

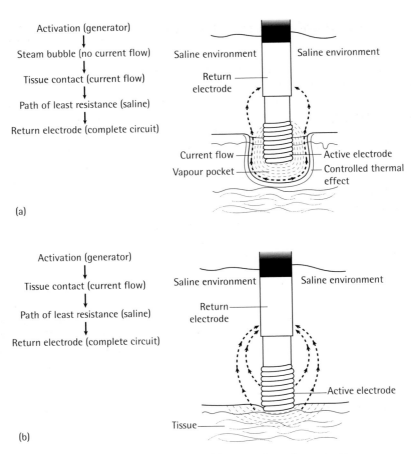

Figure 14.1 *Heat production and tissue effects. (a) Mechanism of vaporization. (b) Mechanism of desiccation.*

Energy is delivered from the generator to the tissue through the active electrode. When activated in the vaporization mode, electrical energy flows and rapidly heats up the active electrode to 'boil' the surrounding saline medium producing a steam bubble ('vapour pocket' $>100°C$). This vapour bubble creates a high resistance microenvironment that surrounds and insulates the active electrode, preventing completion of the circuit until tissue contact occurs. Once the vapour pocket touches uterine tissue, electrical current flows and causes instantaneous cellular rupture (i.e. vaporization). The energy then seeks the path of least resistance through the saline distension media, to the return electrode (situated 2 mm proximally to the active tip) and back to the generator, completing the circuit. Different power outputs and electrode designs will produce different heating responses and a variety of controlled and predictable tissue effects – vaporization, blended cut and desiccation (Fig. 14.1). The preset system values can be adapted between certain limits, to the preference of the surgeon, but such refinements are generally unnecessary.

CHOICE OF OPERATING HYSTEROSCOPE

A continuous flow system is required for therapeutic applications so that clear visualization is ensured. The 3.5 mm Versascope (Plate 5) is designed specifically for use with the Versapoint system, but standard 4–5.5 mm hysteroscopes can be used.

The advantage of the Versascope pertains to its small size, enhancing atraumatic access and reducing patient discomfort as well as its ease of orientation using a 0° hysteroscope with full peripheral viewing and manipulation provided by a deflected (10°) outer sheath and 360° rotating collar. The sheath is disposable, reducing risks of cross-infection, and its unique working channel is designed to expand with introduction of up to 7 Fr (2 mm) instrumentation, once the hysteroscope has been successfully sited within the uterine cavity.

The disadvantages of Versascope, relate to visualization within the uterus. Although high-resolution optics provide precise imaging, the size of the picture obtained is limited by the small 1.8 mm diameter of the hysteroscope. Furthermore, there is no separate outflow channel, continuous irrigation being enabled once the electrode has expanded the working channel, which can then act as a restricted outflow. Despite these limitations, an adequate view is usually obtained to perform procedures suitable for the outpatient setting. A larger, rigid 5–5.5 mm continuous flow hysteroscope provides better irrigation and distension of the uterus and is preferred by the authors if there is a friable vascular endometrium or vascular >2 cm submucous fibroids. It should be noted that a 0° lens allows the electrode tip to be seen at all times, whereas visibility may be lost at full extension with a 30° instrument. In view of the small radial diameter of the active electrode, a greater emphasis is placed upon manoeuvrability of the tiny distal tip in relation to pathology to be treated. This ability is generally less good in standard hysteroscopes as there is no rotating collar.

A further problem that can occasionally arise with the disposable Versacope is damage to the synthetic working channel so that the electrode becomes 'jammed' to one side between the sheath and scope tip. This limits manoeuvrability and can confuse orientation. It is usually a result of multiple passes of the electrode down the working channel. This should be avoided.

TECHNIQUE AND SAFETY CONSIDERATIONS

Electrode selection

Table 14.1 provides a guide to electrode selection and power set-up according to type of surgery. Although different electrode configurations, power settings and current waveforms may optimize desired tissue effect, we should be careful not to create a 'pseudoscience' around outpatient electrosurgical operating. The different tissue effects produced by the tiny active 'spring' and 'twizzle' electrodes are subtle, and the default settings will invariably complete the job satisfactorily. This becomes further apparent when one considers the predictable nature of the uterine pathology likely to be encountered, and the relatively simple procedures suitable for outpatient operating.

Nevertheless, some operators prefer to work at lower power settings but, because of the cooling effect of the surrounding saline solution, 50 W is typically the lowest feasible power setting in the VC mode to obtain any useful effect. Proponents allude to reduced pain and bubble formation at lower settings. However, such unwanted effects are also heavily dependent upon operative technique (see below).

Table 14.1 *Choice of Versapoint electrode*

Operation	Electrode	Recommended uses
Spring	This has the largest active electrode area (1.2 mm $\times$ 1.6 mm) and is the most versatile electrode. It uses the highest default power settings (VC1 130, DES 24) providing rapid tissue vaporization (yellow) and desiccation (blue) with greater lateral tissue damage (typically <2 mm). It is suited to tissue debulking and ablation but also provides an excellent cut	Resection and vaporization of polyps, fibroids, adhesions and septae. Ablation of endometrium within the uterus or residual cervical stump following subtotal hysterectomy
Twizzle	This thin wire, with an active electrode area of 0.6 mm $\times$ 3.0 mm, is the best cutting instrument. The default power settings are between those of the spring and ball electrodes (VC1 100, DES 50) providing rapid vaporization (yellow), precise, needle-like cutting and desiccation (blue). Direct vision and control are required given its design (longer length and thin diameter) and rapid vaporization properties	Resection of polyps, fibroids, adhesions and septae, especially if fine. This electrode tip can be bent at 90° to aid access to polyp stalks
Ball	This is the smallest (1 mm spherical diameter) and least useful electrode. It uses the lowest default power settings (VC1 50, DES 24), providing vaporization with minimal lateral tissue damage (yellow) and desiccating haemostatic effects (blue)	Coagulation, endometrial ablation

Note: The generator provides three different modes of operation waveform: the *VapourCut* (non-modulated current – default settings VC1, 2 and 3 where VC 3 corresponds to the mildest energy flowing into the tissue), *Blend* (modulated current – default settings BL1 and BL2) and *Desiccate* (modulated resembling 'coagulation', DES). Optimal power settings (1–200 W) vary according to the electrode.

General approach

Specific operative procedures are detailed in the proceeding chapters. A general approach to the use of Versapoint follows here.

Pretreatment of pathology (e.g. gonadotrophin-releasing analogues for submucous fibroids) is rarely required and goes against a 'see and treat' outpatient approach. If pathology is known to be present, administer a local anaesthetic block to the cervix. Then insert the electrode down the working channel of the chosen continuous flow hysteroscope and focus the tip at the optimal working distance (<2 cm from the distal end of the hysteroscope with both active and return plates visible). Do not forcibly insert the electrode down the operating channel as this is like to damage it. Retract the electrode within the working channel of the continuous flow system chosen before inserting the hysteroscope and entering the uterine cavity, which should be distended with saline at a satisfactory inflow rate.

The active electrode should be aligned with the pathology. The necessary manoeuvrability needed to access and remove the entire lesion should be confirmed by performing a 'dry run' (by gently moving the entire hysteroscope without activating the electrode). The yellow pedal should be depressed to select and activate the vapour or blended cut modality and the surgery completed. Only tissue in contact with the active electrode within the electrical pathway will be desiccated or vaporized. Although prolonged activation times (>30 seconds) should be avoided (and are rarely necessary or practical), equally repetitive short energy bursts should be avoided apart from when any fine strands of tissue are being removed at the end of the procedure. There is a balance between frequent anatomical review of surgical progress and undue prolongation of outpatient procedures. The therapeutic time window for outpatient procedures is 20 minutes. After this time, patient awareness of discomfort becomes more prominent, compromising tolerability.

Prolonged activation times may increase the likelihood of air embolization and damage to the electrode, which is not allowed sufficient cooling time. Repetitive 'stop-start' energy bursts lead to excessive bubble formation, which is a nuisance, creates excess debris and prevents the formation of a single plane of cleavage. Therefore a smooth operation, generally employing a minimalist 'shearing' or 'paint brush' technique is the best approach. This approach also allows better appreciation of penetration depth and better control of tissue effects, thereby reducing risks of inadvertent perforation and avoiding disorientation, which can occur from the creation of endometrial artefacts. Avoid deep myometrial penetration, as this will cause pain. Haemostasis can be achieved with any of the electrodes by depressing the desiccate (blue) pedal, although this is rarely required as bleeding is usually minimal.

The 'dos and don'ts' of intrauterine bipolar electrosurgery and tips for success are listed in Information Box 14.2 and the advantages and disadvantages of such a system are given in Information Boxes 14.3 and 14.4.

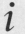 **Information Box 14.2 Tips for successful use of outpatient bipolar uterine electrosurgery**

- *Avoid electrode damage.* Optimal performance of the electrode is achieved by careful, non-forcible insertion and gentle application within the uterus. The non-activated electrode can be used to probe and manipulate tissue (e.g. to locate the base/remaining pathological tissue to be treated). However, such manoeuvres should be kept to a minimum and performed gently.
- *Avoid electrode overheating.* Electrode damage from excessive heating occurs with prolonged (>30 seconds) activation times, activating when there is no tissue contact to complete the circuit, excessive bubble formation and incomplete immersion of the entire bipolar electrode tip assembly within the conductive saline medium. Also avoid burying the electrode in tissue beyond the junction of the active electrode and ceramic insulator, as this may damage the product during use. If excessive heating or physical forces cause damage to the electrode tip, foreign body fragments may result, possibly requiring extended surgery for removal.
- *Avoid surgical complications.* The risk of inadvertent uterine perforation and haemorrhage is minimized principally by good operative technique (see text), keeping

the electrode under direct vision at all times and not forcibly extending the electrode whilst active.

- *Ensure good visualization.* A continuous flow system providing adequate uterine distension is required (see text) to prevent the accumulation of bubbles and to continuously remove bubbles, blood and other debris from the operative field.
- *Planning and selection.* The majority of patients and most frequently encountered uterine pathology are suitable for outpatient electrosurgical treatment. Non-tolerable, incomplete and failed surgery is minimized with experience of the limitations of the equipment and setting. As a general point, multiple, large and vascular pathology may be better treated under general anaesthetic, given the longer operating time required, the option of converting to a larger diameter operating hysteroscope if visualization is compromised, and resecting loops if accessibility is problematic.
- *Minimize discomfort.* The patient should be adequately prepared and an efficient, gentle technique employed (see text). Use the lowest effective power settings (e.g. VC3) and avoid unnecessary myometrial penetration as this will stimulate pain.
- *Therapy time.* It is best to set a 20-minute therapeutic time window for outpatient operating. Patient co-operation will decline after this time from discomfort related to positioning and the procedure itself.
- *Efficiency of movement.* Non-tolerable, incomplete and failed surgery is minimized by using smooth and gentle movement of the hysteroscope to produce a controlled, shearing or 'painting' effect at the distal tip, avoiding repeated short energy bursts and burying the electrode within tissue, which produces a 'Swiss cheese' effect. This will create a single plane of cleavage, if you are resecting pathology, and avoid the need to locate multiple remaining adherent tissue strands. Such residual attachments are vaporized by short energy bursts under high magnification.

---

i Information Box 14.3 Advantages of bipolar electrosurgery intrauterine system

---

- *Outpatient.* Electrodes can be used with small-diameter operative hysteroscopes, which avoid the need for cervical dilatation.
- *Compatibility.* The 5 Fr (2 mm) electrodes can be used with all small-diameter hysteroscopes with an operating channel of sufficient diameter.
- *Tissue effects.* Superb electrosurgical cutting properties producing effects more akin to a high power monopolar output. Laser-like cutting, ablation and coagulation effects are produced according to generator settings and electrode type.
- *Versatility.* The tissue effects produced by a choice of power outputs and electrode configurations allow almost all intracavity structural pathologies to be removed (polyps, fibroids, septae, synechiae). Ablative and or metroplastic uterine operations can also be performed.
- *Operating safety.* Controlled predictable tissue effects are produced with superb electrosurgical cutting properties in a saline-conducting medium. The generation of localized intense heat allows tissue to be rapidly vaporized with almost no blood loss, and avoids production of 'chips' and other debris, which may obscure vision and extend procedure

times. Continuous fluid irrigation provides good visualization and cooling of the electrode during use.

- *Fluid safety.* Use in physiologic saline medium reduces risks from fluid overload.
- *Electrical safety.* Dedicated bipolar generator avoids stray current passing through the patient's body. Electrical injuries from inadvertent activation should not occur unless the tip is bathed in its saline-conducting environment allowing completion of the circuit.
- *Infection safety.* Single use electrodes and Versascope sheath prevents cross-contamination.
- *Cost.* The electrodes are for single use only, but the cost is not prohibitive as is the case with laser fibres, and the suitability for use in an outpatient setting is economically efficient compared with traditional inpatient operating.

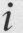 ## Information Box 14.4 Disadvantages of bipolar electrosurgery intrauterine system

- *Limited visibility.* Its small size facilitates outpatient surgery, but inadequate fluid irrigation systems can lead to poor visualization, especially if pathology is large, multiple or vascular.
- *Bubble formation.* Bubbles produced by tissue vaporization, are a normal by-product of electrosurgical procedures in liquids. This can be a nuisance as bubbles may interrupt surgery by temporarily interfering with vision. A passive outflow is normally sufficient, but consider attaching suction (active outflow) if excessive.
- *Restricted operating.* The small size and linear shape of the electrodes limit manoeuvrability so that access to the required operating site can become problematic (e.g. fundal or large, pedunculated polyps) and render treatments incomplete or impossible. Case selection is thus important. Grade I/II submucous fibroids cannot be enucleated safely under direct vision given the shape of the electrode. However, there is evidence to suggest that removal of the intracavity component and restoration of the uterine cavity may give comparable clinical outcomes (see Chapter 16).
- *Indications.* With the innovative design, wide applicability and ease of use of bipolar surgery, there is a danger that overzealous operating and tenuous indications for surgery may arise. In the absence of specific evidence for clinical effectiveness of particular procedures (e.g. treatment of hypoplastic uteri, removal of tiny polyps <1 cm), they should be undertaken only within a research context.
- *Gas embolism*.* Gas (CO_2 and water vapour) bubbles are formed as tissue is vaporized, and a continuous flow fluid management system is required to continuously remove them from the operative field. Excessive bubble formation is usually found in association with vaporization of large fibroids, which is inappropriate for the outpatient setting. Entry into the uterus of less soluble room air should be minimized by using the lowest, effective inflow pressure, avoiding a steep Trendelenberg tilt, purging inflow tubing, not dilating, but occluding the cervix and using a Y-connector to reduce air entrapment during bag changes. Reinsertion of the hysteroscope and instrument changes should be minimized and procedures kept short. Such occurrences have been reported only with

prolonged inpatient myomectomies. However, even when undertaking short outpatient procedures with small diameter hysteroscopes, the operator should not be complacent when using high-power, bipolar vaporization.

- *Cost.* The electrodes are single use only. Cost-efficiency has been demonstrated compared to inpatient operating under anaesthesia. However, certain procedures (e.g. removal of simple pedunculated polyps) may be better performed with cheaper reusable surgical instruments.

* *Diagnosis of pulmonary gas embolism.* Breathlessness and chest pain associated with a decrease in end-tidal CO_2 and O_2 saturation and a respiratory acidosis will be noted on arterial blood gas measurement.

Management of pulmonary gas embolism. 100 per cent O_2 should be administered in the recovery position, a saline bolus given intravenously and aspiration of the right cardiac chamber, if cardiac output reduced.

Evidence Box 14.1 Outpatient bipolar hysteroscopic electrosurgery

Versapoint technology has been assessed for feasibility and safety in small observational outpatient studies. The effectiveness and cost-effectiveness of outpatient uterine electrosurgery has been examined in controlled, but non-randomized studies. Two randomized controlled trials have been performed. One showed no differences in pain control and patient satisfaction between local anaesthetic and conscious sedation regimens. The other (as yet unpublished – personal communication Clark TJ *et al.*) has shown cost-effectiveness of outpatient bipolar polypectomy compared with traditional inpatient procedures. Competing manufacturers are now producing bipolar electrodes based on the Versapoint prototype (e.g. Storz bipolar vaporization electrode).

KEY POINTS

- The Gynecare Versapoint bipolar diathermy system for use in saline is a significant technological advance facilitating a wide variety of hysteroscopic procedures to be performed in the outpatient setting.

- The system provides a variety of tissue effects and its performance is more akin to a monopolar device, yet retains all the inherent safety features of bipolar electrosurgery.

- Problems with fluid overload are eradicated for the most part because the system is designed for use in an isotonic saline medium and the duration of surgery is limited (<20 minutes) in the conscious patient during outpatient procedures.

- The system is ideal for surgical correction of pathology at the time of hysteroscopic diagnosis in keeping with the 'see and treat' philosophy promoted in this book.

FURTHER READING

Bettocchi S, Ceci O, Di Venere R *et al.* Advanced operative office hysteroscopy without anaesthesia: analysis of 501 cases treated with a 5 Fr bipolar electrode. *Hum Reprod* 2002;**17**:2435–8.

Fernandez H, Gervaise A, de Tayrac R. Operative hysteroscopy for infertility using normal saline solution and a coaxial bipolar electrode: a pilot study. *Hum Reprod* 2000;**15**:1773–5.

Gynecare Versapoint bipolar electrosurgery system. (Available at www.jnjgateway.com/public/GBENG/VERSAPOINT_epi.pdf, accessibility verified 10 September 2004.).

Hunter DC, Cooper DW, Phillips G. Gas embolism during VersaPoint hysteroscopic myomectomy. *Gynecol Endosc* 2001;**10**:261–4.

Vleugels MPH. Normal saline field bipolar electrosurgery in hysteroscopy: report of the first 163 cases. *Gynaecol Endosc* 2001;**10**:349–53.

15

Endometrial polyps

DEFINITION (HYSTEROSCOPIC)

Endometrial polyps are discrete outgrowths of endometrium, attached by a pedicle, which move with the flow of the distension medium. They may be pedunculated or sessile, single or multiple and vary in size (0.5–4 cm).

EPIDEMIOLOGY

The presence of endometrial polyps is being increasingly recognized following the introduction of transvaginal ultrasound (TVS) and outpatient hysteroscopy. The prevalence of endometrial polyps in women presenting with abnormal pre- or postmenopausal bleeding is around 25 per cent, although rates between 10 and 40 per cent have been reported. The prevalence of polyps in asymptomatic women is uncertain, but generally thought to be 10 per cent. Small uterine polyps can regress spontaneously, whereas larger polyps are more likely to persist and are associated with abnormal uterine bleeding. Tamoxifen and cervical polyps are independent risk factors for endometrial polyps. The role of other factors such as age, menopause and use of hormone replacement therapy (HRT) is less clear as published data are conflicting.

PATHOLOGY

Endometrial polyps are focal endometrial outgrowths containing a variable amount of glands, stroma and blood vessels, which influence their macroscopic appearance. A practical classification of endometrial polyps is given in Information Box 15.1. Glandular and vascular polyps are more likely to present with unscheduled bleeding or discharge. Most polyps do not appear to be subject to the normal cellular mechanisms that regulate the endometrium. Consequently they are relatively insensitive to cyclical hormonal changes

Information Box 15.1   Practical classification of polyps

- *Typical (functional) polyp.* Appearance similar to those of the surrounding endometrium with proliferative or secretory changes. May be predominantly glandular ('mucous polyp'), or fibrotic ('fibrous polyp'). They are dysregulatory tumours. Often asymptomatic.
- *Hyperplastic polyp.* These are non-cyclic, usually respond to oestrogen and have a vascular, cystic appearance.
- *Cancerous polyp.* To classify a polyp as cancerous (i.e. arising *de novo*), the base/stalk is benign and surrounding endometrium free of cancer. Atypical hyperplastic or malignant polyps often have surface and vascular irregularities and are more likely to be friable, haemorrhagic and necrotic.
- *Atrophic polyp.* Thought to result from retrogressive changes of a previously hyperplastic or functional polyp. Found in postmenopausal women.
- *Pseudopolyp.* Small (<1 cm), sessile, with a structure similar to that of the surrounding endometrium and cycle with adjacent endometrium. More prevalent in the secretory phase and disappear with menstruation.
- *Megapolyp.* Large, cystic polyps filling the uterine cavity and may protrude through the cervix. Usually found in association with tamoxifen therapy and composed of irregular, dilated glands, thick-walled blood vessels and a fibrotic stroma.

leading them to persist and cause unscheduled vaginal bleeding. Endometrial polyps contain hyperplastic foci in 10–25 per cent of symptomatic cases and 1 per cent are frankly malignant. The risk of polyps harbouring serious endometrial disease is increased after the menopause and with the use of tamoxifen.

PRESENTATION

It is unlikely that the increased endometrial surface area caused by the presence of polyps causes excessive menstrual blood loss. However, different expression of sex steroid receptors in the endometrium overlying polyps may result in light, unscheduled bleeding ('spotting') and vaginal discharge, or heavier bleeding if hyperplastic or malignant. The presence of endometrial polyps is frequently found in association with unscheduled bleeding on HRT or tamoxifen and can be a cause of postmenopausal blood loss.

DIAGNOSIS

Blind endometrial sampling (dilatation and curettage (D&C)) will miss 10 per cent of endometrial polyps. Uterine imaging is more sensitive in diagnosing focal intrauterine lesions. Transvaginal ultrasound can detect polyps directly (Fig. 15.1) or indirectly because of abnormally thickened endometrium, although accuracy is limited. Intrauterine injection of saline contrast markedly increases the diagnostic performance of TVS in diagnosing intracavity pathology (Fig. 15.2) so that it is equivalent to that of hysteroscopy, which is generally considered to be the gold standard test.

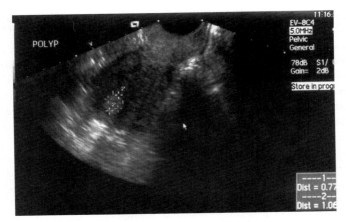

Figure 15.1 *Diagnosis of endometrial polyps: transvaginal ultrasound. An endometrial polyp is detected within the endometrial cavity as a smooth-margined echogenic mass of variable size and shape (sessile or pedunculated) with a fairly homogeneous texture and without distortion of the endometrial–myometrial junction.*

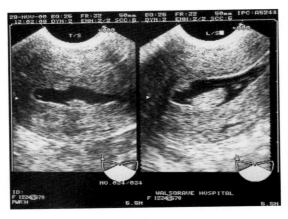

Figure 15.2 *Diagnosis of endometrial polyps: saline contrast transvaginal ultrasound. The endometrial polyp is seen as a hyperechoic and homogeneous mass arising from the posterior uterine wall. (Courtesy of Mr K Cietak.)*

HYSTEROSCOPIC CHARACTERISTICS

A polyp is defined hysteroscopically by the presence of a discrete, focal outgrowth of endometrium (Plate 17). Pedunculated polyps will be seen to move with the flow of disten-sion media or with pressure applied from the endoscope, and have a subjectively 'soft feeling' allowing indentation to be made. These characteristics, along with an absence of prominent, stretched, superficial vasculature, distinguishes a polyp from a submucous fibroid. Polyps can be pedunculated or sessile, single or multiple. Large 'mega' polyps are not uncommon in women taking tamoxifen. A hyperplastic or malignant polyp should be suspected if polyps are irregular, vascular, friable or necrotic especially when diagnosed in postmenopausal women.

The accuracy of hysteroscopy in excluding premalignant or malignant disease of the endometrium is limited. Although hysteroscopy is the gold standard for detecting endometrial polyps, there are scarce data supporting its ability to predict the nature of polyps (i.e. benign or malignant), and so excision biopsy is required. In addition, an endometrial biopsy should be performed to exclude global endometrial disease, which is more commonly found in association with polyps.

INDICATIONS FOR TREATMENT

Traditional management of endometrial polyps is removal by blind curettage or avulsion under general anaesthesia. Fewer than 10 per cent of UK gynaecologists perform endometrial polypectomy in the outpatient setting, and fewer still perform endoscopic procedures. D&C is known to miss polyps in around 10 per cent of cases. It is not surprising therefore, that blind procedures, even after hysteroscopic localization, often fail or result in incomplete polypectomy and subsequent recurrence. Removal under direct vision in the outpatient setting represents optimal management (Fig. 15.3).

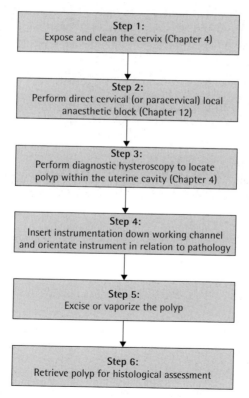

Figure 15.3 *Procedural steps required to perform hysteroscopic polypectomy.*

Over 90 per cent of UK gynaecologists remove polyps once detected. No studies have been conducted addressing the role of expectant management. Thus it is recommended that endometrial polyps be removed once diagnosed for three reasons:

- *Treating symptoms of abnormal uterine bleeding.* Polypectomy is associated with subjective improvement in all types of abnormal uterine bleeding patterns and associated with a high satisfaction rate.
- *Obtaining histology to exclude endometrial hyperplasia or cancer.* This is recommended in all cases and is mandatory if risk factors for hyperplasia and cancer are present (e.g. abnormal bleeding, increasing age, postmenopausal status, HRT/tamoxifen use, hypertension, obesity and suggestive abnormal appearances on hysteroscopy).
- *Optimizing reproductive outcomes.* Removal of larger polyps >2 cm has been reported to enhance fertility, increase pregnancy rates in association with *in vitro* fertilization and reduce pregnancy loss.

HYSTEROSCOPIC POLYPECTOMY

Women should be counselled regarding potential diagnoses prior to undergoing hysteroscopy. This also allows the clinician to discuss and obtain consent for potential 'see and treat' therapies such as polypectomy, especially if suspected from the preceding history or ultrasound examination. The equipment set-up required for outpatient hysteroscopic polypectomy is detailed in Information Box 15.2.

 Information Box 15.2 Basic requirements for set-up for outpatient hysteroscopic polypectomy

- Operative hysteroscopy set-up (see Chapter 3)
- Open-sided speculum (e.g. Cusco's)
- Tenaculum forceps
- Cervical dilation set
- Grasping forceps (polyp, sponge)
- Continuous flow hysteroscope* with a minimum 5 F (1.67 mm) operative channel
- Saline* (3-l bag recommended) ± pressure cuff and inflow/outflow tubing ± suction apparatus
- Mechanical instruments (hysteroscopic semi-rigid scissors and graspers)
- Versapoint coaxial electrodes (spring and twizzle tip)
- Foley balloon catheter (uterine tamponade or splinting)
- Video endoscopy system
- Video recording facility (optional)

* The choice of distension medium and angulation of hysteroscope will depend upon personal preference and applied technique. We find that the advantages of easier orientation with a 0° lens outweigh the expanded field of view produced by off-set lenses. Saline is the safest and most versatile medium.

The approach and techniques applicable for use in the outpatient setting are shown in Figs 15.4–15.6. Steps 1–3 in Fig. 15.3 have been dealt with in previous chapters. Technical options for carrying out steps 4–6 are discussed below.

Steps 4–5: Instrumentation and polypectomy

The advantages and disadvantages of various outpatient techniques are listed in Table 15.1. Care when inserting instruments down operating channels is required to avoid damage to fine instruments or perforation of collapsible working channels (e.g. Versascope). The electrode should be retracted within the operating channel prior to negotiating the endo-cervical canal to prevent equipment damage and inadvertent tissue trauma. Confirm that the hysteroscope is well within the body of the uterus before exposing the electrode tip. If resistance is encountered whilst attempting this, the operator should check that the internal cervical os has been completely traversed.

Mechanical instruments are inherently safer as they avoid inadvertent thermal damage. However, the ancillary instruments (graspers, scissors, biopsy cups) are delicate and easily damaged if undue forces are applied. Fibrous polyps are difficult for such instruments to slice through and the mobile nature of pedunculated polyps makes excision and orientation difficult. Bipolar diathermy electrodes overcome these problems and are preferred for all but the simplest of lesions (Plate 18). Following excision, ablating the area exposed on the uterine wall from where the polyp originated, may reduce the risk of polyp regeneration and subsequent recurrence. The *en bloc* and sequential slicing hysteroscopic techniques are illustrated in Fig. 15.5 as well as vaporization of pathology.

Step 6: Specimen retrieval

DIRECT VISION

The polyp can be cut into several small pieces and retrieved with grasping forceps under direct vision. This approach avoids both cervical dilatation and blind instrumentation of the uterus. However, visualization may be compromised by chips of tissue and free debris (also by bleeding if scissors are used) and the procedure is invariably prolonged as a result of repeated reinsertion of ancillary instruments and/or hysteroscope. The completeness and quality of the specimen available for histological assessment may also be suboptimal.

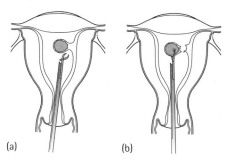

(a)   (b)

Figure 15.4 *Outpatient hysteroscopic polypectomy (mechanical). (a) Hysteroscopic scissors are used to excise the pedicle. (b) The polyp is removed using hysteroscopic grasping forceps or heavier 'blind' instruments (requires cervical dilatation).*

Table 15.1 *Polypectomy: Outpatient techniques*

Technique	Instrument	Advantages	Disadvantages
Blind polypectomy ('directed' to hysteroscopically identified locations)			
Blind curettage or aspiration	Miniature curette or endometrial biopsy device	Simple technique. Success of procedure not dependent upon satisfactory visualization. Cheap instrumentation.	Only suitable for small polyps. Difficulty locating polyp frequently results in failure. Painful as vigorous abrasion required and if procedure prolonged. Risk of incomplete (partial) polypectomy and recurrence.
Blind avulsion	Polyp forceps	Simple technique. Success of procedure not dependent upon satisfactory visualization. Very useful for removal of large pedunculated, fundal polyps and when suboptimal views are obtained because of bleeding/debris from friable, vascular polypoidal endometrium. Cheap instrumentation.	Cervical dilatation required to introduce polyp forceps. Difficulty locating or grasping polyps frequently results in failure. Painful if procedure prolonged. Risk of incomplete (partial) polypectomy and recurrence.
Hysteroscopic polypectomy			
Mechanical	Hysteroscopic scissors, snares and graspers	Direct vision facilitates complete removal of polyp and so risk of persistent symptoms, polyp recurrence and inadequate histological specimens is reduced. Risk of uterine trauma reduced compared with blind instrumentation.	Technically more demanding and so additional training required. Miniaturization of equipment avoids the need for cervical dilatation, but also limits what is technically possible. 'Fiddly' because of miniature size and manipulation of instruments limited by uterine anatomy. Difficult to excise fibrous or pedunculated polyps with mechanical instruments. Bleeding may occur in vascular polyps. Removal of specimen often requires cervical dilatation.
Bipolar diathermy	Bipolar intrauterine system	Direct vision facilitates complete removal of polyp and so risk of persistent symptoms, polyp recurrence and inadequate histological specimens is reduced. Diathermy to the polyp base may also prevent recurrence. Risk of uterine trauma reduced compared with blind instrumentation.	Technically more demanding and so additional training required. Miniaturization of equipment avoids the need for cervical dilatation, but also limits what is technically possible. May not be feasible to remove fundal polyps and those at the level of the isthmus. Removal of specimen often requires cervical dilatation. Higher initial expense resulting from use of disposable electrodes and operating sheaths.

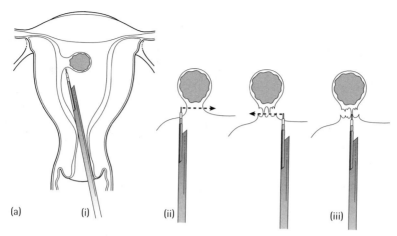

(a) General approach. (i) The Versapoint electrode is orientated with respect to the polyp. Both active and return plates should be visible. (ii) The electrode is activated in close proximity to the tissue. The operating distance is fixed and smooth. Superficial back-and-forth 'painting' motions are utilized avoiding a 'stop-start' approach. (iii) Utilize short-energy bursts under higher magnification (i.e. close proximity) in order to target and excise any remaining strands of fine tissue.

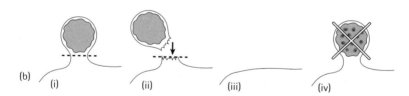

(b) En-bloc technique (recommended). (i) Excise base. (ii) Cauterize base. (iii) Specimen retrieval is performed blind and requires cervical dilatation. (iv) Avoid puncturing holes in tissue ('Swiss cheese approach') or penetrating the myometrium.

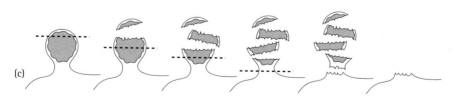

(c) Sequential slicing technique. Progressive 'slicing' allows removal of the specimen under direct vision with hysteroscopic instruments, but is time consuming.

Figure 15.5 *Outpatient hysteroscopic polypectomy (electrosurgery – Versapoint).*

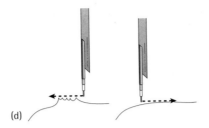

(d)

(d) Vaporization technique. The spring or ball tip can be used to vaporize sessile polyps/poly-poidal endometrium (and fibroids) utilizing smooth, superficial back-and-forth 'painting' motions. Consider biopsying the lesion prior to vaporization (no specimen). Extensive vaporization and ablation of the endometrium is inappropriate in young women requiring fertility.

Figure 15.5 (Continued)

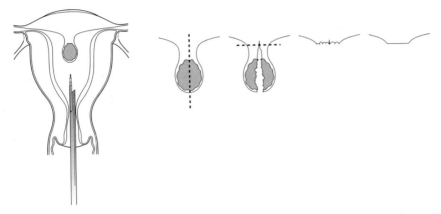

Figure 15.6 Outpatient hysteroscopic fundal polypectomy (electrosurgery – Versapoint). Bisection of the polyp (and bending the needle tip 90°) will facilitate access to the base of a fundal polyp. Additional longitudinal sections may be required with large fundal polyps. Blind avulsion followed by cautery to any basal remnant may be easier with pedunculated fundal polyps.

BLIND

An alternative method (favoured by the authors) is to excise the polyp at the base and remove it en bloc. The cervix needs to be dilated to between Hegar 5 and 8 and this is easily achieved with an adequate local cervical anaesthetic block. Polyp forceps are inserted and the specimen retrieved blindly. This is easy to achieve and quick in 95 per cent of cases and provides a complete, good-quality specimen for the pathologist. However, in a minority of situations (<5 per cent) it can be difficult to locate the specimen thereby prolonging the procedure. One approach is to leave the polyp attached to the uterine wall by a tiny tissue fragment, aiding subsequent location by polyp forceps. This approach does not seem to confer any advantage in terms of speeding retrieval and if it fails then the polyp may regrow unless the blood supply has been sufficiently compromised. It is for these reasons that we recommend excising the polyp to float free within the cavity. In the unusual situation where the specimen cannot be removed, then the cervix should be dilated and the patient should be reassured that the specimen may pass or be broken down spontaneously, but that they may experience a prolonged vaginal discharge as a result (up to 6 weeks).

VAPORIZATION

Vaporization of pathology will obviate the need for specimen retrieval. However, it is prudent to take a directed biopsy of the lesion prior to vaporization.

TROUBLESHOOTING

Outpatient hysteroscopic polypectomy should not be undertaken if there is inadequate visualization and should be discontinued if this occurs during the procedure because of bleeding or if there is substantial patient discomfort. Patient discomfort is more likely to be a problem if:

- the procedure is prolonged beyond 20 minutes;
- there is penetration into the underlying myometrium;
- polyps are sited in the sensitive cornual region of the uterus.

With experience, the operator not only becomes more skilled and quicker in performing surgery, but more importantly recognizes the limitations of the outpatient hysteroscopic procedure and selects cases that are feasible. For example, it can be difficult to resect polyps with a fundal insertion, as the base cannot easily be accessed without bisecting the polyp and removing it in a time-consuming piecemeal fashion. Polyps at the isthmic level can also be difficult to remove hysteroscopically because of inadequate uterine distension when the hysteroscope is situated in the cervical canal. Large pedunculated polyps can present problems as they can 'flop' over the line of excision obscuring the operative field. A reductive two- or more-stepped procedure may be required in this situation. By avoiding outpatient hysteroscopic polypectomy in these situations or by developing techniques to overcome these potential difficulties (see Figs 15.5 and 15.6) the success rate will increase to over 90 per cent.

Information Boxes 15.3 (selection criteria) and 15.4 (troubleshooting) outline key points to consider in order to optimize the success of operative outpatient hysteroscopy. Information Box 15.5 deals with the nuances of hysteroscopic polypectomy using modern bipolar electrosurgery (Versapoint).

Information Box 15.3 Optimizing success of operative outpatient hysteroscopy (polypectomy and myomectomy): selection criteria

- *Patient understands and is able to consent to procedure.* This is a standard requirement for any intervention.
- *Patient tolerated diagnostic hysteroscopy well.* This is a useful screening procedure to predict likely patient tolerance and avoids later complaints as well as wasting of expensive single use instrumentation.
- *No or minimal active uterine bleeding.* This will ensure better visualization. Avoid surgery when there is heavy menstrual flow. If bleeding is heavy postmenopausally, then frank malignancy is likely and blind endometrial biopsy will usually confirm the diagnosis.

- *No malignant features.* A hysterectomy, following histological confirmation, will be required and so conservative surgery is inappropriate. However, if disease is focal, then hysteroscopically directed biopsy (representative or excision) is indicated.
- *Focal pathology <4 cm in diameter.* No arbitrary isolated size cut-off exists in reality because feasibility is dependent upon a number of factors. However, accessibility, visualization and tolerability are increasingly compromised and operative time prolonged thereby reducing chances of success. Polyps of this size can usually be more easily blindly located and avulsed.
- *Focal lesions are pedunculated.* Identification of a discrete stalk eases excision of pathology as orientation is simplified and the amount of tissue to resect is minimized. Broad-based, sessile lesions are more suitable for vaporization using specific energy sources, although tissue for histological examination will be unavailable.
- *Focal lesions located within uterine body but not fundal.* Accessibility and adequacy of uterine distension may problematic when pathology is situated in the uterine isthmus. Resection of 'end-on' fundal lesions can be complicated because the base is difficult to identify and access without sectioning the focal lesion, which may lead to reduced visualization (from bleeding and released debris), compromise the completeness, quality and interpretability of any specimens obtained, and unduly prolong the procedure affecting patient acceptability.
- *Procedure feasible to complete within 20 minutes.* From anecdotal experience, once the duration of a procedure exceeds 15–20 minutes, patient tolerability rapidly declines. This observation probably results from a combination of factors – an acceptability limit is reached for remaining comfortably in the lithotomy position and a pain threshold is reached from the cumulative effect of any unpleasant sensory stimuli. It is also an indirect indication that the procedure is not going well or is too complex and inappropriate for the office setting.

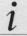 ### Information Box 15.4 Optimizing success of operative outpatient hysteroscopy (polypectomy and myomectomy): troubleshooting

- *Patient anxiety.* Clear, realistic and comprehensive explanation about the proposed procedure backed up with written information. Fully inform patient of alternative options (e.g. general anaesthetic) and promote advantages of outpatient setting. Create a private and relaxed environment and reinforce general good patient acceptance/satisfaction.
- *Poor patient tolerance.* See above. Patient selection (see Information Box 15.3) is important as is communication, dedicated nursing support and an efficient, gentle operative approach. Curtail or stop the procedure at patient request. Anticipate likely instrumentation to be required to avoid delays. Consider use of lower power settings if diathermy is employed (see Chapter 14) and do not penetrate the myometrium.
- *Suboptimal visualization.* Use a continuous flow fluid medium of adequate diameter. If outflow is compromised, then consider dilating the cervix further. If uterine distension is poor, then increase fluid inflow, and apply forceps to maintain distension if the cervix is patulous or has been overdilated (see Chapter 4). Use 3-l fluid bags or 1-l bags through

Y-giving sets so that inflow is not interrupted. Try to remove focal pathology *en bloc* because a 'piecemeal' approach generates unwanted intrauterine tissue debris.

- *Adverse uterine anatomy.* Acute degrees of flexion and version of the uterus are generally overcome by application of tenaculum forceps to straighten the cervical canal and by paying careful attention to patient positioning (see Chapter 4) to optimize access and manipulation within the uterine cavity.
- *Adverse anatomy of focal lesion.* Large pedunculated polyps may be better avulsed blindly followed by ablation of the base, or excised in sections under direct vision because the base may be obscured as the polyp can 'flop' over during excision. Sessile polyps and fibroids are best ablated using thermal energy. Highly vascular, necrotic or friable lesions may be malignant and difficult to excise *en bloc.* A small tissue sample will usually suffice to allow the diagnosis to be verified prior to definitive treatment.
- *Adverse location of focal lesion.* Fundal 'end-on' polyps should be vaporized if non-suspicious, small and sessile. More pedunculated lesions may need to be blindly avulsed (normally easy to grasp if large) or sectioned/bisected, in order to reach the base and allow complete removal. Isthmic polyps should be blindly curetted off or removed under direct vision after the cervical canal has been dilated adequately, so that operative instrumentation can be manipulated within the canal. High inflow rates are invariably required to achieve this.

 ## Information Box 15.5 Polypectomy using bipolar electrosurgery: operating tips

- *Working distance.* The active electrode should be within 2 cm of the end of the hysteroscope allowing good visualization, an appreciation of distance and optimum control. Focusing the electrode prior to insertion of the hysteroscope should be undertaken unless the hysteroscope is already *in situ.*
- *Orientation.* Although 5–6 mm diameter hysteroscopes provide better fluid distension, the specifically designed 4 mm Versascope system with its 10° angulation and rotator collar, facilitates orientation of the electrode in relation to pathology. Laterally and posteriorly sited pathology can be accessed more easily by rotation of the electrode to the appropriate lateral and posterior position respectively.
- *Probe.* The electrode can be used as a probe to gently manipulate the partially excised polyp so that the amount, depth and location of remaining tissue to be excised can be ascertained. This should be done gently, without the passage of electrical current, to avoid damage to the active electrode.
- *Electrode damage.* Do not activate the electrode unless the active electrode is fully immersed in saline, completely out of the working channel and close to the target tissue, so as to avoid damage to the electrode tip.
- *Bubble formation.* Stop electrode activation if production of steam bubbles obscures viewing and allow them to settle. Consider lower fluid inflow, increased outflow or alternative lower power settings if bubble formation remains problematic.

- *Electrode activation.* Avoid unduly prolonged electrode activation cycles ($>$0.5–1 minute) as this may damage the tip and increase the chances of air embolization. However, repeated short burst times prevent the creation of a smooth plane of cleavage and can unduly prolong the procedure.
- *Types of electrode.* There is little to choose between the spring and twizzle tip for polyp treatment (see Chapter 14). Both provide an excellent cut. The tip of the twizzle needle can be manually bent at 90° to facilitate access to the tissue base, which can be especially useful for fundal pathology. The spring provides a larger surface area for vaporization procedures.
- *Planning.* Orientate the electrode and perform a 'dry run'. Then activate the electrode and confidently and smoothly excise the tissue. In contrast to fibroids, most polyps can be almost completely excised with a single activation. The final tissue strands can be excised by using short energy bursts, targeted under close magnification.
- *Movement of electrode.* Once orientated, the working distance should be kept constant (i.e. electrode must be kept still) and the hysteroscope moved so that smooth and superficial back-and-forth 'painting' motions are produced. Avoid deep penetration, which results in holes being punched in the tissue, and pain if the myometrium is breached. This 'Swiss cheese' approach causes debris release and tissue fragmentation such that the operator can become disorientated.
- *Non-detachment of polyp.* Correct movement of the electrode will avoid the situation where delicate strands of tissue remain, anchoring the mostly detached polyp. To aid targeting and excision of these fine tissue threads requires short static energy bursts under high magnification (i.e. close proximity) or placing the electrode just distally and withdrawing the activated electrode proximally over the tissue.
- *Safety.* Avoid extending the electrode whilst activated, as inadvertent perforation may result. Such occurrences should be extremely uncommon if a gentle technique is observed and direct vision is scrupulously maintained. Furthermore, the short length of the active electrode (1–3 mm) and the outpatient setting mitigate against breaching of the uterine wall.

POSTOPERATIVE CARE

Women should recover in a dedicated area with their companions, and nursing staff should be in attendance. Women should be offered a drink and can be discharged within 1 hour if they are well. A small number of women may experience a vasovagal episode (see Chapter 4) as a result of surgery and, in this unusual situation, access to a wheelchair and bed is useful. Lying down, simple analgesia and oral fluids are invariably all that are required to aid a rapid recovery within minutes.

SPECIAL SITUATIONS: CERVICAL POLYPS AND HYSTEROSCOPY

Cervical polyps are commonly visualized during speculum examination in both symptomatic and asymptomatic women (e.g. those undergoing cervical screening) if they are ectocervical or endocervical and prolapsed through the external cervical os. They are easily treated by mechanical avulsion using appropriate polyp forceps or chemical cautery (e.g. silver nitrate application). Some advocate hysteroscopy in women with abnormal uterine bleeding and cervical polyps for two reasons:

- they are independent risk factors for the presence of coexistent endometrial polyps (2–5-fold increase)
- causative intracervical polyps will otherwise be overlooked.

A rational, less invasive strategy in women under 40 years at low risk of serious endometrial disease, is to avulse the cervical polyp and perform a subsequent hysteroscopy if symptoms persist.

Intracervical polyps may be removed blindly following cervical dilatation and fractional curettage or polyps forceps. Hysteroscopic removal using polyp snares has been described, although the usefulness of such approaches is limited because the cervical canal is difficult to distend, restricting visualization and manipulation of endoscopic instruments.

Evidence Box 15.1 Uterine polypectomy

Blind polypectomy is associated with incomplete removal in 10–60 per cent of cases, but this is not the case with removal under direct vision. Technical feasibility of the outpatient hysteroscopic approach in terms of safety, practicality and potential efficacy in treament of abnormal uterine bleeding and infertility has been established in small observational controlled series. An as yet unpublished randomized controlled trial conducted in our centre has shown that treatment efficacy (abnormal uterine bleeding at 1 year) is the same for outpatient hysteroscopic polypectomy compared with traditional inpatient hysteroscopic localization followed by blind curettage and/or avulsion under general anaesthetic. However, cost-effectiveness was much greater for the outpatient approach. As this trial was underpowered, a larger trial is necessary to confirm these findings. Qualitative research is also required to ascertain patient preferences.

KEY POINTS

- Endometrial polyps are common in women of all ages and associated with abnormal uterine bleeding.
- Outpatient hysteroscopy is the gold standard tool for diagnosing endometrial polyps and it facilitates simultaneous removal.
- The development of bipolar intrauterine electrosurgery has further enhanced the ability to perform outpatient hysteroscopic polypectomy, replacing the traditional standard of D&C under general anaesthesia.

FURTHER READING

Anastasiadis PG, Koutlaki NG, Skaphida PG, Galazios GC, Tsikouras PN, Liberis VA. Endometrial polyps: prevalence, detection, and malignant potential in women with abnormal uterine bleeding. *Eur J Gynaecol Oncol* 2000;**21**:180–3.

DeWaay DJ, Syrop CH, Nygaard IE, Davis WA, Van Voorhis BJ. Natural history of uterine polyps and leiomyomata. *Obstet Gynecol* 2002;**100**:3–7.

Clark TJ, Godwin J, Khan KS, Gupta JK. Ambulatory endoscopic treament of symptomatic benign endometrial polyps: A feasibility study. *Gynaecol Endosc* 2002;**11**:91–7.

Clark TJ, Khan KS, Gupta JK. Current practice for the treament of benign intrauterine polyps: a national questionnaire survey of consultant gynaecologists in UK. *Eur J Obstet Gynecol Reprod Biol* 2002;**103**:65–7.

Vilodre LC, Bertat R, Petters R, Reis FM. Cervical polyp as risk factor for hysteroscopically diagnosed endometrial polyps. *Gynecol Obstet Invest* 1997;**44**:191–5.

16

Submucous (intracavity) fibroids

DEFINITION (HYSTEROSCOPIC)

Submucous (intracavity) fibroids consist of firm, smooth and irregular sessile or pedunculated, intracavity formations, covered by a thin, pale and transparent layer of endometrium revealing superficially large blood vessels, distorting the regular contour of an otherwise normal endometrial cavity.

EPIDEMIOLOGY

As with other structural uterine lesions, the presence of submucous fibroids is being increasingly documented with the widespread use of pelvic ultrasonography and outpatient hysteroscopy.

The prevalence of uterine fibroids will vary according to population demographics (age, race, presenting symptoms, etc.), but is estimated from ultrasound studies to be between 20 and 30 per cent in a typical asymptomatic western population. Approximately one-third of such fibroids will have a submucous (intracavity) component and are more likely to be associated with abnormal uterine bleeding symptoms.

PATHOLOGY

Uterine fibroids or leiomyomas, are smooth muscle tumours and are the commonest benign tumours in females. They originate within the myometrium and remain completely within this layer (intramural) or expand to deviate the serosal layer (serosal) or mucosal layer (submucous) so that they are visible within the uterine cavity. These solid tumours are well demarcated by a pseudocapsule and their growth is dependent upon stimulation by oestrogen. Consequently they are prevalent in women of reproductive age and can expand in pregnancy, but tend to shrink after the menopause or in response to ovarian suppressant drugs.

The mechanism by which submucous fibroids cause abnormal uterine bleeding, especially menorrhagia, is uncertain, but thought to relate to an expanded and distorted endometrial surface, increased vascularity and local factors. Impaired implantation dynamics are thought to account for a possible association with poor reproductive performance. Malignant change (leiomyosarcoma) can occur, but is rare (1 in 1000), especially before the menopause.

PRESENTATION

Fibroids are common in asymptomatic women and so their presence in association with certain presenting complaints does not necessarily imply causation. That said, many symptoms are attributed to the presence of submucous fibroids and these include:

- abnormal uterine bleeding – excessive and/or prolonged menstrual loss, intermenstrual and postcoital bleeding, unscheduled bleeding on hormone replacement therapy (HRT) and postmenopausal bleeding;
- pelvic pain and dysmenorrhoea;
- reproductive impairment – subfertility, recurrent miscarriage, preterm labour.

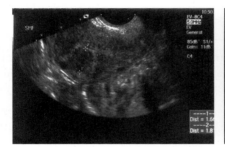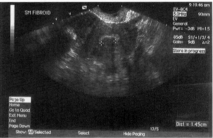

Figure 16.1 *Diagnosis of submucous fibroids: transvaginal ultrasound. Submucous fibroids are distinguished from polyps by their relatively hypoechoic echotexture, with sound attenuation in some cases. They are detected as solid structures of mixed echogenicity, emanating from the myometrium, disrupting the inner circular muscle layer and protruding into the uterine cavity and covered by inact epithelium.*

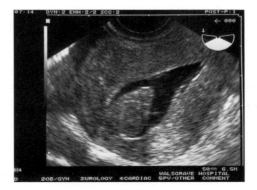

Figure 16.2 *Diagnosis of submucous fibroids: Saline contrast transvaginal ultrasound. A submucous fibroid is seen arising from the fundal myometrium. (Courtesy of Mr K Cietak.)*

DIAGNOSIS

Uterine ultrasound is an excellent diagnostic modality for detecting and locating uterine fibroids with a high degree of accuracy. The advantage of ultrasound over diagnostic hysteroscopy relates to the ability to measure any intramural component of submuous fibroids, which is of use in planning surgery (see below). Submucous fibroids are diagnosed sonographically when deviation of the endometrium is seen (Fig. 16.1). The predictive ability of ultrasound is improved further with the addition of saline contrast (Fig. 16.2) so that accuracy is equivalent to the gold standard set by hysteroscopy. Magnetic resonance imaging (MRI) is no more accurate than ultrasound, which limits its cost-effectiveness, so that is best reserved to characterize large suspicious-looking fibroids.

HYSTEROSCOPIC CHARACTERISTICS

The typical features of a submucous fibroid as seen hysteroscopically are shown in Plate 19. Submucous fibroids are often described as pedunculated (polypoidal) or sessile (flat, no discrete pedicle) hysteroscopically. The operator also gets an impression of the degree of likely intramural extension and this can be estimated or more accurately defined with ultrasound. To categorize the degree of intramural extension, the classification of the European Society of Gynaecological Endoscopy is most often used (Information Box 16.1).

The firm nature of submucous fibroids is inferred from their immobility (polyps move with the flow of distension media) and rigidity when touched with the tip of the hysteroscope (polyps can be moved and indented). Cystic degenerative change can soften them revealing cystic spaces during resection. Degenerative change can impart unusual appearances making them difficult to distinguish from malignancy. However, sarcomatous change is rare, but should be suspected if the fibroid is large, the surface is irregular and the lesion is unusually vascular and very friable. Directed biopsy is mandatory if malignancy is suspected.

TREATMENT

Menorrhagia is often refractory to medical treatments if associated with multiple uterine fibroids or significant cavity distortion from submucous fibroids. If fertility is not a factor, then inpatient transcervical resection of submucous fibroids or hysterectomy is frequently performed.

Information Box 16.1 Classification of submucous fibroids of the European Society of Gynaecological Endoscopy

- *Type 0.* Pedunculated submucous fibroids without intramural extension (i.e. entirely intracavity)
- *Type I.* Sessile submucous myoma and the intramural port is <50 per cent (i.e. mainly intracavity)
- *Type II.* Intramural extension of >50 per cent (i.e. greatest diameter extracavity)

INDICATIONS FOR OUTPATIENT SURGERY

Outpatient hysteroscopic myomectomy is indicated if deemed feasible especially when isolated smaller, predominantly intracavity lesions are encountered in association with menorrhagia, intermenstrual, HRT-related or postmenopausal bleeding. Resection of pathology and normalizing the shape of the uterine cavity results in relief of abnormal uterine bleeding symptoms in over 80 per cent of women. Furthermore, initially ineffective or contraindicated intrauterine treatments may be instigated at the time of surgery or subsequent to it, dependent upon treatment response (e.g. Mirena and thermal balloon ablation of the endometrium). Hysteroscopic myomectomy may also be useful in restoration of the normal uterine cavity to optimize reproductive outcomes in appropriately selected women (see Chapter 18). Guidelines published by the Royal College of Obstetricians and Gynaecologists recommend that intrauterine pathology such as submucous fibroids or polyps found during ultrasonic or hysteroscopic investigation, should be removed hysteroscopically (see Further Reading, page 204).

HYSTEROSCOPIC MYOMECTOMY

PREOPERATIVE PREPARATION

Women should receive comprehensive and clear information both verbally and in writing. The indication and rationale for treatment should be discussed along with alternative treatment options. Future fertility requirements and the need for histological samples should be confirmed. Clearly, patient preparation is easier if they are already known to have submucous fibroids from previous diagnostic work-up. However, all women should be made aware from preprocedural verbal and written information, of the possibility of immediately treating such pathology following diagnosis. Women should also be counselled regarding potential complications (i.e. haemorrhage, perforation, need for two-stage procedure). Most women are agreeable to this 'see and treat' ethos; however, some women may prefer to digest the information further before consenting to treatment, and this should be established before diagnostic hysteroscopy is commenced.

Preoperative simple analgesics (see Chapter 12) should be administered if surgical treatment is known to be necessary or considered highly likely. Routine analgesics are not required for most women undergoing diagnostic hysteroscopy. Preoperative administration of gonadotrophin-releasing hormone (GnRH) analogues in order to enhance surgical feasibility (size, vascularity, etc.) is not necessary for smaller lesions suitable for outpatient treatment. Similarly, antibiotic prophylaxis should be employed only for specific medical indications. Rationalization of treatments in this way, along with judging operative feasibility will avoid unnecessary cost and morbidity.

FEASIBILITY

Of all outpatient surgical interventions, the successful completion of hysteroscopic myomectomy is dependent upon careful case selection. Criteria predictive of operative feasibility are given in Information Box 16.2.

Information Box 16.2 Factors influencing the feasibility of outpatient hysteroscopic myomectomy

PATIENT

- *Patient preference.* Preoperative informed consent obtained. Offered inpatient therapy.
- *Patient tolerability.* Response to diagnostic hysteroscopy is best predictor of compliance.
- *Coexistent medical problems.* Cardiorespiratory and orthopaedic conditions may preclude adequate positioning for required time.
- *Minimal intrauterine bleeding.* Non-menstrual phase of cycle, adequate visualization.

LESION

- *Benign disease.* Biopsy if malignancy suspected.
- *Size <4 cm.* Note that fibroids <4 cm in diameter may not be feasible if other adverse factors present also.
- *Vascularity.* Electrosurgery preferable. Coagulate large superficial vessels.
- *Location.* Fundal and isthmic fibroids can present problems (see text). Vaporization or piecemeal resection may be indicated.
- *Grade* (see text). Pedunculated fibroids are easier to remove compared with sessile lesions with an intramural component.
- *Number.* Multiple fibroids ('leiomyomatosis') will increase procedure time and may impair visualization. Consider a two-stage procedure.

TIME

- *Complete within 20 minutes.* This duration represents the limit of most patients' tolerance (discomfort from procedure and positioning).

NB: Preoperative ultrasonography is helpful in determining the size, nature and number of submuocus fibroids. The degree of intramural extension and resectability can also be determined (see text).

TECHNIQUES

The basic set-up equipment is given in Information Box 16.3 and the fundamental operative steps are shown in Fig. 16.3.

Several operative approaches are described. Choice of technique will depend upon available instrumentation, type of fibroid and personal preference. A combination of electrosurgical and mechanical methods is often employed. Techniques applicable for use in the outpatient setting are described below and illustrated in Figs 16.4–16.6.

Blind myomectomy

This method is only suitable for removal of pedunculated (grade 0) submucous fibroids. It requires cervical dilatation and insertion of a grasping instrument (polyp forceps, sponge forceps) that is opened within the cavity and used to grasp the fibroid. Gentle traction will

---

i Information Box 16.3   Basic requirements for set-up for outpatient hysteroscopic myomectomy

- Operative hysteroscopy set-up (see Chapter 3)
- Open-sided speculum (e.g.Cusco's)
- Tenaculum forceps
- Cervical dilatation set
- Grasping forceps (polyps, sponge)
- Continuous flow hysteroscope* with a minimum 5 F (1.67 mm) operative channel
- Saline* (3-l bag recommended) ± pressure cuff and inflow/outflow tubing ± suction apparatus
- Mechanical instruments (hysteroscopic semirigid scissors and graspers)
- Versapoint coaxial electrodes (spring and twizzle tip)
- Foley balloon catheter (uterine tamponade or splinting)
- Video endoscopy system
- Video recording facility (optional)

* The choice of distension medium and angulation of hysteroscope will depend upon personal preference and applied technique. We find that the advantages of easier orientation with a 0° lens outweigh the expanded field of view produced by off-set lenses. Saline is the safest and most versatile medium.

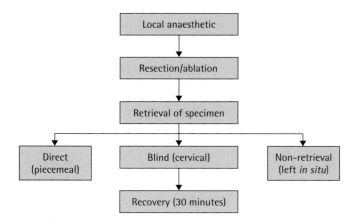

Figure 16.3 *Hysteroscopic myomectomy: operative steps.*

confirm that the fibroid has been adequately seized and it is then avulsed with a combination of twisting and retraction.

Hysteroscopic myomectomy

Resection of fibroids in sections using large-diameter electrosurgical loops is not a feasible option in the outpatient setting.

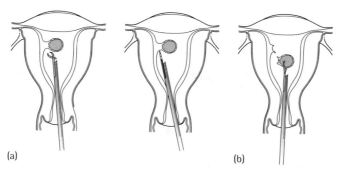

Figure 16.4 *Technique of outpatient hysteroscopic myomectomy: small pedunculated submucous fibroid (Type 0). (a) Hysteroscopic scissors or Versapoint electrodes are used to excise the base of the fibroid. (b) The fibroid is removed using hysteroscopic grasping forceps. Larger fibroids require debulking by progression shaving (electrosurgery only) or insertion of heavier 'blind' instruments after cervical dilatation.*

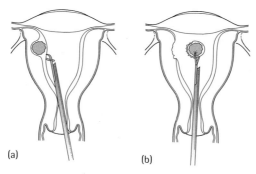

Figure 16.5 *Technique of outpatient hysteroscopic myomectomy: small submucous fibroid (Type 1). (a) Hysteroscopic scissors are used to incise the superficial capsule and undermine the fibroid. Versapoint electrodes can also be used. (b) The extruded fibroid is removed using hysteroscope grasping forceps or insertion of heavier 'blind' instruments.*

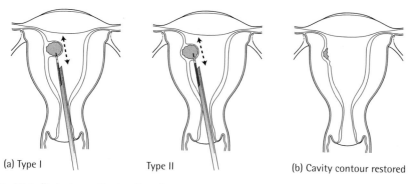

Figure 16.6 *Technique of outpatient hysteroscopic myomectomy: small sessile submucous fibroid (Type 1 and 2). (a) The Versapoint electrode is run systematically over the surface of the intracavity portion of the fibroid. The fibroid may begin to extrude (migrate) into the cavity. (b) Vaporization is stopped once the fibroid is shaved flush with the endometrium.*

MECHANICAL

Hysteroscopic grasping instruments are too fragile to avulse submucous fibroids unless the fibroids are small (<1 cm). Such fibroids are unlikely to be of clinical significance, but tissue obtained in this way may be histologically examined. A more versatile technique (appropriate for pedunculated and sessile fibroids) involves introducing hysteroscopic scissors and incising the superficial fibroid capsule. The fibroid is then undermined and partially or completely detached. Hysteroscopic grasping forceps are then used to extract the fibroid.

ELECTROSURGICAL

Outpatient versus inpatient techniques

The approach using miniature coaxial bipolar electrodes differs in three important ways from standard resection with electrical loops:

- Resection is performed in an antegrade fashion, i.e. from os to fundus.

- Resection is performed *en bloc* rather than by a reductive shaving technique. The production of fibroid 'chippings' is thus avoided, visualization improved and procedure time shortened.

- The intramural component of the fibroid is not resected unless it is pushed out (once the superficial capsule is cut) in response to changes in uterine pressure or myometrial contractions.

Pedunculated (Type 0) fibroids

We prefer to use the spring tip Versapoint bipolar electrode to resect the fibroid *en bloc* (the cost of laser surgery is prohibitive as an outpatient modality) (see Fig. 16.4). If the superficial endometrium overlying the fibroid is exceptionally vascular, preliminary coagulation of large vessels can be performed utilizing the desiccation waveform ($\geqslant 50$ W). However, sealing of blood vessels in this way is normally not required. The complete pedunculated fibroid is then resected at its base (connection with uterine wall myometrium) using the cutting current at $\geqslant 130$ W (Plate 20). At these power outputs and waveforms, the electrode will pass through the fibroid so that mechanical force is not required or indeed desirable. A progressive shaving motion is required as described in Chapter 15. As resection is nearing completion, the distal limit of the cleavage plane developed between the fibroid and myometrium can become obscured. In this situation, the deactivated electrode can be used to gently probe and identify it, guiding the remaining resection. The fibroid is then removed with grasping forceps (polyp/sponge forceps). In the unusual outpatient situation where the specimen is too large to be removed, it should be bisected using Versapoint prior to blind removal.

An alternative, although more time-consuming and less elegant reductive technique, involves progressively shaving the fibroid and removing the fragments piecemeal with hysteroscopic grasping forceps or removing them blindly with polyps forceps. If the resected fibroid appears benign and cannot easily be retrieved from the cavity, then it can be left *in situ*. The patient should be informed that she may experience a heavier than normal and prolonged (up to 6 weeks) vaginal discharge and may even pass partially liquefied ('caseated') tissue. Although a nuisance, the risk of sepsis is minimal and spontaneous resolution is the rule.

Coagulation of basal vessels is rarely necessary, as the procedure is quick and the pathology relatively small. If bleeding is encountered, then rescheduling surgery should be considered unless visualization can be restored by optimizing fluid irrigation. Options include pre-treatment with GnRH analogues prior to further outpatient surgery, or employing a larger diameter operating hysteroscope under anaesthesia.

Pedunculated (Type I/II) fibroids

Surgical treatment of sessile fibroids or those with a substantial mural extension poses more difficulties compared with intracavity fibroids with a distinct pedicle (see Figs 16.5 and 16.6). Complete resection of the intracavity portion should be attempted in all subjects. However, it is inappropriate to attempt resection of the intramural component of the fibroid using miniature outpatient instrumentation, both from a feasibility and safety standpoint. This is because the small cutting surface and reduced manoeuvrability of the Versapoint coaxial electrodes precludes intramural resection. Limiting surgery to the intracavity portion of sub-mucous fibroids minimizes the risk of air and gas emboli as well as inadvertent uterine perforation and damage to visceral structures.

Intramural resection necessitates use of a resectoscope loop along with general anaes-thesia and preferably ultrasound or laparoscopic guidance. However, there is evidence that confining removal to the intracavity component of the fibroid and restoring the normal cavity contour results in effective resolution of abnormal bleeding symptoms and does not predispose to recurrence of the smooth muscle tumour within the cavity. It is the intracav-ity distortion that is most associated with abnormal bleeding patterns and therefore the main aim of treatment should be the restoration of a smooth intrauterine cavity. It is likely that the blood supply to the residual intramyometrial fibroid tissue is compromised by the procedure, thereby preventing regrowth by inducing necrosis.

The operative approach involves resection of the intracavity component and/or systema-tically vaporizing the intracavity fibroid by running a spring tip Versapoint coaxial elec-trode superficially over the fibroid until the endometrial:myometrial junction is encountered and the uterine cavity normalized. The intense heat generated at the small-diameter active electrode allows tissue to be rapidly vaporized with almost no blood loss, similar to the effect produced by more expensive laser fibres. This technique often results in a substantial area of endometrial ablation and so is only appropriate in the treatment of abnormal uterine bleed-ing if future fertility is not a consideration. In many instances, the intramural component of the fibroid will extrude into the cavity following incision of the overlying capsule, and this can be safely vaporized/resected under direct vision. Hysteroscopic forceps can also be used to encourage this migration toward the accessible endometrial surface. Blind forays into the myometrium with activated electrodes must be avoided as significant patient morbidity can result. If a vaporizing approach is undertaken, consideration should be given to perform-ing a hysteroscopically directed biopsy of the fibroid to allow histological examination.

FLUID MANAGEMENT

To overcome the relative vascularity of fibroids, good irrigation is required and this is generally achieved with a high rate of inflow (>150 ml/min), a high instillation pressure (80–150 mmHg) and adequate outflow. A passive outflow is sufficient when smaller-diameter hysteroscopes are used in the outpatient setting. Application of negative suction (e.g. vacuum of −30 to −40 mmHg) is not generally necessary or feasible given the rates of inflow. We favour the use of a 3-l pressure bag compressed by a cuff and both inflow and outflow stopcocks open to maximize flow and reduce intrauterine pressure. In order to optimize patient compliance, the lowest pressure compatible with clear vision should be employed. If heavy bleeding is encountered, uterine distension pressure is increased by gradual closure of the outflow stopcock.

Measurement of fluid inflow and outflow and calculation of the fluid deficit (i.e. that absorbed by the patient) represents good practice. Procedures should be stopped or rapidly curtailed if fluid loss exceeds 1000–1500 ml. However, the risk of fluid overload is negligible in the outpatient setting. This is because resection of large fibroids requiring prolonged operating times and high fluid requirements is not practicable. Furthermore, modern outpatient electrosurgery is based on bipolar circuits and requires a physiological (isotonic) saline conducting medium.

To account for fluid loss accurately and to keep the surgical area clean and dry, outflow ports should be connected to tubing that feeds and empties into a calibrated, waterproof collecting pouch, bucket or suitable receptacle. Specifically designed surgical drapes are available for this purpose.

Complications

Major complications of hysteroscopic myomectomy with traditional monopolar cutting loops occur in 1–5 per cent of procedures and include haemorrhage, genital tract trauma and fluid overload. The incidence of such complications is much lower with the use of bipolar diathermy in an outpatient setting. This is because the use of saline as the distension medium reduces life-threatening fluid overload arising from hyponatraemia. In addition, improved visualization resulting from excellent haemostatic properties, avoidance of haemorrhage resulting from cervical dilatation, and instantaneous tissue vaporization eliminating the production of resection chips, may reduce haemorrhage and genital tract trauma. Furthermore limiting resection to fibroid material visible within the uterine cavity ensures uterine integrity.

Polyps versus fibroids

In general polyps are easier to remove compared with submucous fibroids because they are endometrial in origin and are less vascular. Furthermore, if vision is lost, blind avulsion of the partially attached polyp is possible whereas only the most pedunculated fibroids will allow this. The solid nature of submucous fibroids does, however, facilitate smooth resection along a well-defined cleavage plane because they remain relatively fixed. In contrast, the softer consistency of most glandulocystic polyps renders them mobile ('a moving target'), which can impede resection.

Postoperative care

Women should be given a drink and observed for 30 minutes in a designated recovery area. Simple analgesics should be given as required. Prior to discharge, women should be given a contact number and arrangements to receive a follow-up phone call made by the nurse the next day. Follow-up is indicated if surgery was complicated or incomplete (multistage procedure required, usually as an inpatient). If menorrhagia is persistent, then further ultrasound or hysteroscopy should be performed to exclude recurrence or new fibroids and other conservative intrauterine therapies considered (e.g. Mirena, thermal balloon ablation).

If heavy bleeding is encountered, then a Foley balloon catheter can be inserted at the time of surgery and 10–30 ml of fluid instilled to compress the vascular bed and halt further haemorrhage. Uterine tamponade is usually only required for 1–2 hours, at which time the balloon can be removed and the patient discharged. Admission for observation with or without further management is warranted in the unusual situation where further tamponade is required.

Evidence Box 16.1 Hysteroscopic diagnosis and treatment of submucous fibroids

Diagnostic test studies have demonstrated the ability of transvaginal ultrasound to detect, characterize and locate uterine fibroids with a high degree of accuracy. Hysteroscopy is, however, the gold standard for the diagnosis of submucous fibroids, although recently published systematic reviews (see Further reading) of published evidence have shown saline infusion sonography to have comparably high accuracy. In contrast to sonography, outpatient hysteroscopy offers the opportunity for treatment at the time of diagnosis. The feasibility (failure rates of 0–12 per cent), efficacy and potential cost-effectiveness of outpatient hysteroscopic myomectomy (bipolar electrosurgery) in the treatment of abnormal uterine bleeding have been demonstrated in observational series. Improvement of menstrual symptoms and rates of satisfaction have been reported in 80 and 90 per cent of patients, which compares favourably with traditional inpatient transcervical resection. Longer-term follow-up is required to determine rates of further hysteroscopic or abdominal surgery for recurrence of symptomatic intracavity fibroids, as in women treated with traditional loop resectoscopes, rates have been reported to be between 15 and 32 per cent at 2–4 years. In addition to hysteroscopy, the usefulness of outpatient fibroid treatment using ultrasound energy under magnetic resonance imaging guidance is being examined, although this development is at an experimental stage.

KEY POINTS

- Submucous fibroids are common and associated with abnormal uterine bleeding.
- Outpatient hysteroscopy is the gold standard tool for diagnosing submucous fibroids, and unique amongst diagnostic modalities in allowing simultaneous treatment.
- The development of bipolar intrauterine electrosurgery has revolutionized uterine surgery and facilitated outpatient hysteroscopic myomectomy.
- Outpatient hysteroscopic myomectomy has been shown to be safe, simple and feasible in an outpatient setting because the technique is of short duration (mean duration <30 minutes) and does not require special expertise to set up, or cervical dilatation.
- Experimental studies are required to demonstrate long-term effectiveness and efficiency of outpatient hysteroscopic myomectomy based on encouraging observational efficacy data published to date.

FURTHER READING

Clark TJ, Mahajan D, Sunder P, Gupta JK. Hysteroscopic treatment of symptomatic submucous fibroids using a bipolar intrauterine system: a feasibility study. *Eur J Obstet Gynecol Reprod Biol* 2002; **100**:237–42.

Emanuel MH, Wamsteker K, Hart AA, Metz G, Lammes FB. Long-term results of hysteroscopic myomectomy for abnormal uterine bleeding. *Obstet Gynecol* 1999;**93**:743–48.

Farrugia M, McMillan L. Versapoint in the treatment of focal intra-uterine pathology in an outpatient clinic setting. *Ref Gynecologie Obstetrique* 2000;**7**:169–73.

Hart R, Molnar BG, Magos A. Long term follow up of hysteroscopic myomectomy assessed by survival analysis. *Br J Obstet Gynaecol* 1999;**106**:700–5.

Myers ER, Barber MD, Gustilo-Ashby T, Couchman G, Matchar DB, McCrory DC. Management of uterine leiomyomata: what do we really know? *Obstet Gynecol* 2002;**100**:8–17.

17

Outpatient endometrial ablation

Technological advances have facilitated endometrial ablation in non-anaesthetized patients in an outpatient setting. This development has enabled comprehensive 'menorrhagia' clinics based on a hysteroscopy service to be set up in order to diagnose and treat menstrual disorders efficiently. Inpatient operating can be restricted to hysterectomy or major myomectomy. This chapter describes the rationale and evidence for use of these new endometrial auto-ablative systems along with relevant technical and clinical aspects in the context of an outpatient hysteroscopy service. An example of a successful outpatient approach is given and where necessary the preceding chapters on management of menorrhagia, service delivery and pain control should be consulted.

RATIONALE

Destruction of the entire endometrium prevents cyclical endometrial regeneration and suppresses menstruation, thereby inducing amenorrhoea. In practice, the entire endometrial surface is not removed and islands of endometrium remain functional, although menstrual blood loss is significantly reduced to a level acceptable to most women. 'First-generation' hysteroscopic methods include endometrial ablation and resection and have been extensively evaluated against the gold standard of hysterectomy and shown to be effective, minimally invasive alternatives associated with fewer complications. However, hysteroscopic surgical skills are required to achieve optimal treatment results and minimize the risk of serious complications.

'Second-generation' devices have been developed more recently in an attempt to achieve deep endometrial destruction without the need for hysteroscopic surgical skills, so that treatment outcomes and safety considerations are less operator dependent. Most of these global auto-ablative systems are 'blind' procedures that are not reliant upon direct visualization with large-diameter operative hysteroscopes and fluid distension of the uterine cavity. Thus the main limitations of hysteroscopic approaches, namely poor visualization owing to bleeding and risks of fluid overload, are avoided. Traditional contraindications are overcome such as in women with haemodynamic instability, coagulopathies or in those on anticoagulant therapy, and the need for routine unpleasant and expensive endometrial preparatory drugs is removed.

As visualization is no longer a prerequisite for endometrial ablation, it has been possible to develop miniature devices that are easy to use. This has opened the door for operating in the outpatient setting under local anaesthetic, expanding patient choice and potentially increasing cost-effectiveness of treatment. Several second-generation devices have been marketed (Table 17.1) designed to deliver destructive energy to the endometrium and superficial myometrium. Most second-generation procedures have been performed under general anaesthetic, but many have been used in conscious patients using local anaesthetic with or without intravenous sedation. The potential feasibility of devices for outpatient operating is discussed below and summarized in Table 17.1.

INDICATIONS AND PATIENT SELECTION

Endometrial ablative therapy is indicated in women with menorrhagia of benign aetiology refractory to medical therapy and who have completed childbearing (Fig. 17.1). This is not to say that these surgical procedures should be denied to women who do not wish medical treatment. However, women should be encouraged to try medical therapy as a first line as this

Table 17.1 *Outpatient endometrial ablation: 'second-generation' devices*

Device	Duration of abalation	Outpatient procedure	
		Suitability	Evidence
Electrodes			
NovaSure	1 minutes	✓✓✓	✓✓✓
Vesta	4 minutes	✓✓	✓✓
Freezing			
Her Option cryoablation	10 minutes	✓✓	✓✓
Hot saline			
EnAbl system	15 minutes	✓✓✓	✗
HydroThermAblate	10 minutes	✓✓	✓✓
Laser			
GyneLase ELITT	7 minutes	✓✓	✓
Microwave			
MEA	3 minutes	✓✓	✓✓
Thermal Balloons			
Cavaterm	10 minutes	✓	✗
MenoTreat	15 minutes	✗	✗
Thermablate EAS	2.5 minutes	✓✓✓	✓
Thermachoice III	8 minutes	✓✓✓	✓✓✓
Photodynamic therapy	(experimental)	–	✓

NB: outpatient procedure refers to ablation under local anaesthesia without formal theatre facilities and minimal recourse to conscious sedation.

is relatively safe, inexpensive and effective. Although hysterectomy is an effective treatment for excessive menstrual bleeding, it is invasive, costly and can be associated with substantial morbidity. It is therefore good practice, when a surgical solution is deemed necessary, to offer all women with dysfunctional uterine bleeding minimally invasive endometrial ablative therapy. In the presence of specific uterine pathologies such as submucous fibroids and polyps, hysteroscopic resection should be offered prior to endometrial ablation if indicated. As with any therapeutic intervention, there are absolute and relative contraindications to the use of second-generation endometrial ablation and these are discussed in Information Box 17.1.

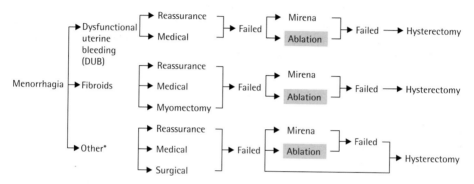

*Other cause of menorrhagia, e.g. polyps, adenomyosis.

Figure 17.1 *Management of menorrhagia: place of outpatient endometrial ablation in the care pathway.*

i Information Box 17.1 Contraindications to endometrial ablation with second-generation devices

- Active genital tract infection
- Pregnancy/planned future pregnancies
  - careful consideration in younger, nulliparous women
- Endometrial disease
  - hyperplasia/cancer (NB: Ablation should not be performed in postmenopausal women)
  - abnormal bleeding following ablation should be assessed with hysteroscopy and biopsy as subsequent endometrial assessment can be difficult
  - if hormone replacement therapy (HRT) indicated, then combined HRT mandatory as there may be residual endometrium
- Previous uterine surgery inducing myometrial weakness
  - classical Caesarian section, transmural myomectomy, metroplasty
  - care if previous endometrial ablation procedure
  - consider preoperative transvaginal ultrasound (TVS) myometrial thickness measurement with previous uterine surgical procedures (avoid ablation if <8–10 mm)

- Cavity length >12 cm
  - some devices have 10 cm as the upper limit (check manufacturers' details)
  - MEA up to 14.5 cm
  - uterine sound <6 cm may suggest a false passage or relatively hypoplastic uterus, which may preclude safe treatment (e.g. balloon expulsion, device insertion, etc.)
- Irregular cavity
  - congenital defects – HTA can be used in subseptate uteri
  - submucous fibroids >2 cm – MEA, HTA may be appropriate up to 5 cm
  - success rates may be lower in all devices in menorrhagia associated with uterine fibromatosis, despite cavities <12 cm
- Essure contraceptive micro-inserts
  - ablation systems that employ radiofrequency (RF)/microwave energy should not be used. Outside of bench research, clinical safety data for other techniques is lacking to date.
  - Intrauterine contraceptive devices (IUCDs) should be removed (can be fitted later if desired)
- Preprocedural uterine trauma
  - suspected or actual perforation or wall damage following diagnostic hysteroscopy, endometrial sampling or cervical dilatation
- Severe adenomyosis
  - difficult to diagnose clinically and if suspected (e.g. known endometriosis, TVS, hysteroscopic myometrial biopsy), then Mirena levonorgestrel intrauterine system (LNG-IUS) may be a better minimally invasive option
  - dysmenorrhoea can be expected to improve in 60–80 per cent of women in most ablative series
  - if dysmenorrhoea worsens, then exclude cervical stenosis/haematometra (hysteroscopy ± cervical dilatation) and consider possible adenomyosis
- Allergies to component parts
  - check with manufacturers – available thermal balloons now made of silicone so sequelae of common latex allergy are avoided

Despite the simplicity of auto-ablation of the endometrium, potential for procedure-related morbidity and reproductive complications exists (Information Box 17.2) and so the procedure should not be promoted in asymptomatic women as a cosmetic 'life-style treatment,' as has been suggested by some.

FURTHER CONSIDERATIONS

Endometrial ablation versus Mirena

Although studies are underway directly comparing second-generation endometrial ablation and the Mirena levonorgestrel intrauterine system (LNG-IUS), rates of treatment satisfaction for dysfunctional uterine bleeding reported in separate studies are comparable. Indications for use are similar and clinicians should help women make informed decisions.

Information Box 17.2 Side effects and complications

Serious (rare, require surgical intervention)
- Uterine perforation leading to intra-abdominal visceral or vascular injury
- Haemorrhage
- Haematometra/post-ablation tubal sterilization syndrome

Minor (self-limiting or easily treated)
- Cervical laceration

- Nausea and vomiting

- Pelvic pain/cramping

- Difficulty with defaecation or micturition

- Prolonged vaginal discharge, uterine or urinary tract infection

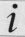 **Information Box 17.3 Counselling for endometrial ablation**

- Consider and discuss alternative medical and surgical treatment options (pros and cons)
- Consider and discuss contraindications (including contraceptive issues)
- Describe what the procedure involves and the entire patient experience
- Discuss inpatient versus outpatient setting
- Inform about possible procedural and post-procedural side effects
- Inform about treatment outcomes – reduction in menstrual loss, satisfaction and amenorrhoea rates

For many women a 'one-off' ablative treatment is more acceptable than an intrauterine, hormonal, foreign body. However, many other women hold no such preferences and in these women the safety and contraceptive aspects of LNG-IUS treatment should be highlighted.

Inpatient versus outpatient setting

The majority of women will be suitable for outpatient operating with these devices and should be adequately counselled (Information Box 17.3) and offered a choice of settings. Patients at risk from general anaesthesia (medical problems, obesity etc.) should be positively encouraged to opt for an outpatient alternative. In general over 90 per cent of women will opt for the outpatient setting, although this will depend upon the appropriateness of the ablative technique used and how women are counselled, as well as local population factors.

WHICH DEVICE?

The choice between the second-generation procedures will depend upon many factors. Paramount amongst these should be evidence of safety, reliability and effectiveness combined with other desirable qualities such as simplicity and suitability for outpatient operating. Costs and local factors (e.g. patient demographics, clinic set-up, facilities and skills, ease of transportation etc.) will also play an important role. However, this is a new and rapidly developing field, with a confusing array of available technologies and a limited evidence base for many techniques. Competing instrument manufacturers frequently promote their products based on potential benefits in the absence of rigorous clinical validation using patient-centred outcomes. Most patients would judge treatment success based on sustained improvement in their health-related quality of life rather than other surrogate outcome measures such as rates of 'eumenorrhoea'. Similarly amenorrhoea may not necessarily be perceived as a health benefit by women but rather as a threat to femininity and sexuality, or it may induce anxiety because of fear of pregnancy. Those women desiring amenorrhoea would be better suited to hysterectomy, and published rates of amenorrhoea, whilst interesting, may not be the best measure of 'success'.

Microwave endometrial ablation (MEA) and Thermachoice are by far the most rigorously evaluated and widely used technologies available and other systems need to be judged against them. A recent health technology assessment commissioned by the National Institute of Clinical Excellence (NICE) in the UK has evaluated MEA and thermal balloon ablation (Thermachoice and Caveterm), and the Food and Drug Agency in the US has evaluated several systems (see Further reading, page 228). However, study heterogeneity precludes reliable comparison between technologies. Direct head-to-head comparisons in clinical trials using patient-centred and economic outcomes are required to inform the debate. Moreover, randomized controlled trials are needed to compare the cost-effectiveness of outpatient versus inpatient treatment. This is because, although these new ablative systems are automated and mostly independent of the operator, treatment outcomes are not necessarily transferable from the inpatient operating theatre setting to the outpatient treatment facility.

In an attempt to provide clarification, currently available second-generation ablative systems and procedures feasible for outpatient use are described below along with their relative merits.

ELECTRODES

NovaSure impedance-controlled endometrial ablation system (Novacept, Palo Alto, California, USA)

MODE OF ACTION

- Bipolar electrical ablation of the endometrium by thermal therapy under impedance control. The bipolar current generated by the device produces a tapered depth of ablation with shallower ablation in the cornual regions/lower uterine segment.

SYSTEM

The system comprises a disposable bipolar electrode array, portable radiofrequency (RF) controller, connecting cord, desiccant, foot switch and power cord. The ablation device is a conformable (three-dimensional), bipolar, gold-plated porous mesh mounted on an expandable frame through which steam, blood and endometrium from desiccated tissue are continuously removed by suction generated by an integral vacuum pump. In this way intimate apposition is maintained between the electrode array and endometrium. The controller contains a constant power output generator (maximum delivery 180 W) and controls the depth of ablation by monitoring tissue impedance (resistance). A 'cavity integrity assessment system' is an additional inbuilt automatic safety feature. The predeployed device is 7 mm in diameter within its protective outer sheath.

PROCEDURE

The uterus is sounded to determine cavity length followed by insertion of the device into the uterine cavity. The outer sheath is retracted deploying the fan-shaped bipolar electrode, which conforms to the shape of the intrauterine cavity. The power delivered by the RF generator is predetermined based on the configuration of the electrode array. This is specific to the cavity size determined by uterine length (sound) and width (integral measuring device – cornu-to-cornu distance) measurements, which are imputed to allow automatic power output calculation. Mean endometrial ablation time is 90 seconds (range 60–120 seconds). Once the RF controller has automatically terminated energy delivery, the device is closed and withdrawn from the cavity.

SUITABILITY FOR OUTPATIENT USE

The short mean procedure time (4 minutes from device insertion to removal) favours outpatient use, although positioning the device correctly ('seating time') can prolong the procedure. Data from subgroups within randomized trials have shown the feasibility of outpatient use, but no such procedures have been reported using local anaesthesia alone, without the addition of intravenous conscious sedation.

ADVANTAGES COMPARED WITH OTHER SYSTEMS

The rapid, destructive process is based on physical tissue characteristics (impedance of ablated superficial myometrium), and not temperature or time, so a reproducible depth of ablation may be achieved regardless of endometrial thickness, obviating the need for endometrial preparation.

DISADVANTAGES

Care is needed to manoeuvre the device to ensure optimal deployment of the electrode array and uterine placement.

OUTCOMES

A small, double-blind randomized trial comparing Novasure (n = 83) with thermal balloon ablation (n = 43) reported significantly higher rates of amenorrhoea (43 per cent *vs* 8 per cent) and satisfaction (90 per cent *vs* 79 per cent) at 12 months' follow-up. A single non-blinded randomized trial comparing Novasure (n = 175) with rollerball ablation (n = 90) reported comparable rates of amenorrhoea (41 versus 35 per cent) at 12 months' follow-up, and rates of amenorrhea/hypermenorrhoea of 80 per cent. Satisfaction rates of >90 per cent were found at 12 months. No uterine perforations or serious complications were reported in the Novasure arm, but there were three in the rollerball arm. A small observational series suggested that for procedures using conscious sedation, intra- and postoperative pain may be less with Novasure than with Thermachoice, although both were well tolerated.

FURTHER READING

Bongers MY, Bourdrez P, Mol BW, Heintz AP, Brolman HA. Randomised controlled trial of bipolar radio-frequency endometrial ablation and balloon endometrial ablation. *Br J Obstet Gynaecol* 2004; 111:223–32.

Cooper J, Gimpelson R, Laberge P *et al.* A randomized, multicenter trial of safety and efficacy of the Novasure system in the treatment of menorrhagia. *J Am Assoc Gynecol Laparosc* 2002; 9:418–28.

Laberge PY, Sabbah R, Fortin C, Gallinat A. Assessment and comparison of intraoperative and postoperative pain associated with Novasure and Thermachoice endometrial ablation systems. *J Am Assoc Gynecol Laparosc* 2003;10:223–32.

Vesta (Vesta Medical Inc, Mountain View, California, USA)

MODE OF ACTION

- Electrical ablation of the endometrium by thermal therapy with regional control so that ablation depth is shallower in the cornual regions.

SYSTEM

The system comprises a handset containing a distensible multi-electrode balloon, electrosurgical generator and control box. The silicone balloon contains 12 electrodes, each under individual thermistor control. The control box distributes and monitors current from the electrosurgical generator. The predeployed device is 8 mm in diameter within its protective outer sheath.

PROCEDURE

The cervix is dilated to Hegar 8–9 and the uterus is sounded to determine cavity length, followed by insertion of the device into the uterine cavity. The outer sheath is retracted exposing the balloon which is inflated, via a syringe, with air to a volume that ensures a good contact with the endometrium (usually 12–15 ml). A syringe is used via a central channel to check for fundal perforations by passing and recovering a small amount of air or fluid (approximately 2 ml). The generator is activated and equilibration of the electrodes occurs over the next 90 seconds ('warm up' period – the system has a 3-minute fail-safe shut-off). Impedance is monitored at the electrodes and high resistance suggestive of perforation or non-contact with endometrium leads to system shutdown. The control box automatically begins a 4-minute treatment cycle when all electrodes have reached the preset temperature levels (cornual electrodes 72°C, remainder 75°C). The balloon is then deflated and removed.

SUITABILITY FOR OUTPATIENT USE

Outpatient use is facilitated by the relatively short procedure time of 7 minutes (mean overall procedure time including paracervical local anaesthetic administration is 23 minutes). In the one phase III trial conducted, over 80 per cent of Vesta procedures were conducted using paracervical blockade with or without conscious sedation in an office or outpatient setting.

ADVANTAGES COMPARED WITH OTHER SYSTEMS

This is one of the more simple and safe procedures, but no distinct advantage has been identified over other forms of endometrial ablation.

DISADVANTAGES

Device malfunction has been reported in 10 per cent of cases resulting in inability to complete the treatment. Data regarding safety and effectiveness are limited.

OUTCOMES

A single non-blinded randomized trial comparing Vesta (n = 122) with hysteroscopic resection/ablation (n = 112) reported comparable rates of amenorrhoea (31 versus 35 per cent) at 12 months' follow-up, and rates of amenorrhoea/hypomenorrhoea of 80 per cent. Satisfaction rates are unavailable, but 10 per cent of women were found to be disappointed with the results at 12 months. No uterine perforations or serious complications were reported, but in one procedure postoperative hysteroscopy revealed that the balloon had entered and treated a Caesarean section 'diverticulum'.

FURTHER READING

Corson SL, Brill AI, Brooks PG *et al.* Interim results of the American Vesta trial of endometrial ablation. *J Am Assoc Gynecol Laparosc* 1999;**6**:45–9.

Corson SL, Brill AI, Brooks PG *et al.* One-year results of the vesta system for endometrial ablation. *J Am Assoc Gynecol Laparosc* 2000;**7**:489–97.

FREEZING

Her Option Uterine Cryoblation Therapy System (Cryo-Gen, Inc, San Diego, California, USA)

MODE OF ACTION

- Cryogenic endometrial ablation based on the Joule–Thomson principle in which pressurized gas (cryogen) is expanded through a small orifice to produce extreme cooling producing an 'ice ball' – temperatures of –100 to –120°C are developed). Tissue that comes into contact with the portion of the 'ice ball' that is <–20°C is destroyed.

SYSTEM

The system consists of a console, cryoprobe and single-use disposable control unit (CU) which covers the cryoprobe during use. The console contains the compressor system (continuously circulates a pressurized gas mixture consisting of a mixture of common refrigerants during operation), user interface (displays the cycle, temperature, heating or thawing mode and total time in each mode) and microprocessor. The cryoprobe comprises a handle and a probe shaft to which are attached plastic transport hoses connecting it to the compressor system housed within the console. The 'Freeze' and 'Heat' buttons are located on the sterile CU so that the distal metal tip (containing the heater wire and thermocouple) can transfer heat at the completion of a freeze cycle enabling removal of the unit from the 'ice ball'. The cryoprobe/CU diameter is 5.5 mm.

PROCEDURE

The cervix is dilated to Hegar 6 if necessary and the uterus sounded, followed by insertion of the device into the uterine cavity. Active freezing is initiated by pressing the 'Freeze' button on the CU. Freezing continues until the user presses the freeze button to pause freezing, presses the heat button to begin heating, or until the safety time limit of 10 minutes is reached. The user presses the 'Heat' button to cease the freeze. The heater cycles automatically to maintain temperatures on the probe surface of 37°C until the user pushes the 'Freeze' button to start a second freeze cycle. Cryoablation is performed under transabdominal ultrasound guidance with the Her Option system to determine treatment effect. Tissue necrosis to a depth of 9–12 mm can be expected. The technique described involves insertion of the cryoprobe tip into one cornual area and a 4-minute freeze cycle followed by repositioning of the cryoprobe into the contralateral cornual region and a second freeze cycle of 6 minutes' duration. Once the RF controller has automatically terminated energy delivery, the device is closed and withdrawn from the cavity.

SUITABILITY FOR OUTPATIENT USE

Outpatient procedures should be relatively simple, so the need transabdominal ultrasound guidance with procedure times of up to 10 minutes may limit applicability in this setting. However, low temperatures may exert an analgesic effect, reducing anaesthetic requirements, and in the one phase III trial conducted, 39 per cent (72/186) were conducted using paracervical blockade with conscious sedation.

ADVANTAGES COMPARED WITH OTHER SYSTEMS

Avoidance of extrauterine tissue damage may be reduced and adequacy of treatment assessed by the ability to visualize the advancing ice front in real time by ultrasonography, thereby facilitating judging the depth of tissue penetration.

DISADVANTAGES

Competence in imaging and/or interpreting ultrasound is required. Device malfunction has been reported in 25 per cent of cases, resulting in inability to complete the treatment in 3 per cent of all attempted procedures. Data regarding safety, reproducibility and effectiveness are limited.

OUTCOMES

A single non-blinded randomized trial comparing Her Option cryoablation (n = 193) with rollerball ablation (n = 86), all with endometrial pretreatment, reported lower rates of amenorrhoea for cryoablation (20 versus 45 per cent) at 12 months' follow-up, but comparable rates of amenorrhoea/hypomenorrhoea of 80 per cent. Satisfaction rates of >80 per cent were found at 12 months. No uterine perforations or serious complications were reported.

FURTHER READING

Duleba AJ, Heppard MC, Soderstrom RM, Townsend DE. A randomized study comparing endometrial cryoablation and rollerball electroablation for treatment of dysfunctional uterine bleeding. *J Am Assoc Gynecol Laparosc* 2003;**10**:17–26.

Townsend DE, Duleba AJ, Wilkes MM. Durability of treatment effects after endometrial cryoablation versus rollerball electroablation for abnormal uterine bleeding: two-year results of a multicenter randomized trial. *Am J Obstet Gynecol* 2003;**188**:699–701.

HOT SALINE

Hydrothermablator (Boston Scientific, Natick, MA, USA)

MODE OF ACTION

- Thermal ablation of the endometrium by transfer of heat from heated liquid circulating freely under low pressure within the uterine cavity.

SYSTEM

The device consists of a microprocessor-based control system that controls the fluid temperature, irrigation and treatment time. A 1-l bag of 0.9 per cent saline hangs from an integral pole above the control unit, which also has a fluid reservoir mounted on it 115 cm (45 in) above the level of the uterus. The hydrostatic pressure is modulated by evacuation pump within the control unit to produce a net intrauterine pressure of 50–55 mmHg, below that required for transtubal passage (70 mmHg). Recirculating fluid volume is continuously monitored by the system. A standard 3 mm or smaller hysteroscope is housed within an insulated 7.8 mm continuous flow outer sheath which contains inflow and outflow ports.

PROCEDURE

The cervix is dilated to accept the 7.8 mm sheath (Hegar 8–9) with care to avoid overdilatation and retrograde loss of fluid (a cervical sealing tenaculum may be necessary), as the control system will halt the procedure if 10 ml of fluid is lost from the closed loop recirculation. An initial diagnostic hysteroscopy is then performed with saline at room temperature to confirm correct placement within the uterine cavity and absence of contraindicated pathology, as well as to verify the integrity of the closed loop circulation. Heating to 90°C is then begun. The heating phase takes 3 minutes and treatment phase 10 minutes, during which time endometrial blanching is observed through the hysteroscope video system. A 1-minute cooling phase follows and the control unit prompts the user to withdraw the hysteroscope and sheath.

SUITABILITY FOR OUTPATIENT USE

The procedure requires cervical dilatation and exceeds 10 minutes, which is less favourable for outpatient use. In the one phase III trial conducted, 40 per cent of the procedures were conducted in the outpatient setting and 45 per cent under local paracervical blockade with or without the addition of conscious sedation.

ADVANTAGES COMPARED WITH OTHER SYSTEMS

Circulating free fluid will conform to the shape of the uterine cavity allowing efficient coverage and treatment of the entire endometrial lining, less accessible areas and potentially uterine anomalies such as subseptate uteri and small submucous fibroids ($\leqslant$4 cm). In contrast to blind mechanical devices, direct visualization throughout the procedure may reduce perforation risk.

DISADVANTAGES

Inadvertent burns of unconfined fluid is a potential serious side effect. The phase III trial reported 2/187 (1 per cent) first-degree burns on the thigh and buttocks and attributed to prolonged contact with inflow tubing, and insulation has been increased as a result. Inadvertent thermal injury to the cervical epithelium was recorded in 13 per cent of patients, although effects appear transient and no apparent clinical significance.

OUTCOMES

A non-blinded randomized trial comparing HydroThermAblator (n = 187) with hysteroscopic rollerball ablation (n = 89) reported similar rates of amenorrhoea (40 per cent versus 51 per cent) at 12 months' follow-up and rates of amenorrhoea/hypomenorrhoea of 80 per cent. Satisfaction rates are unavailable, but improvement in unvalidated quality of life scores was comparable. No uterine perforations were reported but two serious complications were reported in the HTA arm (inadvertent burns – see above) and one in the roller ball arm (cervical laceration followed by septicaemia).

FURTHER READING

Corson SL. A multicenter evaluation of endometrial ablation by HydroThermAblator and rollerball for treatment of menorrhagia. *J Am Assoc Gynecol Laparosc* 2001;**8**:359–67.

Goldrath MH. Evaluation of HydroThermAblator and rollerball endometrial ablation for menorrhagia 3 years after treatment. *J Am Assoc Gynecol Laparosc* 2003;**10**: 505–11.

LASER

GyneLase endometrial laser intrauterine thermal therapy or 'ELITT' (ESC/Sharplan Laser Ltd, Needham, MA, USA)

MODE OF ACTION

- Laser destruction of the endometrium by thermal therapy. Light is absorbed and transformed to heat, causing controlled tissue coagulation.

SYSTEM

The GyneLase system used in the ELITT procedure is composed of a compact tabletop with a 20 W, 830 nm diode laser that emits laser beams through three separate parallel channels, to a disposable Teflon handset via fibre connectors. The handset comprises three integrated optical-light diffusers that can be adjusted to conform to the shape of the uterine cavity. The folded handset is 6 mm in diameter.

PROCEDURE

The endocervical canal is dilated to 7 mm, and the folded light diffuser handset is inserted into the uterus until the fundus is reached. The side diffusers are then adjusted forming a 'butterfly-wing contour' that conforms to the shape of the intrauterine cavity. The laser is then activated for a 7-minute preprogrammed cycle that automatically terminates at the end of the cycle. No user setting or handset manoeuvring is required. The extended wings are then refolded and the handset is removed from the uterus.

SUITABILITY FOR OUTPATIENT USE

The procedure time is reasonably short at 7 minutes, but routine dilatation required, and use of ultrasound control, if device deployment is problematic, is less favourable. A small number of procedures (<25) have been conducted using intravenous conscious sedation with or without local anesthesia (paracervical block).

ADVANTAGES COMPARED WITH OTHER SYSTEMS

The laser beam is diffused throughout the uterine cavity without the need for direct contact with the endometrium so that less accessible areas of the uterus, such as the cornua, may be treated.

DISADVANTAGES

Cervical dilatation and/or preparation (e.g. osmotic dilators) is required to Hegar 7 to insert the device to prevent breakage of the optical fibres. Ultrasound is required to confirm correct intrauterine positioning when insertion/placement is difficult or uncertain. There are minimal clinical data available regarding safety and effectiveness.

OUTCOMES

A single observational study of 100 cases, all with endometrial pretreatment, reported an amenorrhoea rate of 70 per cent at 6 and 12 months' follow-up, and a rate of amenorrhoea/hypomenorrhoea (spotting) of 90 per cent. Satisfaction rates of over 90 per cent were found at 12 months. No uterine perforations or serious complications were reported.

FURTHER READING

Donnez J, Polet R, Rabinovitz R, Ak M, Squifflet J, Nisolle M. Endometrial laser intrauterine thermotherapy: the first series of 100 patients observed for 1 year. *Fertil Steril* 2000;**74**:791–6.

MICROWAVE

Microwave endometrial ablation or 'MEA' (Microsulis plc, Waterlooville, Hampshire, UK)

MODE OF ACTION

- Low-power, high-fixed frequency microwave energy used to ablate the endometrium by thermal therapy.

SYSTEM

The MEA system consists of a reusable applicator, operating console, microwave cable, data transmission cable, foot switch and power cord. The applicator is a reusable aluminium instrument covered with a fluoroplastic sheath to allow for chemical or autoclave cleaning. It comprises a main body and 8.5 mm diameter, graduated shaft (or dielectric 'waveguide') along which the microwave energy propagates and is then released at the distal ceramic tip of 7 mm length. A solid black band extending 35 mm below the tip is used to indicate the tip position with respect to the endocervical canal, proximal to which is a solid yellow alerting band. The applicator includes two thermocouples measuring the tip temperature adjacent to the endometrium and the shaft temperature. The applicator is connected to the MEA system by two cables. The coaxial cable carries the microwave energy from the microwave module to the applicator. The data cable carries temperature data from the applicator, allowing for continuous temperature monitoring of tissue in the treatment field as data for monitoring the number of applicator uses. The console contains the control unit (including user touch screen, start button and emergency stop button), microwave generator and power module. The microwave frequency chosen for the MEA system is 9.2 GHz and the operating power is 42 W. This preset frequency and power results in a 5–6 mm depth of thermal necrosis.

PROCEDURE

The uterus is sounded and the cervix dilated to Hegar 9 to accommodate the microwave applicator, which is inserted through the cervix until the tip abuts the fundus, and the marking on the applicator shaft is checked to confirm it corresponds to the soundings previously taken. The applicator is energized by a foot pedal. The temperature sensor embedded at the applicator tip shows a rapidly rising temperature and within 45 seconds the endometrial temperature will have reached therapeutic levels (70–80°C). The microwave applicator is then moved gently from side to side to ensure even heating of the fundal areas including cornual regions. Once the fundal area has been completely treated, shown by the temperature acquired in the therapeutic band, then the applicator is slowly withdrawn in 2–3 mm decrements, maintaining a gentle side-to-side sweeping or 'painting' motion to ensure even heating of the whole uterine cavity (Fig. 17.2). During this process the temperature will be seen to fluctuate on the console computer screen that displays the treatment temperature band. The speed of applicator movement is dependent on this visual information – if the temperature falls below the therapeutic band, then the applicator is held still momentarily until that area is treated; the rising temperature will confirm that the treatment is complete in that area and the applicator is then moved again. As an additional safety feature, mechanisms within the system prevent significant increases above the temperature band.

   As the applicator tip reaches the internal cervical os, the black band on the applicator shaft starts to appear at the external cervical os indicating that the power should be switched off to avoid treating the cervical canal. The applicator is then withdrawn and the

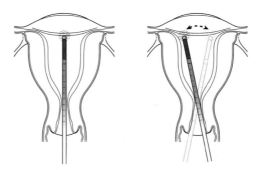

Figure 17.2 *Microwave endometrial ablation schema.*

treatment is complete. The total treatment time is approximately 3 minutes for an average-sized uterus. The treatment time is dependent, however, upon the cavity length (e.g. cavities of up to 11.5 cm may be treated but will take 6 to 7 minutes to complete treatment). The microwave system can generate a printout of the patient's temperature profile, which can be included in the patient's notes.

SUITABILITY FOR OUTPATIENT USE

MEA is a simple, easily learned, rapid procedure with a short recovery time and is thus suited to the outpatient setting. From conception of MEA to the present, procedures have been performed under local anaesthetic blockade with or without the need for conscious sedation as well as general anaesthesia. A randomized controlled trial (RCT) has compared general versus local/sedative approaches for MEA (in a formal theatre environment rather than outpatient treatment room). This found local anaesthetic treatment to be an attractive alternative in 70 per cent of women and highly acceptable in 87 per cent, although less than under general anaesthesia (97 per cent). Treatment under local anaesthesia did not offer additional safety or immediate/short-term postoperative recovery benefits, and this led the authors to conclude that MEA under local anaesthesia/conscious sedation should be limited to those women with a strong preference or those with medical factors favouring avoidance of general anaesthesia. Service delivery will, however, depend upon local factors such as patient demographics, theatre capacity, clinic set-up and experience.

ADVANTAGES COMPARED WITH OTHER SYSTEMS

Of all the available second-generation ablative devices, only Thermachoice can compete with MEA as regards validation of clinical safety, effectiveness and cost-effectiveness. Observational and experimental studies have been published and over 15 000 women have been treated worldwide. Perhaps the main advantage of MEA is the putative ability to treat enlarged (up to 14.5 cm) and irregular cavities and those containing small submucous fibroids or polyps. Amenorrhoea rates appear higher than Thermachoice, but overall rates of patient satisfaction are comparable.

DISADVANTAGES

The diameter of the applicator requires cervical dilatation up to Hegar 9, which can be difficult to achieve in a conscious patient without inducing discomfort and risks uterine trauma. One RCT reported device malfunction in 8 per cent of cases and procedure abandonment in 4 per cent, although this was attributed to use of a prototype generator. Reusable applicators (30 procedures) may be cost-effective, but decontamination services are required to prevent cross-contamination.

OUTCOMES

The MEA literature contains the RCT of highest methodological quality comparing MEA (n = 116) with hysteroscopic endometrial resection (n = 124). The trial was non-blinded and all women underwent endometrial preparation. All reported comparable rates of amenorrhoea (40 per cent) and satisfaction rates of (75 per cent) at 12 months' follow-up. These results were sustained at 2 years' follow-up. A single uterine perforation, but no other serious complications, was reported in both trial arms.

FURTHER READING

Cooper KG, Bain C, Parkin DE. Comparison of microwave endometrial ablation and transcervical resection of the endometrium for treatment of heavy menstrual loss: a randomised trial. *Lancet* 1999; **354**:1859–63.

Garside R, Stein K, Wyatt K, Round A, Price A. The effectiveness and cost-effectiveness of microwave and thermal balloon endometrial ablation for heavy menstrual bleeding: a systematic review and economic modelling. *Health Technol Assess* 2004;**8**:1–155.

Wallage S, Cooper KG, Graham WJ, Parkin DE. A randomised trial comparing local versus general anaesthesia for microwave endometrial ablation. *Br J Obstet Gynaecol* 2003;**110**:799–807.

FLUID-FILLED THERMAL BALLOONS

Cavaterm Plus System (Wallsten Medical, Morges, Switzerland)

MODE OF ACTION

- Thermal ablation of the endometrium by transfer of heat from heated liquid circulating within an intrauterine balloon.

SYSTEM

The Cavaterm Plus system consists of a single use, adjustable silicone balloon housing a heating element, thermocouples and an umbilical cable that connects to a battery-operated, central electronic computerized unit, which powers the heating elements, and monitors intrauterine pressure, balloon temperature, fluid circulation and treatment time. The predeployed balloon catheter is 6 mm in diameter.

PROCEDURE

The uterus is sounded so that the balloon length can be adjusted to the cavity length. The balloon catheter is primed ready for use, by a syringe to purge air from the system and deflates the balloon. The cervix is dilated to Hegar 6 and the catheter inserted to the fundus when the balloon is inflated using a syringe containing 30 ml of 5 per cent dextrose, until a stable pressure of 230–240 mmHg is obtained. The pressure allows optimal contact between the balloon and tissue, ensuring an even heat penetration through the tissue, thereby destroying the endometrium and underlying myometrium to a depth of 6–8 mm. Heating commences up to the preset temperature of 78°C, and pressure is maintained by further fluid inflation/deflation of the balloon. An integral drain tube within the catheter acts as a safety valve by preventing excess pressure from overinflation. Once the treatment time of 10 minutes has been completed, the pump is manually deactivated and the balloon deflated and removed from the uterus.

SUITABILITY FOR OUTPATIENT USE

The high uterine pressures (>200 mmHg) may induce more intraoperative pain, and the procedure time (10 minutes' cycle) is at the upper limit of what patients can reasonably be expected to tolerate. Although the manufacturers advocate use under local or general anaesthesia, all data published to date have pertained to general anaesthesia only.

ADVANTAGES COMPARED WITH OTHER SYSTEMS

This is one of the more simple and safe procedures. Conformity to uterine size and shape may be enhanced by the adjustability of the balloon length compared with other thermal balloons, but no distinct advantage has been identified over other forms of endometrial ablation.

DISADVANTAGES

It is a longer procedure than most and may be unsuited to outpatient work.

OUTCOMES

A single blinded randomized trial comparing Cavaterm (n = 37) with the Nd:YAG laser (n = 33) reported comparable rates of amenorrhoea (29 versus 39 per cent) at 12 months' follow-up and rates of amenorrhoea/hypomenorrhoea of 70 per cent. Another small randomized trial comparing Cavaterm (n = 18) with Novasure (n = 37) reported higher rates of amenorrhoea with Cavaterm (43 versus 11 per cent) at 12 months' follow-up, but comparable rates of amenorrhoea/hypomenorrhoea of 70 per cent. Satisfaction rates of 80–90 per cent with Cavaterm were found at 12 months and no uterine perforations or serious complications were reported in either trial.

FURTHER READING

Abbott J, Hawe J, Hunter D, Garry R. A double-blind randomized trial comparing the Cavaterm and the Novasure endometrial ablation systems for the treatment of dysfunctional uterine bleeding. *Fertil Steril* 2003;**80**:203–8.

Hawe J, Abbott J, Hunter D, Phillips G, Garry R. A randomized controlled trial comparing the Cavaterm endometrial ablation system with the Nd:YAG laser for the treatment of dysfunctional uterine bleeding. *Br J Obstet Gynaecol* 2003;**110**:350–7.

Thermablate EAS (MDMI Technologies Inc., Richmond, BC, Canada)

MODE OF ACTION

- Thermal ablation of the endometrium by transfer of heat from heated liquid circulating within an intrauterine balloon. Fluid is heated externally in contrast to other thermal balloon therapies where heating occurs inside the balloon.

SYSTEM

The device consists of a disposable cartridge that contains a silicone reservoir and a silicone balloon connected by an insulated tube and a handheld, reusable treatment control unit (TCU) which controls all treatment parameters (time, pressure, and temperature). The TCU operates an electromechanical heating and pumping/draining system that is designed to deliver treatment in 128 seconds. The TCU has an LCD display providing information relating to the procedure (warming-up cycle, balloon leak test, treatment cycle and completion of treatment). The predeployed balloon catheter is 6 mm in diameter.

PROCEDURE

The cartridge is filled with a biocompatible fluid, which is heated to 173°C in the reservoir before the treatment commences. Once the balloon has been inserted into the uterine cavity and the user depresses the trigger button, a pneumatic pump applies pressure to the reservoir and fluid is forced into the balloon. A pressure of 180–200 mmHg is applied to the treatment fluid. During treatment the pressure is pulsed periodically to help mix the fluid within the balloon. This ensures a uniform temperature distribution in the balloon and promotes a uniform treatment of the uterus. The temperature of the fluid in the balloon is approximately 155°C when it first enters the uterus, and declines to 115°C by the end of the 128-second treatment period. The temperature of the endometrium is elevated significantly during treatment causing tissue necrosis (4–5 mm depth), whereas the temperature of the myometrium is only mildly elevated and is therefore left unharmed.

SUITABILITY FOR OUTPATIENT USE

External fluid heating to high temperatures facilitates faster endometrial cauterization and a short procedure time (2.5 minutes), which is favourable for outpatient use for which it has been designed. To date there are minimal available data about feasibility, safety and effectiveness under local anaesthesia.

ADVANTAGES COMPARED WITH OTHER SYSTEMS

It is an extremely compact, transportable and automated system with a short duration of therapy combined with simplicity of use.

DISADVANTAGES

Safety and effectiveness data are lacking.

OUTCOMES

Combined data from two small observational series (16 and 54 patients respectively) reported rates of amenorrhoea of 25 per cent at 6 months' follow-up and rates of amenorrhoea/hypomenorrhoea of 80 per cent. Satisfaction rates of 90 per cent were found at 6 months and no uterine perforations or serious complications were reported in either study.

FURTHER READING

Mangeshikar PS, Kapur A, Yackel DB. Endometrial ablation with a new thermal balloon system. *J Am Assoc Gynecol Laparosc* 2003;10:27–32.

Yackel DB, Vilos GA. Thermablate EAS: a new endometrial ablation system. *Gynecolog Surg* 2004;1: 129–32.

Thermachoice III (Gynecare Inc, Somerville, New Jersey USA)

MODE OF ACTION

*   Thermal ablation of the endometrium by transfer of heat from heated liquid circulating within an intrauterine balloon.

SYSTEM

The Thermachoice III uterine balloon system comprises a disposable 4.5 mm diameter, graded dual lumen catheter with a silicone balloon at its distal end containing the heating and circulating elements. Fluid is instilled into the balloon via a proximal fluid-filled port using a 30 ml syringe. The plastic catheter connects via an umbilical cable and pressure line (with circulation connector) to a control unit that monitors, displays and regulates intrauterine balloon pressure, temperature, fluid circulation and duration of treatment. The system continually monitors fluid temperature and intrauterine pressures and will automatically deactivate at pressures <45 mmHg or >200 mmHg as a safety feature.

PROCEDURE

In the majority of parous women, cervical instrumentation (grasping forceps, sounding, dilatation) is not required for device placement, and vigorous preprocedural endometrial curettage, previously described in the literature, is unnecessary. The balloon catheter is primed ready for use by a syringe to purge air from the system and deflate the balloon. It is then inserted into the uterine cavity to the level of the fundus and the cavity length noted from the graduated catheter. The balloon is then inflated with sterile 5 per cent dextrose until the pressure is stabilized between 160 and 180 mmHg. This pressure allows optimal contact between the balloon and tissue ensuring an even heat penetration through the tissue, thereby destroying the endometrium and underlying myometrium to a depth of 3–10 mm (Fig. 17.3). Intrauterine pressure fluctuation occurs as a result of contraction and relaxation of stimulated myometrial smooth muscle. The amount of intrauterine fluid required will depend upon cavity size, but is between 10 and 15 ml on average. No more than 30 ml of dextrose should be instilled and the procedure abandoned if therapeutic pressure not reached.

The system is then switched on so that fluid within the balloon is heated to a preset temperature of 87°C, which takes 30–45 seconds on average (depending upon the amount of fluid instilled). The system then begins a standard 8-minute treatment cycle. If the pressure fluctuates and drops <160 mmHg (as is often the case), the addition of further dextrose water as 'top ups' to maintain the intrauterine pressure between 160–180 mmHg should be considered at the discretion of the operator. Although this goes against manufacturer's

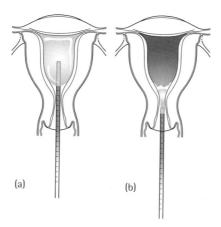

(a)   (b)

Figure 17.3 *Thermachoice endometrial ablation schema. (a) Before: the catheter is inserted into the uterine fundus and the balloon is inflated to the required pressure (160–180 mmHg) and the treatment cycle begun. (b) After: the balloon is deflated and removed, leaving the ablated endometrial cavity.*

instructions, a trend towards improved treatment outcome has been demonstrated with pressures >160 mmHg. In practice only occasional small 'top up' injections are required to correct small drops in pressure. The need for large 'top ups' (>2 ml) in response to rapid pressure drops is unusual and may lead to rebound pressure increases or temperature drops outside the preset parameters, resulting in system deactivation. In such a situation the procedure should be abandoned and uterine perforation or system malfunction considered. On completion of the treatment cycle, the balloon is deflated and removed. Throughout all stages of the procedure, there are both visual and audible prompts from the control unit console to direct the operator.

SUITABILITY FOR OUTPATIENT USE

The simplicity, safety, avoidance of cervical dilatation, uterine pressures (<200 mmHg), short duration (8 minutes) and rapid recovery time suits the Thermachoice procedure to the outpatient setting. Many procedures (subgroups within larger series) have been performed under local anaesthesia with or without the need for conscious sedation. More recently, the feasibility and success of a truly 'outpatient/office' approach, without endometrial pretreatment or scheduling, sedation or the need for formal theatre facilities, has been reported. Only 1 in 50 patients could not tolerate the procedure with analgesics and cervical anaesthesia alone, and the simple protocol described is transferable to most settings.

ADVANTAGES COMPARED WITH OTHER SYSTEMS

Thermachoice is one of the most simple, safe and widely used procedures with over 250 000 women treated worldwide. Of all the available second-generation ablative devices, only MEA can compete with Thermachoice as regards validation of clinical safety, effectiveness and cost-effectiveness. Observational and experimental studies have been published with long-term follow up and, along with MEA and Cavaterm, recommended for use in the UK by NICE.

DISADVANTAGES

The overall procedure time is 10–15 minutes, which may be longer than some competing devices, but this time is still within tolerable limits. The probability of successful treatment has been shown to be reduced to a variable extent by the shape (irregular/fibroids), size (>10 ml fluid required, pressures <140 mmHg), axis (retroversion) and endometrial thickness (>4 mm) of the uterus. In an attempt to optimize treatment and overcome these adverse prognostic factors, the updated Thermachoice III has been launched. It incorporates a more conformable silicone balloon and impellar to circulate fluid to provide more even heat coverage.

OUTCOMES

A non-blinded randomized trial comparing Thermachoice (n = 125) with hysteroscopic rollerball ablation (n = 114) reported lower rates of amenorrhoea with (15 versus 27 per cent) at 12 months' follow-up but comparable satisfaction rates (over 90 per cent). An uncontrolled, observational series of 300 women reported rates of amenorrhoea/hypomenorrhoea for Thermachoice of 63 per cent at 12 months. No uterine perforations or serious complications were reported in either study and a recent European survey of over 5000 procedures reported an intraoperative complication rate of <0.25 per cent.

FURTHER READING

Amso NN, Fernandez H, Vilos G *et al.* Uterine endometrial thermal balloon therapy for the treatment of menorrhagia: long-term multicentre follow-up study. *Hum Reprod* 2003;**18**:1082–7.

Clark TJ, Gupta JK. Outpatient thermal balloon ablation of the endometrium. *Fertil Steril* 2004; **82**:1395–1401.

Meyer WR, Walsh BW, Grainger DA, Peacock LM, Loffer FD, Steege JF. Thermal balloon and rollerball ablation to treat menorrhagia: a multicenter comparison. *Obstet Gynecol* 1998;**92**:98–103.

OTHER METHODS

Hysteroscopic 'first-generation' techniques

Although traditional hysteroscopic endometrial rollerball ablation and resection under local anaesthesia and conscious sedation have been reported, the outpatient setting has not become established. They remain firmly inpatient techniques because of practical and safety issues. Versapoint negates many of the outpatient limitations of traditional hysteroscopic approaches and outpatient endometrial ablations have been reported. However, application is limited by the geometry of the minute distal electrodes, which make producing and ascertaining a uniform depth of thermal destruction difficult, with resultant prolonged procedure times.

Other second-generation devices

No published local anaesthetic (outpatient) data are available for the MenoTreat (Atos Medical, Horby, Sweden) thermal balloon system. It does not appear suitable for use without regional or general anaesthesia as the procedure time is over 10 minutes and the device diameter is 11 mm requiring dilatation and high intrauterine pressures (200 mmHg).

Two future potential outpatient methods include endometrial destruction using photodynamic therapy (light activation of a locally administered photosensitizer generating highly reactive oxygen intermediates causing cellular oxidation and subsequent irreversible tissue injury and necrosis) and the EnAbl system (InnerDyne Medical, Sunnyvale, CA), a 6.7 mm intrauterine device that circulates hot saline. Photodynamic therapy has been reported without the need for anaesthesia. However, clinical studies for both procedures are still at an experimental stage.

PERFORMING ENDOMETRIAL ABLATION IN AN OUTPATIENT SETTING

From a technical standpoint, outpatient endometrial ablation using second-generation systems is easier than other outpatient procedures described in this book. However, it has the potential to provoke most patient discomfort, impairing compliance, reducing feasibility and threatening the viability of an outpatient ablative service. However, correctly set up and managed, outpatient treatment is invariably successful, highly rewarding and greatly appreciated by women. Non-operative skills come to the fore and these include honest and comprehensive preoperative counselling, perioperative communication and postoperative pain management. An example of a successful approach using the Thermachoice system is described (Information Box 17.4). Although other ablative techniques will have their own individual nuances, the procedures are similar, so that the general approach outlined should be applicable to other technologies.

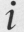 **Information Box 17.4 Outpatient Thermachoice: a suggested protocol for an outpatient 'office' procedure**

PREOPERATIVE

- *Inform all women not to fast* for the procedure thereby preventing hypoglycaemia, dehydration and propensity to vasovagal attacks.
- *Premedicate* 1 hour prior to the procedure.
- *Simple analgesics.* Diclofenac 100 mg rectal suppository + two co-dydramol tablets orally. If non-steroidal anti-inflammatory drugs are contraindicated, then alternatives (e.g. oral opiate tramadol hydrochloride 100 mg) should be administered.
- *Anti-emetic.* Ondansetron 4 mg orally.
- *Antibiotics.* Augmentin (amoxycillin + clavulonic acid) 375 mg. (NB: The risk of uterine/pelvic infection is low [1:200] and so routine prescription unnecessary.)

OPERATIVE PROCEDURE

- *Position* in the dorsolithotomy position and designate a nurse to stay with the patient throughout the procedure to offer support and distraction, providing a 'vocal-local'.
- *Local anaesthesia.* Directly infiltrated the cervix such as three 2.2 ml vials of the local anaesthetic Citanest (Astra, UK – prilocaine 3 per cent + felypressin 0.03 units/ml) into four quadrants: the 3, 6, 9 and 12 o'clock positions. Inject the majority of local anaesthetic (1.5 ml) at the deepest possible point in each quadrant, using a 35 mm, 27 G dental syringe, approximating the level of the internal cervical os, and distribute the remainder evenly throughout the length of the cervix on withdrawal.
- *Do not use intravenous sedation or narcotic analgesia.* No anaesthetist needs to be present.
- *Perform* a standard diagnostic hysteroscopy (and/or transvaginal ultrasound scan) to exclude intrauterine pathology/anomalies distorting the uterine cavity, which contraindicate the procedure, and to ascertain likely compliance with the procedure ('patient screening').
- *Significant intrauterine polyps or fibroids* should be blindly avulsed or excised under direct endoscopic vision if necessary, before endometrial ablation is performed.
- *Perform an endometrial biopsy* if no result is available within the last 6 months (ideally take before the date of procedure to minimize discomfort and maintain compliance).
- *Perform the Thermachoice* procedure according to manufacturer's instructions (see above).

POSTOPERATIVE

- *Return the woman to a designated recovery area*, where she can lie supine or sit and recuperate (e.g. day-case ward).
- *Administer 5–10 mg of morphine* as the peak postoperative pain follows 1 hour following completion of surgery. (Alternatively give in the treatment room.)
- *Administer additional simple analgesia* as required.
- *Discharge home after a minimum stay of 2 hours* once she has tolerated oral diet, passed urine and has adequate pain control.

- *Discharge with an information leaflet* describing expected postoperative symptoms and instructions to take simple analgesics regularly for the first 24 hours (diclofenac 50 mg t.i.d. and/or co-dydramol, two tablets four times daily).
- *Arrange nurse telephone contact* the following day to check on progress.

NOTES

This is one suggested approach, which has evolved over time after continual modification and has been demonstrated to work very well, avoiding risks associated with intravenous sedation and the need for formal theatre facilities. Alternative pharmacological agents (e.g. analgesics, anti-emetics and local anaesthetics) and dosing schedules can be used if preferred. Although this approach is described in the context of Thermachoice, it is also a suitable template for use with other appropriate second-generation ablative procedures.

CONCLUSION

Outpatient menorrhagia treatment should not be restricted to medical therapies, but include endometrial ablation, hysteroscopic surgical interventions and placement of LNG-IUS devices. Many second-generation ablative devices are currently available for the treatment of excessive menstrual bleeding. Over the next few years the place of individual systems will become clearer. Some systems will undoubtedly fall by the wayside, others will become increasingly established and some superseded by future developments. The avoidance of general anaesthesia and the ability to offer outpatient treatment, thereby expanding management options and patient choice, will be a prime factor driving future system usage and development.

Evidence Box 17.1 Outpatient endometrial ablation

The evidence supporting or refuting the available endometrial ablative devices in terms of feasibility and effectiveness has been detailed above. Data pertaining to the outpatient, local anaesthetic setting are scarce. Head-to-head randomized trials comparing settings and/or devices are required to help determine the best ones in particular populations along with qualitative research examining the overall patient experience.

KEY POINTS

- Endometrial ablation is an effective treatment for dysfunctional uterine bleeding refractory to medical therapy.
- The simplicity, safety and comparable effectiveness of newer auto-ablative systems, so called 'second-generation' devices, means they have replaced traditional 'first-generation' hysteroscopic methods.

- The design of second-generation systems along with short operating and recovery times has made operating in an outpatient hysteroscopy clinic setting feasible, expanding patient choice and health service capacity.
- The success of an outpatient endometrial ablation service is dependent upon the development and institution of appropriate treatment protocols.

FURTHER READING

Abbott JA, Hawe J, Garry R. Quality of life should be considered the primary outcome for measuring success of endometrial ablation. *J Am Assoc Gynecol Laparosc* 2003;**10**:491–5.

Cooper J, Gimpelson RJ. Summary of safety and effectiveness data from FDA: a valuable source of information on the performance of global endometrial ablation devices. *J Reprod Med* 2004;**49**: 267–73.

Garside R, Stein K, Wyatt K, Round A, Price A. The effectiveness and cost-effectiveness of microwave and thermal balloon endometrial ablation for heavy menstrual bleeding: a systematic review and economic modelling. *Health Technol Assess* 2004;**8**:1–155.

Lethaby A, Hickey M. Endometrial destruction techniques for heavy menstrual bleeding: a Cochrane review. *Hum Reprod* 2002;**17**:2795–806.

National Institute for Clinical Excellence. Fluid-filled thermal balloon and microwave endometrial ablation techniques for heavy menstrual bleeding. *Technology Appraisal Guidance* 78, April 2004. [Available at www.nice.org.uk/TA078guidance]

Subfertility and miscarriage

Investigation of women with infertility or recurrent pregnancy loss involves assessment of the entire reproductive tract and relevant endocrine systems. The role of hysteroscopy in both diagnosis and treatment is somewhat limited, as it is restricted to assessment of the uterine cavity and correctable anatomical anomalies within the uterus. These account for <5 per cent of underlying causes of infertility and recurrent pregnancy loss. Despite this, outpatient hysteroscopy can usefully be employed in selected women.

DIAGNOSTIC HYSTEROSCOPY

Structural anomalies such as polyps and submucous fibroids are common in the general female population, and their relative importance in causation of unexplained infertility is unclear. Congenital and acquired uterine anomalies are less common, but the degree of any adverse impact they exert on fertility is similarly contentious. Hysteroscopy is the gold standard for assessment of the cervical canal and uterine cavity for structural anomalies. However, other imaging techniques such as transvaginal ultrasound (TVS), saline infusion sonography (SIS) and hysterosalpingography (HSG), can also provide some assessment of the uterine cavity for the presence of structural anomalies while providing additional information that is more likely to explain the cause of subfertility. For example, TVS can assess the adnexae for relevant pathology (polycystic ovaries, endometriomas and hydrosalpinges) and HSG provides important information about tubal structure and patency. Advocates of hysteroscopy argue, however, that modern hysteroscopy is a simple and safe outpatient procedure, and not routinely employing it compromises evaluation of the uterine cavity.

As well as equivocation over the role of uterine anomalies in subfertility, there is considerable uncertainty about the effectiveness of any surgical intervention in producing favourable

Information Box 18.1 Indications and rationale for diagnostic hysteroscopy in management of subfertility

COEXISTENT SYMPTOMS

- *Oligoamenorrhoea following a history of uterine surgery or pelvic infection.* Adhesions (Asherman's syndrome)
- *Intermenstrual bleeding.* Polyps, submucous fibroids
- *Persistent and severe dysmenorrhoea ± vaginal discharge.* Cervical stenosis, extruded submucous fibroid, endometritis
- *Menorrhagia which has not responded to medical treatment.* Submucous fibroids

ABNORMAL IMAGING

- *'Filling defects' seen on HSG or anomalies on TVS/SIS.* Polyps, submucous fibroids, adhesions, congenital anomalies

Abbreviations: HSG, hysterosalpingography; SIS, saline infusion sonography; TVS, transvaginal ultrasound.

fertility outcomes. The Royal College of Obstetricians and Gynaecologists (RCOG) of the United Kingdom recommends that hysteroscopy should not be considered as a routine investigation for infertility, while there is no evidence linking treatment of uterine abnormalities with enhanced fertility.

In spite of these considerations, selected women may benefit from intrauterine assessment, especially if you take into account the improved optics and relatively simple and non-invasive nature of outpatient microhysteroscopy today (Information Box 18.1).

DIAGNOSTIC HYSTEROSCOPY AND INFERTILITY

The previously described standard technique for assessment of the uterine cavity and endometrium is recommended. However, certain points need to be emphasized:

- *A reassuring and gentle approach is especially important.* This is because the investigation of infertility is an emotive area and the woman is likely to have already undergone several intimate and invasive procedures. In addition, the cervical canal of nulliparous women may be narrower than the canal encountered in parous women.
- *Particular attention should be paid to the vaginal vault and course of the endocervical canal.* This is important in order to avoid missing congenital anomalies such as duplicate genitalia or 'additional' uterine chambers of a bicornuate or uterine septum. Intracervical polyps, adhesions and atresia may be diagnosed.
- *The shape and size of the cavity should be carefully assessed.* In addition to the apparent 'heart-shaped' appearance of arcuate and bicornuate uteri, the hypoplastic uterus often appears 'T-shaped' as a result of the contracted tubular body.

- *Close inspection of the tubal ostia.* The number of ostia visualized should be recorded, as only a single ostia may be visualized with unicornuate uteri or uteri with rudimentary horns. Close inspection of the tubal ostia will prevent cornual polyps from being overlooked and a 'pinpoint' appearance of the tubal ostia may suggest proximal tubal blockage, especially at higher intrauterine pressures (>70 mmHg), when distension media should be seen exiting through the ostium, revealing the interior of the proximal intramural segment, if patent.

- *Carefully assess the nature, extent, location and size of structural anomalies.* In addition to recording the presence of septae, adhesions, polyps and fibroids, detailed description is required so that the need and feasibility of subsequent corrective surgery can be assessed.

- *Consider endometrial biopsy.* Endometrial biopsy will be indicated at the time of hysteroscopy in women with menorrhagia in association with risk factors for endometrial hyperplasia (obesity, polycystic ovaries, anovulation, >40 years of age). It is also useful to confirm the presence of functional endometrium when the cavity appears unexpectedly atrophic or there is uncertainty regarding cavity visualization in the presence of congenital or acquired uterine distortion.

DIAGNOSTIC HYSTEROSCOPY AND RECURRENT PREGNANCY LOSS

Diagnostic hysteroscopy is useful in excluding congenital malformations (e.g. uterine hypoplasia, septae) and intracavity fibroids or adhesions, which may be associated with unexplained recurrent first and second trimester miscarriage (>3) or preterm labour. Cervical incompetence is a dynamic disorder and cannot be diagnosed hysteroscopically, although a patulous cervical canal with substantial backflow of distension media and difficulty distending the cavity may be suggestive. Assessment of the length of the various aspects of the intravaginal cervix should be described so that suitability for particular cervical cerclage techniques in a subsequent pregnancy can be determined.

SURGICAL HYSTEROSCOPY

Indications for outpatient hysteroscopic surgery in the management of subfertility and recurrent miscarriage are given in Information Box 18.2. As always, judgement is required regarding feasibility of outpatient procedures. Severe congenital or acquired uterine anomalies will require more extensive hysteroscopic procedures, often in combination with concurrent laparoscopic visualization. Such procedures will need to be performed on inpatients under general anaesthesia. Newer, unproven treatments such as hysteroscopic transfer of gametes (GIFT – gamete intrafallopian transfer) and embryos as part of an assisted conception programme have been reported using conscious sedation. Widespread application of this technique is unlikely in view of the restricted indications for GIFT and uncertainty over the feasibility and efficacy of the hysteroscopic approach. This approach cannot be recommended outside of a research setting.

Information Box 18.2 Indications for outpatient hysteroscopic surgery in the management of subfertility

- *Selective salpingography.* Selective salpingography is more accurate than traditional HSG for diagnosing proximal tubal blockage (PTB) because it helps distinguish between true anatomic occlusion and apparent occlusion arising from tubal spasm. In addition, simultaneous tubal catheterization (TC – see below) may allow true obstruction to be overcome; i.e. a 'see and treat' approach. The procedure can be performed transcervically under fluoroscopic control or under direct hysteroscopic visualization. Published data are scant regarding the hysteroscopic approach, which may reflect the ease and accessibility of the radiographic approach. Enthusiasts argue that tubal cannulation using the hysteroscopic approach is simpler and reduces radiation exposure.
- *Tubal catheterization.* This procedure may be performed to relieve proximal tubal obstruction (confirmed by selective salpingography) in the absence of other tubal abnormalities (see below). It is successfully achieved in 50–70 per cent of cases of PTB and may avoid the need for tubal surgery or *in vitro* fertilization.
- *Adhesiolysis.* Division of adhesions (see below).
- *Metroplasty.* Resection of complete or partial uterine septae (see below). Expansion of uterine cavity in hypoplastic uterus (see below).
- *Polypectomy.* In the absence of symptoms of vaginal discharge or bleeding, any benefit to fertility following removal is questionable. In one series of 70 subfertile women, 10 per cent were noted to have polyps near the ostia and half of these were associated with PTB on hysterosalpingography (HSG). Thus, following diagnosis, polypectomy is recommended because it is simple, safe, may in some situations improve fertility and is unlikely to have an adverse effect on fertility. Furthermore, removal of the specimen allows histological assessment (see Chapter 15).
- *Myomectomy.* Pedunculated submucous fibroids can be removed with electrosurgery. Resection or vaporization of large, sessile and predominantly intramural fibroids will result in ablation of a substantial area of endometrium. This may compromise fertility and so careful consideration and patient counselling is required before undertaking such a procedure on fertility grounds (see Chapter 16).

TUBAL CATHETERIZATION AND HYSTEROSCOPIC SELECTIVE SALPINGOGRAPHY

The patient should be prepared and positioned in the standard way appropriate for outpatient hysteroscopic intervention. The use of premedication with a non-steroidal anti-inflammatory drug and a cervical anaesthetic block is recommended, as manipulation in the vicinity of the tubal ostia is likely to trigger discomfort. Some recommend use of conscious sedation, although tubal catheterization (TC) can usually be achieved without need for this.

In order to aid access to the tubal ostia (especially when they are located laterally), the woman's hips should be well abducted, a single-tooth tenaculum applied to the anterior lip of the cervix should be employed, and the use of a 4–5 mm rigid hysteroscope with an offset lens or flexible fibroscope is recommended. Carbon dioxide or fluid can be used to distend the uterine cavity. If a fluid distension medium is chosen, then a continuous flow system must be used. The hysteroscope must contain a working channel of sufficient diameter for the chosen cannulation system (normally 2–6 Fr). Various types of cannulation systems have been used, which usually employ obturators and/or guidewires (e.g. Cook UK, Letchworth, Hertfordshire UK; Novy or SS-TC catheter systems). Mechanical dilatation of the tube has been reported using an angioplasty balloon catheter. The chosen catheter is connected via tubing to a syringe containing low-viscosity, water-soluble contrast medium (e.g. Hexabrix 320; Mallinckrodt Medical, Round Spiney, UK; Isobist; Schering, AG Berlin, Germany).

The catheter is aligned with the tubal ostia and gently threaded into the fallopian tube to a distance of about 10 mm beyond the ostium. Approximately 2 ml of water-soluble contrast medium is then injected to confirm tubal patency followed by an abdominal X-ray 15 minutes later. The catheter will pass into the tube where there is no proximal tubal blockage (PTB) and will overcome minor degrees of PTB. Resistance precluding satisfactory advancement of the catheter into the tube and reflux of contrast medium into the uterus indicates that PTB is present. A guidewire is then advanced through the cannula towards the obstruction, and gentle forward pressure applied to overcome the PTB, followed by withdrawal of the guidewire and injection of contrast medium as described above.

INTRAUTERINE ADHESIONS AND ADHESIOLYSIS

Definition (hysteroscopic)

- Isolated or extensive band(s) of filmy or firm, white or grey tissue, which lead to varying degrees of uterine cavity distortion. The uterine walls may be coapted without discrete tissue bands visible, and the uterine fundus and cornual recesses occluded.

ASHERMAN'S SYNDROME

- This is defined as the presence of permanent intrauterine adhesions causing partial or complete obliteration of the uterine cavity and clinical symptoms including menstrual abnormalities (usually amenorrhoea or oligomenorrhoea), infertility (usually secondary) and recurrent pregnancy loss. Other symptoms such as pelvic pain, dysmenorrhoea and dyspareunia are also commonly found in association with menstrual disturbance.

Epidemiology

The most common aetiological factor is uterine surgery, in particular endometrial curettage on a gravid uterus (e.g. evacuation of retained products of conception, termination of pregnancy). Other implicated procedures include endometrial ablation, myomectomy and Caesarean section. Uterine infection (endometritis) is likely to increase the probability of postsurgical adhesion formation or be the primary cause, as in the case of genital tuberculosis. Constitutional factors may also predispose to adhesion formation.

Pathology

Adhesions may originate within the endometrium, myometrium or connective tissue, and the hysteroscopic appearance will vary accordingly (i.e. filmy mucosal, dense myofibrous and fibrous). The gross pathological appearance of the uterine cavity depends upon the amount, severity and location of adhesions in addition to their nature. The cavity may become rigid because of uterine fibrotic change within the myometrium ('uterine fibrosis'), and shortened giving it a hypoplastic appearance. Following release of adhesions, any exposed endometrium is normally benign and functional (>90 per cent). However, it may be atrophic in 5 per cent (may be due to reduced exposure to oestrogen) or conversely hyperplastic (3 per cent).

Presentation and diagnosis

Most women will present with some or all of the characteristic symptoms of Asherman's syndrome described above, with duration dating from a history of uterine surgery. Menstrual disturbance in the form of amenorrhoea or oligomenorrhoea is the most common presenting complaint. A history of subfertility or recurrent pregnancy loss is also highly suggestive. Uterine adhesions may occasionally be detected incidentally in asymptomatic women.

Diagnosis

Uterine synechiae may be suspected during infertility work-up when abnormal shapes and filling defects in the uterine cavity are seen at HSG. TVS and SIS may also reveal an indistinct or irregular and eccentric echogenic endometrial stripe with or without intrauterine fluid collections. Sensitivity of uterine imaging is high, but this is at the cost of high rates of false positive diagnosis. Magnetic resonance imaging (MRI) has not been rigorously evaluated to date.

Hysteroscopy provides the definitive diagnosis. It is important to note the amount of hysteroscope advancement (presumed uterine depth) and to identify a tubal ostia, or failing that endometrial tissue, in order to confirm entry into the uterine cavity. In the absence of these findings, an iatrogenic lesion (false passage) should be suspected, especially if resistance has been encountered or cervical dilatation required.

Hysteroscopic characteristics

Many classification systems based on hysteroscopic features alone or incorporating clinical and pathological features have been produced (see Further reading, page 243). Whether or not such standardized nomenclature is employed, it is important to record the following hysteroscopic features so that surgical treatment can be planned and clinical response to treatment be objectively assessed:

APPEARANCE

Superficial endometrial ('mucous') adhesions exhibit an appearance similar to the surrounding endometrium and are often thin and filmy. Myofibrous adhesions are thicker and often covered with endometrium, whereas purely fibrous adhesions are pale, thick, avascular and devoid of covering endometrium.

SITE AND NUMBER

In the absence of total obliteration of the uterine cavity, adhesions may be single or mult-iple. They may be sited within the cervical canal or within the uterine isthmus, body or fundus. Those within the body may be centrally and/or marginally sited.

VISIBILITY OF TUBAL OSTIA

The ability to see the tubal ostia should be recorded, as visualization helps guide surgery, thereby increasing feasibility. The presence of adhesions and degree of agglutination of the cornual areas should be recorded, as this may effect tubal patency and hence fertility.

UTERINE SHAPE AND SIZE

The nature, amount and severity of adhesions will influence the degree of uterine distortion, which can be minimal in the case of filmy marginal adhesions, to complete cavity obliteration in the case of multiple, dense myofibrous adhesions. The extent of the cavity involved (e.g. $<\frac{1}{3}$, $\frac{2}{3}$, $>\frac{2}{3}$) should be recorded, as should the appearance and size of the uterine cavity e.g. it may appear rigid and hypoplastic (contracted) in the presence of significant uterine fibrosis.

ENDOMETRIAL CHARACTERISTICS

The amount, condition and appearance of the endometrium must be noted. Directed biop-sies are useful to histologically ascertain the functional endometrial status.

Treatment

The general equipment set-up for outpatient hysteroscopic fertility procedures is given in Information Box 18.3. The overall aim of hysteroscopic therapy is to reinstate a functional

---

Information Box 18.3 Basic requirements for set up for outpatient hysteroscopic adhesiolysis and septoplasty

BASIC REQUIREMENTS

- Operative hysteroscopy set-up (see Chapter 3)
- Atraumatic tenaculum forceps
- Cervical dilation set
- Continuous flow hysteroscope* with a minimum 5 F (1.67 mm) operative channel
- Saline* (3-l bag recommended) and inflow/outflow tubing ± suction apparatus
- Mechanical instruments (hysteroscopic semirigid scissors and graspers)
- Versapoint coaxial electrodes (spring and twizzle tip)
- Ultrasound machine (mandatory imaging for all but the simplest of adhesions)
- Foley balloon catheter (uterine tamponade or splinting)
- Video endoscopy system
- Video recording facility (optional)

* The choice of distension medium and angulation of hysteroscope will depend upon personal preference and applied technique.

uterine cavity so that menstruation and fertility is restored. To achieve this, specific surgical aims have to be achieved:

- restore the size of the uterine cavity
- restore the shape of the uterine cavity
- restore (uncover) hidden functional endometrium.

Techniques

HYSTEROSCOPIC ADHESIOLYSIS

Many techniques have been described utilizing mechanical methods (sheath alone or scissors), electroresection with electrodes of various types and laser. Adhesiolysis is continued until a normal panoramic view of the endometrial cavity is obtained and both tubal ostia visualized. A non-aggressive approach is needed to protect newly exposed and surrounding functional endometrium, so that regeneration and re-epithelization is encouraged, which is essential for a good anatomical and functional result. If menstrual cycles are present then scheduling surgery in the early proliferative phase may help visualization.

The outpatient approaches employ one or more of the following techniques:

- avulsion ('target abrasion') using the hysteroscope tip and sheath (filmy adhesions);
- scissors to resect filmy or thin fibrous adhesions;
- Versapoint bipolar electrosurgery to resect well demarcated adhesions of any type.

Adhesions should be broken down or resected systematically, starting inferiorly and working towards the fundus. Central adhesions should be treated first to gain access and orientation before addressing any more marginal lesions (unless they are distinct and filmy). Fundal advancement should cease once the tubal ostia come into view. Resection is complete once the uterine architecture (shape and size) is normalized.

MYOMETRIAL SCORING

This technique is indicated in women with previous failed hysteroscopic adhesiolysis and/or greatly reduced uterine volumes. It involves making six to eight longitudinal incisions into the myometrium extending from the uterine fundus to the isthmus. The incisions are distributed equidistantly and in a radial fashion to a myometrial depth of 4 mm. This procedure is not suitable for an outpatient setting because it usually requires general anaesthesia to facilitate cervical dilatation, instrumentation and simultaneous laparoscopy to check on uterine integrity. The use of Versapoint bipolar electrodes with ultrasound guidance under local anaesthesia has been reported and may be suitable in selected cases.

Selection for outpatient hysteroscopic surgery

Feasibility and safety as well as patient wishes will dictate whether an outpatient 'see and treat' approach is indicated. The overall risk of uterine perforation is estimated to be approximately 3 per cent. Uterine perforation is more likely if:

- the tubal ostia are obscured (landmarks for orientation);
- the adhesions are marginal, dense and vascular (difficult to distinguish denuded myometrium from remaining scar tissue);
- the cavity is substantially fibrotic (poor uterine distension) and distorted.

If the above features are present, then patients should be scheduled for more extensive inpatient surgery. Transabdominal ultrasound guidance is recommended for all but the most minor, filmy or centrally located adhesions. If uterine perforation is suspected then admission for a period of observation with recourse to laparoscopy/laparotomy is required, especially if energy sources have been used. Potential surgical complications are as for any hysteroscopic procedure (see Chapter 4).

Reproductive complications

Women should be counselled that surgical restoration of a normal uterine cavity is an unrealistic aim in severe Asherman's syndrome, and that assisted conception techniques may be still be required to overcome tubal factors. Moreover, it should be noted that reproductive complications following hysteroscopic adhesiolysis are proportional to the severity of the adhesions. Pregnancy following extensive adhesiolysis in a contracted cavity requires close antenatal and postnatal surveillance, as abnormal placentation may increase risks of miscarriage, growth restriction, prematurity, stillbirth, uterine rupture and postpartum haemorrhage (placenta accreta or percreta). These risks are lower with hysteroscopic compared with older open procedures, but women should be advised that adverse maternal and fetal outcomes may ensue. Modern miniature instrumentation (e.g. Versapoint) obviate the need for cervical dilatation, thereby reducing fears relating to iatrogenic cervical incompetence.

Postoperative management

Prophylactic use of antibiotics (e.g. 2 g amoxycillin + clavulonic acid) is not indicated routinely, but should probably be reserved for severe cases requiring extensive inpatient resection. Non-copper-bearing intrauterine contraceptive devices (e.g. for 4–6 weeks) or paediatric (8 F) balloon catheters (e.g. for 72 hours ± broad spectrum antibiotics) are employed by some to keep the raw dissected surfaces apart, thereby preventing re-adherence whilst healing takes place. Uterine splinting in this way is unnecessary in cases suitable for outpatient surgery. The use of postoperative oestrogen therapy (e.g. 30 µg ethinyloestradiol or 0.625 mg conjugated equine oestrogen) × 2–3 months with or without cyclic progestogens is recommended to encourage re-epithelialization of the scarred surfaces. Routine follow-up hysteroscopy after 3 months is advocated by some to monitor response to treatment and need for retreatment. However, it is best reserved following difficult or incomplete restoration of a normal cavity at initial (usually inpatient) surgery or if menstruation is not reinstated (10 per cent of cases).

CONGENITAL UTERINE ANOMALIES

Definition (hysteroscopic)

In both septate and bicornuate uteri, intervening tissue is discovered so that a two-chambered 'double' uterus is produced. A subseptate uterus (incomplete septum) is diagnosed if both tubal ostia are visible on either side of the dividing sagittal septum on panoramic, mid-line view (isthmic level). A septate uterus (complete septum) is diagnosed when only one tubal ostium is visible on panoramic view and this cannot be distinguished from a bicornuate uterus.

Epidemiology

The reported prevalence of congenital uterine anomalies is dependent upon the characteristics of the population studied and the tests and diagnostic criteria employed. Despite this heterogeneity, the overall prevalence is estimated to be between 3 and 5 per cent, and higher, but variable, rates have been reported in women with a history of recurrent miscarriage. The septate uterus is the most common (and important) of all structural anomalies with an estimated prevalence of 1 per cent in both fertile and infertile women, rising to approximately 3 per cent in women with a history of recurrent pregnancy loss. Environmental teratogens (e.g. diethylstiboestrol exposure) and genetic factors may be involved in a small number of cases.

Embryology and pathology

The uterus, tubes and upper vagina are formed embryologically from the Müllerian ducts. Congenital structural defects (Fig. 18.1) arise when these ducts fail to develop (e.g. unicornuate

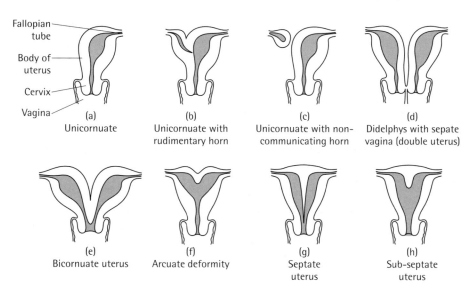

Figure 18.1 *Types of uterine anomalies. Only a septate or subseptate uterus is amenable to hysteroscopic surgery.*

uterus) or fuse properly (e.g. uterine septae). Various systems of classification exist (see Further reading, page 243). However, lateral fusion anomalies are the most commonly encountered and include the anomalies listed in Information Box 18.4.

The remainder of this section relates to the septate or subseptate uterus because this is the most common anomaly, may be associated with poor reproductive outcomes and is amenable to hysteroscopic surgery in the outpatient setting.

Presentation

Uterine septae may be detected at hysteroscopy as an incidental and usually clinically non-significant finding during investigation of women with abnormal uterine bleeding. The finding may however, be of significance if symptoms of abnormal bleeding and/or dysmenorrhoea persist despite adequate medical treatment. The hysteroscopic diagnosis of a uterine septum is potentially of greater significance if found in conjunction with a history of recurrent miscarriage. The relative avascularity and uterine distortion associated with septae are thought to result in defective embryonic implantation and explain the propensity to miscarriage in the first and second trimester. Premature delivery is also associated, and this may be the result of increased uterine pressure and cervical incompetence. The possible relationship between uterine septae and infertility remains the subject of debate.

Diagnosis

Hysteroscopy with or without directed biopsy is the gold standard for diagnosing intrauterine structural abnormalities such as uterine septae. Both a septate uterus and a bicornuate uterus will appear as two distinct uterine horns at hysteroscopy, but as with HSG, hysteroscopy is unable to differentiate between them, because this requires information about the serosal surface of the uterus. This can be acquired from transvaginal ultrasound. In both cases two separate endometrial echoes are clearly seen in transverse and sagittal planes for part of or all the uterine length. However, in contrast to the bicornuate uterus, the

Information Box 18.4 Congenital uterine anomalies

- *Arcuate shaped uterus.* After fusion of the Müllerian ducts, there is incomplete fundal resorption producing a flat-topped uterus without the usual fundal bulge.
- *Septate or subseptate uterus.* The two adjacent and fused Müllerian duct walls fail to break down leaving an intervening 'septum'. The uterus is outwardly normal, but contains a complete or incomplete septum depending upon the degree of resorption failure. The septae consist primarily of fibromuscular tissue with overlying endometrium that may be relatively insensitive to the effect of female sex steroids.
- *Bicornuate uterus.* There is a failure of fusion of all but the lower parts of the Müllerian ducts resulting in separate cornua.
- *Uterus didelphys.* The two Müllerian ducts fail to fuse so that the two halves of the uterus remain separate and each has its own cervix.

septate uterine contour appears convex and flattened with minimal fundal indentation (≤ 1 cm) and the cavity is seen to be divided by an echogenic structure. Diagnostic accuracy is high and may be improved with saline instillation or three-dimensional approaches or MRI. However, laparoscopy remains the most reliable method for assessment of the external uterine contour, and so determines suitability for hysteroscopic metroplasty.

Hysteroscopic characteristics

In both septate and bicornuate uteri a two-chambered uterus is discovered. A subseptate uterus (i.e. both tubal ostia visible on panoramic view) is easily diagnosed, but a complete or near complete dividing septum (i.e. only one tubal ostium visible) and bicornuate uterus can be overlooked. To minimize false negative diagnosis requires:

- a slow and systematic entry into the uterus under direct vision so that an additional entrance into another uterine chamber will be identified;
- suspecting the diagnosis when only one tubal ostia or cornual recess is seen in a narrow, cylindrically shaped uterus.

Approximately 20 per cent of septa are complete, 40 per cent occupy more than half the cavity length and 40 per cent less than half.

Treatment

INDICATIONS FOR SURGERY

Corrective surgery should be considered if septae are found in association with a history of poor reproductive performance, i.e. recurrent pregnancy loss (≥ 3 miscarriages) or extreme prematurity. Other causes amenable to treatment should have been excluded, particularly antiphospholipid syndrome. Women with a long-standing history of unexplained infertility may also be candidates for metroplasty, especially if >35 years old or in whom assisted reproductive techniques are being considered, although they should be counselled regarding the lack of data on effectiveness for this indication. Abnormal uterine bleeding or dysmenorrhoea refractory to medical therapy may also be a reasonable indication for intervention.

ROLE OF OUTPATIENT HYSTEROSCOPY

Outpatient hysteroscopy is useful to diagnose uterine malformations. However, although hysteroscopic correction of uterine defects ('metroplasty') is feasible in the outpatient setting, it is generally best performed using laparoscopic guidance under general anaesthesia. In selected cases, where anaesthesia presents significant risk or where a bicornuate uterus has been excluded with confidence (e.g. previous laparoscopy), careful and limited procedures may be performed, preferably combined with ultrasound imaging. A short précis of the general approach follows.

PREOPERATIVE PREPARATION

The patient needs to made fully aware regarding the limited evidence supporting the effectiveness of surgical intervention and the potential for adverse effects, namely iatrogenic adhesion formation. Consideration should be given to endometrial preparation with gonadotrophin-releasing hormone (GnRH) analogues (although this is generally unnecessary) or scheduling surgery in the proliferative phase in the case of complete septae, in order to minimize bleeding from the overlying endometrium.

SET-UP

As for hysteroscopic adhesiolysis.

INSTRUMENTS

The choice of instruments is the same as for hysteroscopic adhesiolysis. Mechanical dissection using semirigid scissors allows motion independent of the hysteroscope and is safe because thermal damage is avoided. Advocates also suggest that such damage to the endometrium predispose to adhesion formation, although this has not been substantiated. However, incision of thicker, vascular septae can be problematic and operating times prolonged. The cutting properties of Versapoint bipolar electrodes and low cost relative to laser fibres, make this technology particularly suited to septoplasty.

TECHNIQUE

The cornual recesses and both sides of the septum should be identified to facilitate spacial orientation. The septum should be incised mid-way between anterior and posterior uterine walls and the fibromuscular tissue will be seen to retract into the surrounding endometrium. A progressive 'thinning' technique (i.e. sequential bites on alternate sides along one plane) may need to be employed if thick septae are being dissected with mechanical instruments. Dissection should be continued along the central uterine axis until the fundal endometrium is reached. The correct dissection level is confirmed when both tubal ostia can be viewed simultaneously and the hysteroscope can be manoeuvred from one cornual recess to the other without intervening obstruction. Bleeding will occur if the fundal myometrium is penetrated, and dissection should cease immediately. Indeed, a residual <1 cm septum is unlikely to impair reproductive performance, so a conservative approach should be adopted to avoid uterine perforation (especially if the procedure is undertaken in the outpatient setting without laparoscopic guidance). Care should be taken if you are using the Versapoint technology, as dissection by vaporization is rapidly achieved (Plate 21). Surgical complications are as described for hysteroscopic adhesiolysis. An increased risk of uterine rupture during future singleton pregnancies has not been substantiated following uncomplicated hysteroscopic septoplasty, and so elective Caesarean section is not indicated for this reason.

POSTOPERATIVE CARE

Antibiotics, insertion of intrauterine devices and hormonal administration are used by some operators in an attempt to reduce adhesion formation and encourage rapid re-epithelialization. Evidence for benefit is lacking and so such postoperative manoeuvres are probably unnecessary in the case of uterine septae. It seems sensible to delay attempts at conceiving for a short period (e.g. two cycles) to allow healing. Some recommend follow-up examination after 1–2 months using hysteroscopy, TVS or HSG to check the operative result and exclude adhesion formation. Adhesion formation is rare and so such follow-up is only indicated if surgery was complicated or incomplete.

UTERINE HYPOPLASIA

This is a rarer congenital malformation due to incomplete development of both Müllerian ducts and is associated with reproductive failure. It is diagnosed at hysteroscopy when a small, cylindrical uterine cavity (typically uterine length <6 cm) is detected. Often the contracted uterus takes on a 'T-shape', with well formed cornual recesses, but a tubular uterine body, making the ostia difficult to access.

This malformation is amenable to hysteroscopic treatment using bipolar electrosurgery (Versapoint) and small, uncontrolled studies have suggested improved reproductive outcomes. Two metroplastic techniques have been described (similar to myometrial scoring described above) both with the aim of increasing uterine capacity and restoring a triangular uterine shape. One approach involves incising each lateral wall of the uterus (5–7 mm depth, 130 W power output) from fundus to isthmus, and the other describes a deeper myometrial incision (10 mm, 80 W power output) into the fundus between both ostia under transabdominal ultrasound guidance. Although these procedures are simple and rapid, there are no reports of them being attempted in an outpatient setting. Conscious sedation or general anaesthesia is probably required because of anticipated discomfort arising from myometrial incision.

HYSTEROSCOPIC MYOMECTOMY

This technique is dealt with in detail in Chapter 16.

It is generally believed that distortion of the uterine cavity by submucous fibroids may impair implantation and account for infertility and recurrent pregnancy loss in some women. This relationship is contentious and perhaps too simplistic when we consider recent evidence suggesting that intramural fibroids without cavity alteration are associated with reduced *in vitro* fertilization (IVF) pregnancy and ongoing pregnancy rates. Surgery should be restricted to women without other explanations for infertility and pregnancy loss and considered prior to or after failed IVF treatment.

If hysteroscopic resection of submucous fibroids is undertaken as a fertility-promoting procedure, care should be taken to avoid extensive endometrial damage in order to retain as much functional endometrium as possible and avoid adhesion formation. This is achieved primarily by limiting surgery to discrete fibroids with significant cavity distortion, targeting the surgical field precisely and avoiding lateral thermal spread and charring from unnecessary application of dampened coagulation current.

HYSTEROSCOPIC POLYPECTOMY

This technique is dealt with in detail in Chapter 15.

Polyps are common, hysteroscopic removal generally straightforward and adverse effects on reproductive function unlikely. However, their association with infertility is weak unless cornual and causing proximal tubal blockage. Larger polyps are likely to be of more significance and reduced success rates of IVF have been reported if they are >2 cm in diameter, although this evidence is methodologically poor.

Evidence box 18.1 Hysteroscopic interventions for uterine anomalies associated with reproductive dysfunction

The evaluation of hysteroscopic interventions for the treatment of congenital or acquired uterine structural anomalies is problematic. This is because the validity and transferability of available evidence is questionable. All data to date are derived from small, mostly retrospective observational series with inadequate follow-up. Without control of confounding variables, particularly population characteristics and disease spectrum, significant selection bias results, which limits the strength of inferences to take into clinical practice. Hysteroscopic metroplasty and adhesiolysis appear to increase the likelihood of a successful pregnancy (liveborn child) in women with a poor reproductive history (infertility and recurrent miscarriage). The reproductive prognosis is, however, better for recurrent miscarriage than for infertility. Hysteroscopic myomectomy and polypectomy do not appear to have a detrimental effect on reproductive outcome and may be associated with improved fertility and success of *in vitro* fertilization techniques.

KEY POINTS

- Outpatient hysteroscopy is the gold standard tool for diagnosing intrauterine structural lesions and is useful in assessing suitability for surgery in the appropriate setting.

- Hysteroscopic adhesiolysis, metroplasty, myomectomy and polypectomy aim to restore the uterine cavity towards normal and improve reproductive outcome.

- Modern bipolar electrosurgical systems (Versapoint) appear to be an effective alternative to traditional instruments and energy sources.

- Evidence for the effectiveness of such treatment in improving fertility and reducing pregnancy loss is weak.

- Other causes for pregnancy loss and infertility should be excluded before embarking on surgery for uterine anomalies.

- Potentially serious intraoperative complications may occur as well as adverse reproductive outcomes.

FURTHER READING

Al-Inany H. Intrauterine adhesions. *Acta Obstet Gynecol Scand* 2001;**80**:986–93.

Fernandez H, Gervaise A, de Tayrac R. Operative hysteroscopy for infertility using normal saline solution and a coaxial bipolar electrode: a pilot study. *Hum Reprod* 2000;**15**:1773–5.

Homer HA, Li TC, Cooke ID. The septate uterus: a review of management and reproductive outcome. *Fertil Steril* 2000;**73**:1–14.

Lee A, Ying YK, Novy MJ. Hysteroscopy and hysterosalpingography and tubal ostial polyps in infertility patients. *J Reprod Med* 1997;**42**:337–41.

Shushan A, Rojansky N. Should hysteroscopy be part of the basic infertility work-up? *Hum Reprod* 1999;**14**:1923–4.

Fertility control

The outpatient hysteroscopy clinic is playing an increasingly prominent role in many aspects of female contraceptive management. This development has occurred for two main reasons. The first of these reflects advances in methods of fertility control, namely hysteroscopic sterilization and intrauterine contraceptive devices (IUCDs). Outpatient hysteroscopic sterilization provides effective, safe and permanent control of women's fertility in a convenient setting (Chapter 2). The effectiveness and tolerability of IUCDs have improved, and the hysteroscopy clinic setting facilitates fitting of such devices. In particular, effective local cervical anaesthesia can be administered and adverse uterine anatomy can be overcome (e.g. narrow cervical canals or acutely flexed uteri). Fig. 19.1 compares the traditional

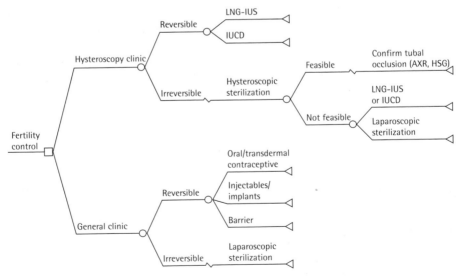

Figure 19.1 *Comparison of contraceptive care pathways: outpatient hysteroscopic versus general gynaecological clinic. AXR: abdominal X-ray.*

contraceptive care pathway in a general gynaecology clinic setting with that offered within an outpatient hysteroscopy clinic set-up.

Second, outpatient hysteroscopy is a useful modality for investigating and managing complications arising from the use of both hormonal and non-hormonal contraceptive methods. These include assessment of the endometrial cavity if there is abnormal genital tract bleeding and retrieval of lost IUCDs.

INTRAUTERINE DEVICES

The available devices are listed in Table 19.1. The main mode of action of copper-bearing devices relates to the direct toxic effect of copper ions upon sperm and ova. The IUCD also promotes a foreign body reaction resulting in endometrial changes that impair fertility. The levonorgestrel-releasing IUCD (Mirena) acts mainly by thickening cervical mucus and preventing endometrial proliferation. In some cycles ovulation may be suppressed and its physical presence may also contribute to the overall contraceptive effect.

COPPER INTRAUTERINE DEVICES (COILS)

Copper-containing IUCDs typically comprise a plastic frame loaded with copper wire and/or copper sleeves. Although insertion of the available copper-bearing IUCDs varies slightly, the general approach (history, examination and insertion) is as described in Chapter 13. Additional important points to consider and discuss with the woman are listed below.

Pelvic infection

Outside of high-risk populations (high disease prevalence), a policy of routine antibiotic prophylaxis to prevent ascending pelvic infection and its sequelae is not supported by the available evidence. Genital tract swabs should be taken in the presence of purulent discharge, cervicitis or pelvic tenderness, insertion of the IUCD should be deferred and antibiotic treatment instigated in accordance with microbiology results. Selective screening of women for genital tract infection (prevalence of asymptomatic chlamydial infection is 3–6 per cent, higher with multiple sexual partners) should also be considered. All women should be informed of pelvic infection risks outside of mutually monogamous relationships.

Table 19.1 *Reversible intrauterine contraceptive devices ('IUCDs')*

Intrauterine device	Type	Failure rate at 1 year	Licensed duration
Multiload Cu 250	Copper (generation II)	1–2 per 100 users	3 years
Nova-T 200	Copper (generation II)	1–2 per 100 users	5 years
Multiload Cu 375	Copper (generation III)	<1 per 100 users	5 years
Nova-T 380	Copper (generation III)	<1 per 100 users	5 years
Gyne T 380	Copper (generation III)	<1 per 100 users	10 years
Gynefix	Copper (frameless)	<1 per 100 users	5 years
Mirena	Hormonal	<1 per 100 users	5 years

Timing of insertion

Although IUCD insertion may be easier during or shortly after menstruation because the cervix is soft and the os open, it can be easily fitted at any time of the menstrual cycle. However, the luteal phase should be avoided unless the possibility of pregnancy can be confidently excluded.

Follow-up

Women should be given written information and shown what the device looks like so that it can be recognized if expelled. They should be instructed and advised to self-examine on a monthly basis in order to check for threads. The patient should be re-examined by her general practitioner 6 weeks after insertion and once a year afterwards, or more frequently if clinically indicated (e.g. threads not felt).

Effectiveness

Failure rates are low (Table 19.1). Ectopic pregnancies are more likely in the event of pregnancy (5–10 per cent).

Side effects

These are shown in Information Box 19.1 and occur in 30 per cent of users. Between 4 and 15 per cent of IUCDs have to be removed at 1 year because of side effects.

GENERAL POINTS

Indications

The IUCD is popular in older, parous women who want to space or have completed their family. However, it is also an acceptable choice of contraceptive for young, nulliparous women in stable relationships, where risk of infection is low. Fitting in the hysteroscopy clinic, with access to local anaesthetics and cervical dilators, is straightforward.

Contraindications

These are as for the levonorgestrel intrauterine system (LNG-IUS) (see Chapter 13).

 Information Box 19.1   Side effects of copper intrauterine contraceptive devices

- *Uterine insertion problems.* Expulsion (2–8 per cent at 1 year) and perforation (1 per 1000 insertions)
- *Menstrual problems.* Increased menstrual loss and worsening dysmenorrhoea
- *Pelvic infection.* Low prevalence (equivalent to background rate) in carefully counselled and selected women. Acute infection with *Actinomyces*-like organisms is rare

Copper IUCD versus LNG-IUS

It should be borne in mind that the IUCD is a cheap, immediately reversible, well-tolerated and effective contraceptive. Although the LNG-IUS has superseded it in women with associated menstrual disturbances, the LNG-IUS is no more effective than the third-generation IUCDs (bearing more copper), is more expensive and has a different side effect profile, which may be less tolerable.

REMOVAL

Removal of IUCDs is not uncommon in hysteroscopy clinics – prior to undertaking intra-uterine surgery and when retrieving 'lost coils'. Although it is advisable to remove IUCDs at the time of menstruation in order to avoid an ensuing pregnancy, this is rarely practical. Ideally, women should be advised to avoid sexual intercourse or use barrier contraception 7 days prior to planned removal. Removal without replacement is not advised otherwise.

FRAMELESS (GYNEFIX)

This is a frameless copper IUCD, which has been available in the UK since 1998. It comprises a polypropylene thread onto which six copper sleeves ($330\,mm^2$) are threaded. A single knot at the upper end of the thread acts as a retention body to anchor the device within the fundal myometrium following insertion. The Gynefix was developed to overcome problems and limitations associated with traditional IUCDs, namely expulsion and placement within irregular cavities, e.g. fibroids (anchoring technology) and poor compliance because of side effects such as pain and bleeding (small size).

Insertion technique

The Gynefix (marks I and II) insertion apparatus consists of the four parts: a plastic uterine sound, a calibrated insertion tube with flange, a plunger (plastic rod + distal stylet, which contains a 'notch' that carries the anchoring knot) and the Gynefix device (which comes preloaded within the insertion tube). The woman is positioned in the standard way, the cervix is cleaned and a tenaculum applied to the anterior cervical lip. The uterus is sounded using the sterile sound provided and the inserter is then introduced to the level of the uterine fundus. The plunger is then gently advanced for 1 cm so that the stylet and anchoring knot penetrate the myometrium. The thread is then released from the notch, while the operator holds the inserter against the fundus. The handle is then withdrawn while the insertion tube is kept pressed against the uterine fundus. The insertion tube is then withdrawn (rotating movements with the mark II device). Gentle traction on the tail of the Gynefix provides confirmation that the anchor is correctly inserted. The thread is then trimmed 2–3 cm below the cervix. Correct positioning can be checked with an ultrasound scan if there is doubt, and the device removed by gentle traction. As fitting differs from other IUCDs, the manufacturers do not recommend prescription and fitting of Gynefix by any doctor who has not received the Gynefix training certificate.

Evidence

Data to date show that the frameless device performs similarly to traditional copper IUCDs (Cu380A) in terms of efficacy, expulsions, acceptability (rates of continued use) and adverse effects. Published rates of insertion failure (<1 per cent) and uterine perforation (0 per cent) are low in specialist centres.

Indications, counselling and follow-up

These are generally as for the copper-framed IUCDs. Women should be advised to abstain from intercourse or from the use of tampons for 5 days. The frameless IUCD may be more suitable in women with previously expelled IUCDs, women with irregular cavities and nulliparous women (small uterine cavities) who may experience more pain with larger IUCDs.

INTRAUTERINE SYSTEM (MIRENA)

Insertion

This is described in detail in Chapter 13.

Efficacy

Studies have shown that the failure rate is about 0.2 per 100 woman-years (two failures per 1000 users per year), even in young women. Expulsion rates, perforation rates and discontinuation rates are as for copper IUCDs. Its licensed duration of use is 5 years. A frameless device may be available soon (Fibroplant levonorgestrel IUS).

Indications

These are as for the copper IUCD. The LNG-IUS is particularly useful in women with excessive and/or erratic menstrual bleeding, dysmenorrhoea and those at risk of endometrial hyperplasia (polycystic ovarian syndrome, obesity). It should also suitable in women with contraindications to the combined oral contraceptive or sterilization procedures (medical conditions posing anaesthetic risks).

Contraindications

These are as outlined in Chapter 13.

Counselling (side effects)

This is as outlined in the section above and Chapter 13. In order to optimize compliance with the LNG-IUS, women should be made aware of its:

- excellent contraceptive properties in terms of its safety, effectiveness, reversibility and local action;
- non-contraceptive benefits such as reduction in menstrual loss and dysmenorrhoea;
- progestogenic side effects (experienced by 20–50 per cent of women as a result of some systemic absorption);

- potential for inducing amenorrhoea (this is one of the main reasons for discontinuation of use because many women may not view absence of menstrual bleeding as a positive health benefit, but rather as a threat to their femininity; women should be informed that amenorrhoea occurs in 20–50 per cent of women after 1 year of use, and is not indicative of pregnancy (failure rates are low), oestrogen deficiency or menopause);

- association with unscheduled light bleeding or discharge for the initial 3–6 months (one in five women may experience more persistent vaginal spotting, but this normally resolves so that rate of unscheduled bleeding is no higher than for the background population).

Follow-up

This should be as for copper IUCDs.

LOST THREADS

Recourse to a general anaesthetic to retrieve IUCDs from the uterine cavity is an anachronism. It is only indicated in the rare situation where outpatient removal has failed. The following approach is recommended:

Urinary pregnancy test

This should be performed if pregnancy is suspected from the history.

Pelvic ultrasound scan

A transvaginal ultrasound should be carried out to exclude expulsion of the IUCD and confirm its location and presence within the uterine cavity (Fig. 19.2).

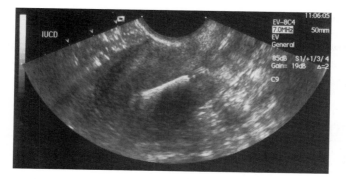

Figure 19.2 *Correctly sited intrauterine device as seen on transvaginal ultrasound. A bright, linear echo is seen within the uterine cavity (IUCD frame) extending from the uterine fundus towards the isthmus where the threads are seen.*

Abdominal X-ray

In the unusual circumstance where perforation into the peritoneal cavity is suspected (suggestive or negative ultrasound scan in combination with a history of acute/chronic pelvic pain or other contemporaneous urinary or gastrointestinal symptoms), an abdominal X-ray is indicated after acquiring a negative pregnancy test. This will show up both copper-bearing IUCDs and the LNG-IUS, which contains barium for this reason.

Exploration of the cervical canal

In 50 per cent of referred cases, a hysteroscopy is not required. The woman should be positioned in the standard fashion and once the cervix has been cleaned, the cervical canal should be gently probed with narrow artery forceps (e.g. long-handled Spencer–Wells forceps). The threads are invariably grasped and the IUCD easily removed and replaced as required.

Hysteroscopic retrieval

A diagnostic outpatient hysteroscopy should be performed, the threads identified and the IUCD removed under direct vision using grasping forceps passed down a working channel (Plate 22). The hysteroscope, grasper and IUCD are removed as a single unit. Even if the IUCD is correctly sited at the uterine fundus, removal and replacement is advisable to avoid further inconvenience to the patient. Occasionally slight cervical dilatation is required to achieve withdrawal of the IUCD from the uterine cavity. The IUCD may be removed if it is partially embedded, but recourse to general anaesthesia may be required to insert heavier instruments. The IUCD can occasionally be embedded entirely within the uterine wall (cavity is noted to be empty or only the threads are visible), and in this situation laparoscopic removal is indicated.

Exploration of the uterine cavity (blind)

An alternative approach is to instrument the uterine cavity blindly using disposable, plastic thread retrievers (e.g. Emmett or Retrievette), specially designed IUCD-retrieving forceps/hooks or polyp forceps (requires cervical dilatation). None of these approaches are recommended where facilities to achieve removal under direct hysteroscopic vision are available.

HYSTEROSCOPIC STERILIZATION

HISTORY

Female sterilization is the most commonly used method of fertility control in developed countries and is widespread in the developing world. Tubal occlusion is most commonly performed transabdominally via laparoscopy. However, since the advent of hysteroscopy, interest has been shown in developing transcervical methods of permanent birth control, thereby avoiding the risks of an incisional approach under anaesthesia. Three techniques to effect tubal blockage (interstitial portion) were developed during the 1970s and 1980s:

- destruction by thermal energy (electrocoagulation or cryosurgery);
- injection with sclerosing agents or tissue adhesives;
- mechanical occlusion with various plugs and devices.

All developed techniques were limited by various factors relating to feasibility, acceptability, safety and effectiveness.

PRESENT

The translation of hysteroscopic sterilization from an attractive concept to a practical reality seems at last to be taking place following the development of the Essure Permanent Birth Control System (Conceptus Inc, San Carlos, CA, USA). Other systems are currently being developed (e.g. bipolar electrodiathermy, mechanical, potentially reversible, atraumatic occlusive screws and intraluminal plugs). However, the Essure system is the only commercially available hysteroscopic method of permanent birth control. Approval for its use has been granted by the Food and Drug Administration (FDA) agency in the US and by National Institute for Clinical Excellence (NICE) in the UK, based on available published data. The remainder of this chapter describes use of this system in the outpatient setting.

ESSURE SYSTEM

Micro-insert

The micro-insert consists of a reinforced (antikinking) dynamic outer coil (nickel titanium alloy) within which is contained a flexible inner coil (stainless steel) along and through which runs a layer of polyethylene terephthalate (PET, Dacron) fibres (Plate 23). The outer coil expands to anchor the micro-insert within the intramural and proximal isthmic portions of the fallopian tube and the PET fibres induce a benign localized tissue response consisting of inflammation and fibrosis, which leads to obliteration and occlusion of the tubal lumen over a 3-month period, and permanent placement of the micro-insert. Permanent contraception is thus achieved.

Delivery components

During insertion, the micro-insert is maintained in a wound-down configuration by a release catheter, which is enclosed by a transparent hydrophilic delivery catheter to improve tracking along the fallopian tube. A guide wire is attached to the inner coil to facilitate device placement, and the entire system is attached to a handle (which consists of a thumbwheel and release button) designed to allow single-handed release of the micro-insert (Plate 23).

Preprocedure

Any woman requesting permanent fertility control must be adequately counselled and written informed consent obtained. A comprehensive medical history is required with particular attention paid to the past medical, obstetric and contraceptive history and known allergies (Information Box 19.2). Studies have demonstrated that around 3 per cent of women attending for sterilization are already pregnant. Therefore, in order to reduce the risk of failing to detect current or imminent (luteal phase) pregnancies and subsequent litigation, the date of the last menstrual period should be recorded and a negative urinary pregnancy test obtained. Continued use of hormonal contraception, or abstinence from sexual intercourse if relying on barrier methods during the menstrual cycle immediately preceding scheduled sterilization should be confirmed. The phase of the menstrual cycle is not generally important (although the proliferative phase may be preferred from a visualization/pregnancy point of view). Operations should be rescheduled if dates coincide with heavy menstrual flow.

 Information Box 19.2 Counselling for hysteroscopic sterilization (This should be backed up by a written information leaflet – see Chapter 20.)

INFORMATION SHOULD BE GIVEN AND SPECIFIC CONSENT SOUGHT UNDER THESE HEADINGS:

- *Appropriateness.* Take a detailed history to ascertain relative and absolute contra-indications to hysteroscopic sterilization (uncertain of desire for permanent birth control, anatomical anomalies, uterine neoplasia, acute or past history of pelvic infection, unexplained abnormal uterine bleeding, history of chronic pelvic pain, severe dysmenorrhoea or dyspareunia, prior tubal surgery, ongoing endometrial, tubal or ovarian pathology, allergy to contrast media, hypersensitivity to nickel confirmed by skin test, and inability to understand or comply with procedure and follow-up).
- *Awareness of alternative contraceptive methods.* Discuss alternative forms of contraception, (appropriateness, advantages, disadvantages, comparative failure rates) with emphasis placed on reversible long-term forms of contraception (injections, implants and coils) and male sterilization (vasectomy) to ensure that the woman is adequately informed of all options.
- *New method of female sterilization approved and licensed in the United Kingdom.*
- *Comparison with traditional laparoscopic sterilization.* Inform the woman about established laparoscopic sterilization under general anaesthesia. Discuss advantages of hysteroscopic sterilization over traditional laparoscopic methods:
  - possibly shorter waiting times
  - avoidance of risks and inconvenience of general anaesthetic and inpatient stay
  - quick
  - no scars
  - rapid return to work/normal daily activities).

Discuss disadvantages compared with laparoscopic sterilization:

- technical non-feasibility higher 10–15 per cent (compared with 1–2 per cent for laparoscopic sterilization)
- post-procedural contraception required for 3 months until mandatory radiographic imaging has confirmed correct bilateral device placement (abdominal X-ray) ±tubal occlusion (hysterosalpingogram)
- in 1–5 per cent tubal blockage will not be demonstrated, resulting in the need for either repeat imaging at 6 months (as tubal blockage may be confirmed as long as both devices are within the tubes) or alternate forms of contraception/sterilization.

Emphasize that sterilization is meant to be a permanent, non-reversible method of contraception. Tubal reconstruction is not possible following hysteroscopic sterilization if the woman regrets her decision at a later date leaving *in vitro* fertilization as the only solution with uncertain success rates under such circumstances.

- *Evidence of effectiveness and safety.* Evidence regarding its effectiveness (post-procedure pregnancy rate) and effect on long-term health is less well known as it is a new procedure compared to laparoscopic sterilization where more is known. Provisional studies show low post-procedural pregnancy rates (no pregnancies recorded in 9620 women-months, mean follow-up 21.4 months). Rates may thus be comparable to the 1 in 200 lifetime failure rate (pregnancy can occur several years after the procedure), quoted for laparoscopic sterilization. No major complications have been reported. The main risks are of device expulsion, uterine perforation, unsatisfactory micro-insert placement and severe pain/bleeding. As with laparoscopic sterilization the risk of ectopic pregnancy is high with ineffective procedures, which can compromise long-term health.

- *Preprocedural information.* No need for fasting (if sedation not used). Premedication required with non-steroidal analgesics (oral or rectal). Need for contraception before the procedure as no precautions can be guaranteed to avoid preprocedure fertilization, which may be undetectable; abstinence advisable during the menstrual cycle immediately preceding sterilization if non-hormonal methods of contraception used. The procedure will have to be postponed if patient is menstruating heavily as visualization is impaired.

- *Procedural information.* Most women will experience period-like cramping pain during and for some time after the procedure. However, pre- and postoperative analgesics and perioperative local anaesthesia ± sedation will minimize any discomfort, which is usually mild and short-lived (home within 1–2 hours return to work within 48 hours). Pain and vaginal bleeding and technical failure are the main complications of the procedure. Reassure women that there are no substantial long-term health risks from sterilization procedures to date.

- *Technical failure.* Appropriate alternative methods should be discussed in advance in case the intended hysteroscopic method cannot be successfully completed (10 per cent of cases). This should include fitting of an intrauterine contraceptive device/system as default, repeating the procedure again where appropriate (in cases of unilateral device placement where poor visualization or tubal spasm prevented bilateral device placement), or choosing an alternate approach to achieve sterilization (laparoscopic tubal occlusion or vasectomy).

- *Post-procedure information.* Discuss:
    - resolution of any period-like pain (<24 hours) and blood-stained vaginal loss (<15 days);
    - still having periods – should not be adversely affected by the sterilization procedure in the long term;
    - need for continued contraception for at least 3 months to allow tubal fibrotic occlusion to take place;
    - radiographic imaging at 3 months to confirm correct device placement/tubal occlusion before all clear is given and contraception can be discontinued.

---

i Information Box 19.3 Basic requirements for set-up for outpatient hysteroscopic sterilization

- Operative hysteroscopy set-up (see Chapter 3)
- Specula (open sided and Sim's)
- Atraumatic tenaculum forceps
- Cervical dilatation set
- Continuous flow hysteroscope with a minimum 5 F (1.67 mm) operative channel
- Saline (3-l bag recommended) and inflow/outflow tubing ± suction apparatus
- Video endoscopy system
- Video recording facility (optional)
- Essure procedure kit

Preoperative analgesia 30–60 minutes prior to the procedure using non-steroidal anti-inflammatory drugs (e.g. diclofenac 100 mg rectal suppository, 500 mg oral mefenamic acid, 20 mg piroxicam buccally) will help reduce visceral pain and optimize rates of successful placement by two- to three-fold. Routine screening for genital tract infection and/or selective or universal use of prophylactic antibiotics is not required unless infection or medical conditions dictate such a policy.

Procedure – positioning and set-up

The patient should be placed in the lithotomy position with slight (15°) downward Trendelenburg tilt. Confirm that the buttocks are right at the end of the couch and her hips are adequately flexed and abducted to optimize the capacity of hysteroscopic movement. Patient positioning is crucial to achieve high procedure completion rates because lateral tubal ostia, especially in association with acute degrees of uterine flexion/version can present problems unless wide degrees of hysteroscopic manipulation are possible. The equipment set-up required for outpatient hysteroscopic sterilization is shown in Information Box 19.3.

Screening hysteroscopy

TECHNIQUE

Clean the cervix with saline or antiseptic solution, followed by a direct cervical or paracervical nerve block with a quick-acting local anaesthetic (e.g. lidocaine 1 per cent, prilocaine 3 per cent). Optimal visualization is very important for this procedure and so attention must be paid to minimizing trauma to the fragile endocervical and endometrial mucosa. With this in mind, there is no need to routinely dilate the cervix, although a tenaculum placed at 12 o'clock on the anterior cervical lip helps with insertion of the 5 mm rigid scope under direct vision with normal saline running. Remember to adjust the direction of the hysteroscope in keeping with the angle of view (30°) as discussed in chapter 4. A 3-l bag of saline (alternatively two 1-l bags plus a Y-connector), fed under gravity or pressure (not to exceed 150 mmHg) is recommended. This will avoid delays resulting from the need to change bags of distension media. Although physiological saline is used, fluid deficit should not exceed 1500 ml.

EXCLUDE PATHOLOGY AND CONFIRM FEASIBILITY

Inspect the uterine cavity to exclude endometrial pathology and confirm the feasibility of the procedure (i.e. adequate visibility, both tubal ostia identified, absence of structural anomalies precluding successful bilateral device placement, e.g. fibroids, polyps and congenital malformations or other adverse anatomical features such as lateral tubal location, acute uterine axis). Note that stenosis of the tubal ostia preventing successful cannulation cannot readily be predicted by visualization alone, although it may be suspected if the woman has a past history of endometritis. As with all outpatient conscious procedures, efficiency is essential to optimize success. In our experience, hysteroscopic sterilization is not particularly uncomfortable for the patient (i.e. no need for sedation), but endometrial fluid absorption (oedema) can compromise visualization of the remaining tubal ostia if the early part of the procedure is unduly prolonged. Thus diagnostic hysteroscopy should be short so as to allow maximum operative time (seize the 'window of opportunity'). Standard fluid absorption monitoring procedures should be followed.

Sterilization procedure

The procedure involves three stages:

- tubal access
- device deployment and anchoring
- withdrawal of delivery system.

TUBAL ACCESS

A plastic split introducer is placed in the 5 Fr (1.7 mm internal diameter) operative channel of a 5 mm 30° hysteroscope. The Essure system is fed along the operating channel via the introducer. Each tubal ostia is visualized with the hysteroscope in very close proximity to it so that as the fragile system appears within the uterus from within the operating channel, it is stabilized and directed towards the tubal opening. Accessing the tube is potentially the most tricky part of the procedure and tubal access is likely to fail or be unduly prolonged

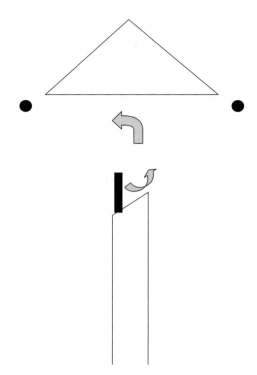

Figure 19.3 *Rotation of the hysteroscope can be used to help direct the micro-insert into laterally sited tubal ostia.*

without closely approximating the hysteroscope and the tube. Lateralized ostia can present difficulties in achieving this, and rotation of the hysteroscope may help (Fig. 19.3).

DEVICE DEPLOYMENT AND ANCHORING

The system is inserted until a black positioning marker on the delivery catheter is reached. The micro-insert is then released by retraction and detachment of the catheter delivery system (Fig. 19.4). This involves rotating the thumbwheel to withdraw the delivery catheter (positioning marker will be seen to move back). This is followed by pressing the release button and further use of the thumbwheel to withdraw the release catheter, thereby allowing expansion of the outer coil. This expansion serves to anchor the micro-insert in the tubal lumen (spans the intramural and proximal isthmic portions of the fallopian tube – Fig. 19.5). Permanent placement of the micro-insert is achieved upon subsequent fibrous tissue ingrowth.

Optimal positioning of the insert occurs when 3–8 mm of the proximal end of the micro-insert is visible at the ostium (three to eight intrauterine coils visible – Plate 24). The most important factors to ensure correct placement of the micro-insert are:

• Stabilize the handle during withdrawal of the delivery catheter (otherwise distal placement is likely because of inadvertent 'feed forward'). Although the system is designed for single operator use, less experienced operators should consider directing

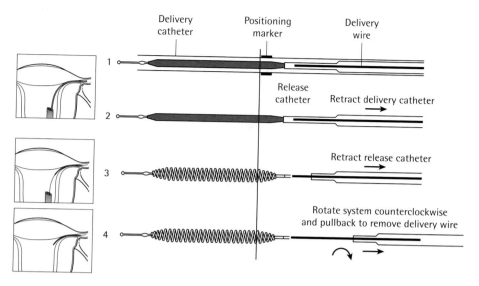

Figure 19.4 *Essure hysteroscopic sterilization system: schematic representation of procedure. (Reproduced with kind permission of Conceptus Inc.)*

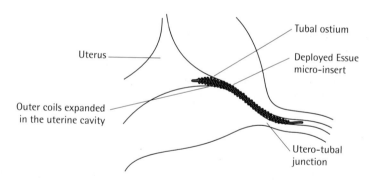

Figure 19.5 *Essure hysteroscopic sterilization system: Illustration showing micro-insert in situ. This cross-sectional view of the uterus and fallopian tube shows the device placed across the uterotubal junction (external).*

an assistant to manoeuvre the thumbwheel and release button, whilst the operator concentrates on system stabilization and tubal visualization.

- Ensure the device is straight and properly positioned prior to withdrawing the release catheter and expanding the outer coil. This is achieved by having <1 cm of the insert trailing within the uterine cavity and having the orange release catheter (immediately behind the insert) in view. A notch, representing the initial part of the wound down outer coil, can be visualized with experience. This should be situated just outside the ostium less than half way between it and the orange release catheter. Fine adjustment can be made at this stage.

WITHDRAWAL OF DELIVERY SYSTEM

Finally, the guide wire is detached and removed by anticlockwise rotation and gentle retraction on feeling its release from the micro-insert.

Procedural tips

In order to facilitate placement of the fragile micro-inserts, the procedure requires good visualization of the tubal ostia and the tip of the hysteroscope to be positioned in very close proximity to them. Most technical problems result from an inability to optimally site the hysteroscope, or the related problem of obscured visualization of the ostia from oedematous or ragged and fragmented endometrium. Information Box 19.4 details potential problems and strategies to overcome them.

 Information Box 19.4 Outpatient hysteroscopic sterilization: troubleshooting (also refer to Chapter 4)

- *Pain.* Minimize by preoperative patient preparation and analgesia; use of local anaesthetic; a delegated nurse to act as a 'vocal-local'; minimum effective distension pressure (<150 mmHg); direct vision to minimize tissue trauma and bleeding; adequate communication; speed and gentle tissue handling. Abandon if a single tubal cannulation attempt takes >20 minutes.
- *Adverse anatomy* (acute uterine axis, lateral tubal ostia, obesity, intracavity anomalies). Careful attention to patient positioning can help minimize failure associated with lateral tubes, acute degrees of uterine flexion/version and obesity. Confirm patient buttocks are right at the end of the couch and hips are adequately flexed and abducted to optimize the capacity for hysteroscopic movement. Use a tenaculum to straighten the acute angulation between cervix and uterus. The operating couch will need to be lowered for acutely retroverted uteri. Consider access to the cervical canal using a Sim's speculum or via vaginoscopy so that manoeuvrability of the hysteroscope is optimized. Rotation of the hysteroscope may be necessary to optimize ease of cannulation (Figure 19.3, page 256). Lowering uterine distension pressure may also help access to lateralized tubal ostia. Intracavity anomalies obscuring tubal ostia will need hysteroscopically removing.
- *Suboptimal view.* Optimize visualization by using the minimum effective distension pressure (a 3-l bag avoids delays that may be necessary using 1-l bags of fluid, which may need changing); adequate assistance to optimize efficiency and avoid ensuing endometrial congestion; direct vision to minimize tissue trauma and bleeding, and adequate patient positioning.
- *Suboptimal view of tubal ostia* (pin-point ostia, covered with filmy endometrial tissue, ragged endometrium or debris, clots). The procedure should be abandoned if both tubal ostia cannot be seen. In cases where ostial visualization is suboptimal or there is some uncertainty regarding their location (e.g. artefactual appearance arising from previous

uterine instrumentation or infection), then gentle probing with the device tip or a 5 Fr instrument is indicated. In such circumstances, it is important to proceed only if minimal resistance is encountered, and also to obtain panoramic views before releasing the device to confirm that it is correctly sited within the tube and not bent back on itself into the uterine cavity. Tubes obscured by endometrial tissue can also be probed gently, and/or hysteroscopic graspers/catheters introduced to clear.

- *Endometrial congestion.* Endometrial oedema can lead to inadequate tubal visualization. Endometrial oedema is more likely to occur with prolonged procedures (especially in the luteal phase of the menstrual cycle) and with high uterine distension pressures. Speed and the use of minimum effective instillation pressures minimize the incidence of this problem. If this problem is encountered it is usually during attempted placement of the second device. In this situation, rather than persevere and risk losing the patient's confidence, an attempt at a later date is advisable (two-stage procedure required in about 5–10 per cent of cases) and this is easily understood and accepted by the patient who can see the procedure on the video screen.

- *Difficult tubal cannulation* (stenosis, tortuosity, spasm or lateral position of tubal ostia). Check optimal patient positioning. Gently probe the ostia by applying constant but very gentle forward pressure to help overcome resistance from tubal spasm/stenosis. Check the device is straight and avoid bending and consequently irreversibly damaging the fragile device (necessitating a new one). Check the angle of entry and adjust the scope/device tip to optimize this. Adjust the scope relative to the micro-insert to stabilize it and keep the scope in close proximity to the ostia to prevent bending. Abandon procedure if any encountered tubal resistance is not easily overcome, as perforation likely.

- *Incorrectly placed device.*
    - *Distally placed* (<3 intrauterine coils visible). Inadvertent forward movement of the micro-insert can easily occur if the system is not stabilized during retraction of the delivery catheter. This can be recognized if the orange segment and notch are not in view and can be corrected by pulling back the system to the proper position before deployment.
    - *Proximally placed* (>8–20 intrauterine coils visible). Document in operative notes for evaluation by X-ray and hysterosalpingography (HSG).
    - *Proximally placed* (>20 intrauterine coils visible or expelled). Do not deploy the system without adequate visualization and proper positioning of the device. Take care not to make sudden jerking movements during all stages of the deployment, and take special care when detaching and withdrawing the delivery wire at the end in order to avoid partial or complete expulsion of the micro-insert. In this situation, graspers can be placed down the operating channel to remove the abnormally situated device.

- *Inadvertent system damage.* If damage to the device is noted, then the most expedient solution is to remove and replace the system with a new one. Deployment problems (see below) often arise from bending and damage to the device system. Such damage can be prevented by:
    - gentle and careful insertion of the system into and down the 5 Fr operating channel;
    - steady, controlled feeding of the delivery catheter down the operating channel so that the device does not inadvertently touch the uterine wall on entry;
    - stabilizing the system at all times to avoid sudden inadvertent movements;

- accurate identification and gentle cannulation of the ostia with the hysteroscope in very close proximity to stabilize the device;
- avoidance of excessive pressure on the device with difficult tubal cannulation;
- keeping the device straight, well aligned and under close direct vision, and performing all manoeuvres according to manufacturers' instructions slowly and gently.

• *Device deployment problems* (inability to retract delivery catheter; inadvertent forward movement of insert; outer coils fail to expand fully; delivery wire fails to detach). If the delivery catheter sticks or fails to retract, then check that it has not been twisted and, if it has, rotate it accordingly followed by gentle retraction. Also, when you externally stabilize the delivery catheter, avoid excess pressure on it, as this can prevent catheter withdrawal. The system must be straightened to facilitate full expansion of the outer (intrauterine) coils. The most common problem is at the very end of the procedure with non-detachment of the delivery wire. This is usually overcome by straightening the system followed by gentle (and patient) anticlockwise rotation in conjunction with light withdrawal tension. Be careful not to pull out the micro-insert if the tension applied is too great and the delivery wire remains incompletely detached.

Post procedure

The operation note should describe the operative findings, the placement procedure and specifically record the ease of placement and trailing lengths of both micro-inserts.

Women should be given a drink and observed for between 30 minutes and 1 hour in a designated recovery area. Simple analgesics should be given as required. An appointment for radiographic imaging (see below) and gynaecological review with results should be made. Prior to discharge, women should be given a contact number and arrangements to make a follow-up phone call made by the nurse the next day. The need for continued contraception should be reiterated.

Radiographic imaging

The manufacturers recommend an abdominal X-ray at 3 months following uncomplicated procedures to confirm satisfactory placement of devices (Fig. 19.6). A HSG is recommended following difficult procedures or those resulting in suboptimal device placement. For example, if fewer than three coils are visible in the uterine cavity, there is an increased risk of micro-insert migration, if more than eight coils are visible, an increased risk of expulsion and encountered resistance during placement increases the risk of perforation into the peritoneal cavity. Recommendations for performing and assessing placement of the micro-inserts radiographically are available from the manufacturers (Essure). In our experience, appearances on abdominal X-ray vary widely and so we prefer to perform an HSG on all women at 3 months to locate the micro-insert and confirm tubal occlusion. This policy is also followed in the USA and is part of FDA-approved labelling for the Essure system.

In the absence of safety data at present, intrauterine procedures involving electro-diathermy (near cornua) and global thermal endometrial ablation are best avoided following micro-insert placement. Formal dilatation and curettage is also best avoided in favour of other sampling methods.

Additional information

Table 19.2 below presents feasibility and efficacy data for use in patient counselling and business case preparation. Table 19.3 compares the two approaches to female sterilization – hysteroscopic (transcervical) versus laparoscopic (transabdominal).

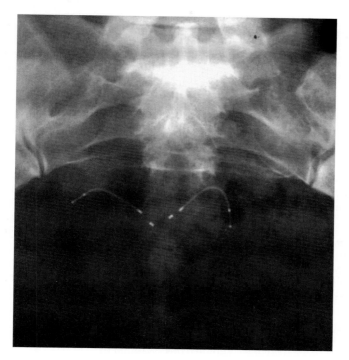

Figure 19.6 *Follow-up abdominal X-ray showing satisfactory placement. Correct placement: both microinserts appear in tubal lumen, spanning uterotubal junction and are symmetrical. (Reproduced with kind permission of Conceptus Inc.)*

Table 19.2 *Feasibility and efficacy data of Essure**

Feasibility	(%, 95% CI)	Comments
Non-feasible	2 (1–4)	Cervical stenosis, uterine polyps, poor visualization
Failed bilateral placement		
First attempt	13 (10–16)	Anatomic (tubal factors 50), poor visualization (20)
Second attempt	9 (7–12)	
Time		
Mean length of procedure	36 minutes	Mean 'hysteroscopy' time 13 minutes
Mean time to discharge	80 minutes	

(Continued)

Table 19.2 (*Continued*)

Efficacy	(%, 95% CI)	Comments
Hysterosalpingogram (HSG) follow-up (3 months) of bilaterally placed micro-inserts		
Bilateral correct placement	92 (90–95)	
Bilateral correct occlusion	96 (94–98)	All correctly placed cases had tubal occlusion at 6/12
Pregnancies	0 (0–1)	Denominator is 449/507 (89 per cent) bilateral placements, 9620 women-months, mean follow-up 21.4 months
Complications		
Patient	3 (2–5)	Vasovagal episodes (0.5 per cent), hypervolaemia, vomiting
Technical	4 (2–6)	Tubal expulsions (3 per cent), tubal perforations (1 per cent)
Symptoms		
Periprocedural (per cent admitted)	45 (41–49)	Cramps (30 per cent), severe pain (4 per cent), nausea (9 per cent). NB: <0.5
Post-procedure bleeding	19 (16–22)	Bleeding >7 days (no overall change in menstrual flow)

*From JM Cooper, 2003.

Table 19.3 *Hysteroscopic sterilization: hysteroscopy versus laparoscopy*

Feature	Hysteroscopy	Laparoscopy	Comment
Favours hysteroscopic approach			
General anaesthesia	No	Yes	Hysteroscopic sterilization (HS) performed using local anaesthesia ± sedation, which avoids potential morbidity associated with general anaesthesia in 'high risk' women, e.g. obesity, smokers, previous abdominal surgery, medical conditions
Surgical incision	No	Yes	Port sites used during laparoscopic sterilization (LS) may be sore or become infected postoperatively. Non-dissolved sutures will require removal
Hospital stay	No	Yes	LS is a day case or inpatient procedure because of the postoperative time needed to recover from general anaesthesia, narcotic analgesia and pain associated with pneumoperitoneum

(*Continued*)

Table 19.3   (*Continued*)

Feature	Hysteroscopy	Laparoscopy	Comment
Surgical morbidity	Low	Low	Potential serious morbidity is greater with laparoscopy. Generally pelvic discomfort from uterine cramping associated with HS is less than abdominal/shoulder tip discomfort resulting from laparoscopy
Favours laparoscopic approach			
Periprocedural pain	Yes	No	HS is well tolerated, but two-thirds of women will experience visceral uterine cramping pain. LS is invariably performed under general anaesthetic
Feasibility	Moderate	High	HS is unsuccessful in 10 per cent of women in whom the procedure is attempted compared with 2 per cent of women undergoing LS (failed pneumoperitoneum, poor visualization, pelvic adhesions), but default mini-laparotomy can be performed if required at the same sitting to overcome this
Failure rate	Low	Low	LS fails in 1 in 200 cases. Failure rate for HS is less well known, but probably comparable
Follow-up	Yes	No	An abdominal X-ray ± hysterosalpingogram required at 3 months following HS to confirm correct micro-insert placement. Additional contraception required until all clear given at 3 months. Women under-going LS must continue to use effective contraception until their next (post-procedure) period. Follow-up may be required following LS to remove non-dissolvable sutures to port sites if used
Evidence	Scarce	Abundant	LS is well established in gynaecological practice and consequently more is known about its effectiveness and side effects. Phase II/III studies published for HS. No pregnancies recorded in 9620 women-months to date

Evidence Box 19.1 Intrauterine devices (IUDs)/hysteroscopic sterilization and contraceptive efficacy

- *IUDs.* Systematic quantitative reviews confirm the feasibility and effectiveness of IUDs. Contraceptive efficacy appears to be comparable between hormonally impregnated devices (LNG-IUS), third-generation copper coils (>250 mm²) and frameless products (Gynefix).
- *Hysteroscopic sterilization and efficacy.* Data from phase II and II studies are available (see Further reading, page 265), which demonstrate the feasibility and safety of the Essure procedure. Although no pregnancies have been recorded so far, follow-up efficacy data are short (mean follow-up 21 months) and longer follow-up results awaited. Randomized controlled data are unavailable to compare patient-centred and economic outcomes with current gold standards (laparoscopic sterilization and vasectomy). No other transcervical procedure efficacy data are available for assessment.

KEY POINTS

- Fertility plans are a prime factor influencing management of common gynaecological conditions.
- Women seeking contraceptive advice should be informed of the pros and cons of all available methods for controlling fertility.
- The outpatient hysteroscopy clinic setting is suited to insertion and retrieval of 'lost' intrauterine contraceptive devices avoiding the need for general anaesthesia.
- Outpatient hysteroscopy is a usefulness modality for investigating and managing abnormal vaginal bleeding and discharge associated with the use of common hormonal contraceptive methods.
- Interest in transcervical methods of permanent birth control has reignited with the development of outpatient hysteroscopy.
- Alternative methods of sterilization should be discussed with women seeking permanent fertility control. These are: female sterilization with hysteroscopic and laparoscopic approaches, and male sterilization, i.e. vasectomy.
- The Essure hysteroscopic sterilization procedure employs a standard outpatient hysteroscopic approach and has approval for use in the UK from the National Institute for Clinical Excellence (subject to consent and continuing audit/research) and the Food and Drug Administration Agency in the USA.
- Alternative hysteroscopic techniques are also being developed and may become more widely available e.g. Adiana procedure (Adiana Inc, Redwood City, CA, USA), which involves bipolar ablation of the proximal fallopian tube followed by placement of a synthetic matrix and subsequent tubal occlusion.

- Hysteroscopic methods of tubal occlusion are still under evaluation and should be used only within the present guidance system for new surgical interventions.
- Feasibility and effectiveness from studies evaluating the Essure system (published phase II and III studies) demonstrate the procedure to be feasible and effective in the short term. Longer-term follow-up data are awaited.
- Women requesting permanent methods of birth control should be thoroughly counselled regarding the pros and cons of all available methods.

FURTHER READING

Cooper JM, Carignan CS, Cher D, Kerin JF. Selective Tubal Occlusion Procedure 2000 Investigators' Group. Microinsert nonincisional hysteroscopic sterilization. *Obstet Gynecol* 2003;**102**:59–67.

Dillon A. *Hysteroscopic Sterilization by Tubal Cannulation and Placement of Intrafallopian Implants*. National Institute for Clinical Excellence Interventional Procedure Guidance 44 (ISBN 1-84257-524-4) 2004. [Available at: www.nice.org.uk/IPG044distributionlist, accessibility verified 12 March, 2004.]

French R, Cowan F, Mansour D *et al.* Hormonally impregnated intrauterine systems (IUSs) versus other forms of reversible contraceptives as effective methods of preventing pregnancy. *Cochrane Database Syst Rev* 2004;**3**:CD001776.

Kerin JF, Cooper JM, Price T *et al.* Hysteroscopic sterilization using a micro-insert device: results of a multicentre Phase II study. *Hum Reprod* 2003;**18**:1223–30.

National Institute for Clinical Excellence Interventional Procedures Programme. *Interventional Procedure Overview of Hysteroscopic Sterilisation by Tubal Cannulation and Placement of Intrafallopian Implant 2003*. [Available at: www.nice.org.uk/IP218overview, accessibility verified 12 March, 2004.]

Royal College of Obstetricians and Gynaecologists. *Male and Female Sterilisation. Evidence-Based Clinical Guideline No. 4*. London: RCOG Press, 2004.

20

Training, safety and medicolegal issues

TRAINING IN OUTPATIENT HYSTEROSCOPY

We hope that this book demonstrates the utility, versatility and untapped potential of the outpatient hysteroscopy clinic setting for the management of many common gynaecological conditions. As is the case in any branch of medicine, proficiency and expertise can only be acquired following an adequate training period. Just as an aptitude for general gynaecological surgery does not automatically translate into mastery of endoscopic surgical skills, so outpatient hysteroscopy and related interventions cannot be expertly practised by all gynaecologists. The nuances and skills required to perform interventions successfully in a conscious patient in an outpatient setting need to be taught effectively. Proven technical capability for performing such procedures in women under general anaesthesia does not always mean that similar success will follow in the outpatient hysteroscopy clinic. Despite this caveat, most gynaecologists are more than capable of setting up and successfully running an outpatient hysteroscopy service for the management of common, benign gynaecological complaints.

Fundamental skills of outpatient hysteroscopy and related interventions

Most of the skills required for undertaking outpatient interventions are generic, but particular emphasis should be placed upon the following aspects:

- *Communication and demeanour.* The ability to impart accurate information in an easily understandable manner, appreciate women's concerns and alleviate any anxiety. The doctor–patient relationship is of paramount importance and maintaining the trust of the patient essential.

- *Technical aspects.* Developing an expedient approach with minimal and gentle tissue handling. The operator must become competent in communicating with the patient whilst maintaining concentration on the procedure in hand.

Training needs

This should be aimed at those medical professionals wanting to develop an interest in outpatient diagnostic and/or operative hysteroscopic surgery. This will include:

- gynaecologists in training
- trained 'established' gynaecologists
- general practitioners/primary care physicians
- nurse hysteroscopists.

It is likely that training in operative work will be primarily for gynaecologists, although other practitioners with an interest and aptitude should be encouraged to further enhance their skills and expand their roles. Training should include both theoretical and practical components (Information Box 20.1).

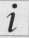 **Information Box 20.1 Training**

THEORETICAL PREPARATION

- Foundation in relevant anatomy and gynaecological pathology
- Indications, contraindications, rationale and peculiarities of outpatient hysteroscopic intervention
- Safety considerations – avoiding, recognizing and managing complications
- Fundamentals of diagnosis – including diagnostic landmarks/features, capabilities and limitations and assessing the utility of testing
- Fundamentals of surgery (including surgical and local anaesthetic techniques), relevant pharmacology, safe use of distension media, electrosurgery and instrumentation, etc.
- Attendance at appropriate courses/reading relevant literature

PRACTICAL PREPARATION

- Observation, assistance and supervised operating in anaesthetized patients in a formal theatre setting*
- Observation, assistance and supervised operating in non-anaesthetized patients in an outpatient setting
- Attendance at postgraduate practical courses or 'workshops' where theoretical and practical skills are demonstrated with an opportunity for 'hands-on' training using inert pelvic trainers and/or animal models
- Attendance at established 'see and treat' centres specializing in outpatient hysteroscopic intervention
- Use of multimedia (e.g. video, DVD, computer software)

*Initial performance under general anaesthesia is only of value if miniature hysteroscopes are used and correct technique is taught. Unfortunately, the trainee using larger-diameter hysteroscopes in the anaesthetized patient may acquire bad habits. These include rough tissue handling and routine cervical dilatation, followed by blind or obscured insertion of the hysteroscope into the uterine cavity. For this reason we believe that training in the conscious outpatient from the start is preferable, especially as clear views relayed upon a video monitor allow the supervising trainer to subtly make or direct technical adjustments as necessary.

Suggested progressive steps in training are shown schematically in Fig. 20.1. Although the steps are somewhat arbitrary it serves as a general template for the trainee. Knowledge is continually acquired along with increasing competence and confidence as the trainee progresses through the steps from the simple to more complex. The breadth of training will depend to a large part upon the service requirements and wishes of the trainee. For example, some operators may want to limit their practice to diagnostic work alone or a selection of operative procedures. Others may want to offer a comprehensive outpatient hysteroscopy service and thus may learn a wide range of procedures.

Accreditation

Formal accreditation in outpatient hysteroscopic intervention has not been established at present in the UK or elsewhere. However, the Royal College of Obstetricians and Gynaecologists is producing a special skills module in outpatient hysteroscopy and the British Society of Gynaecological Endoscopy a nurse hysteroscopy programme. Other colleges and accrediting bodies throughout the world are likely to follow as the ambulatory setting expands and technology advances, so that a uniform standard of practice can be guaranteed

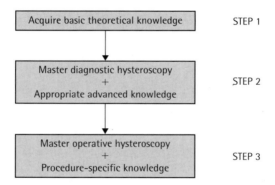

Fig. 20.1 *Template for training and progression in outpatient hysteroscopy.*

 Information Box 20.2 Example of training and accreditation requirements for outpatient hysteroscopy: levels and competencies for hysteroscopic procedures

- *Level 1: Diagnostic and simple operative.* Diagnostic, target biopsy, removal of intrauterine contraceptive device (IUCD)
- *Level 2: Minor operative.* Polypectomy, resection/ablation of small pedunculated fibroids, minor adhesiolysis
- *Level 3: Complex operative.* Endometrial ablation, sterilization, septoplasty

to the general public. A record of supervised procedures will be necessary, and training to different levels may be possible (Information Box 20.2). Maintenance of accreditation, as with endoscopic surgery, may require demonstrating up-to-date practice by attendance at workshops, audit and quality control.

SAFETY

Prior to undertaking outpatient hysteroscopy the gynaecologist must ensure that the indication is valid, that there are no contraindications and that informed consent has been obtained (see above). The operator must be trained to a sufficient level and be capable of performing the procedure or supervised by a competent surgeon. The adequacy and cleanliness of all equipment should be regularly checked between cases. General safety considerations during outpatient hysteroscopic procedures are given in Information Box 20.3.

Information Box 20.3 Outpatient hysteroscopy: general safety considerations

PREOPERATIVE

- Ensure that the patient's general health is satisfactory to tolerate outpatient intervention
- Obtain any history of previous allergic reactions to pharmacological agents

OPERATIVE

- Avoid/minimize blind instrumentation (e.g. cervical dilators)
- Advance the hysteroscope under direct vision at all times
- Confirm correct orientation within the uterine cavity by identification of uterine landmarks (tubal ostia) prior to commencing operative procedures
- Operate under direct vision at all times using good basic surgical technique
- Only undertake procedures in which you are fully trained
- Take particular care with surgical procedures at the thinner cornual regions and if you are using energy sources
- Monitor fluid balance with more complex operative procedures
- Consider limiting extent of procedures in high-risk/older patients
- Complete the procedure on a subsequent occasion (two-stage procedure) if visualization has been lost or patient compliance is compromised
- Stop procedures if complications occur, and document carefully
- Make sure that resuscitation equipment is accessible
- Closely monitor trainees and delegate procedures commensurate with their experience and competence

POSTOPERATIVE

- Discharge the patient after a suitable period of postoperative observation in a dedicated area

MEDICOLEGAL IMPLICATIONS OF OUTPATIENT HYSTEROSCOPIC INTERVENTION

The law

BREACH OF DUTY

The accepted legal test for medical negligence applied by the courts following the judgement by Mr Justice McNair in the Bolam case (see Further reading, page 274), stated that the defendant had to have acted in accordance with the practice accepted as proper by a 'responsible body of medical men'. Therefore, the claimant has to establish that breach of duty occurred because the diagnosis, examination, investigations and/or treatments fell below a reasonable standard, which was expected to be provided by a reasonably competent clinician of equal status. In subsequent cases such as Maynard v West Midlands Regional Health (1984), the courts referred to a 'respectable body of professional opinion'.

CAUSATION

In the Bolitho case in 1987 (see Further reading, page 274), the House of Lords reviewed the test for medical negligence and the use of the adjectives 'responsible, reasonable and respectable'. Following this the court has to be satisfied that the exponents of the body of opinion relied upon could demonstrate that such opinion has a logical basis. The claimant must also establish that her injuries have been caused, on a balance of probabilities, by any failings, i.e. what is more likely than not to have occurred as a result of any failings. If the same injuries would have been likely to occur in any event, then there is no claim in respect to those injuries.

Accordingly, the test for medical negligence is not only whether the diagnosis or treatment accords with sound medical practice but also whether in the opinion of the court that practice stands up to critical and logical analysis. Furthermore, it is a requirement that the experts supporting that practice had directed their minds to the question of comparative risks and benefits and had, on a balance of probabilities, reached a defensible conclusion on the matter.

Relevance to outpatient hysteroscopy

As clinicians we must provide patients with diagnostic and treatment options that are based on principles of good clinical practice. These practice guidelines should ensure that we do no harm. We should also ensure that we provide a quality service based on:

- an evidence-based approach – this book collates that evidence to allow clinicians to follow that approach;
- following guidelines/protocols that may have been devised either locally or on a national basis.

Women presenting with clinical problems should be managed using a systematic approach. Diagnosis requires the careful taking of a clinical history followed by a clinical examination and finally by performing investigations where appropriate. It is important to adhere to this diagnostic pathway in a stepwise manner, as clinical history and examination alone can result in the correct diagnosis in the majority of patients. Clear documented evidence of this is essential in the medical records. The likely diagnoses and their implications in terms of natural history and prognosis should be discussed as well as the potential benefits and risks of treatment. Patients should be given a choice regarding use of anaesthesia where appropriate and the most suitable setting chosen. Treatment options generally include:

- conservative approach – explanation and reassurance, expectant management;
- medical approach – administration of local or systemic drugs;
- surgical approach – operative procedures in the conscious or unconscious patient.

Patients are then in a position to arrive at an informed decision regarding their further management. Legible (black ink photocopies are best) and comprehensive medical records should be kept. Relevant information pertaining to the particular gynaecological condition and options for treatment should be reinforced using clear patient information leaflets (Information Box 20.4).

Consent

If surgical intervention is intended, then obtaining consent is essential. This should clearly detail the risks and benefits of the treatment and should now be in accordance with NHS standards (see Further reading, page 274). Failure to comply with any of these standards may constitute a breach of duty as the clinician may not have acted in accordance with the practice accepted as proper by a responsible body of medical professionals.

 Information Box 20.4 Patient information leaflets

The production and dissemination of high-quality patient information leaflets is highly valued by patients and improves their overall experience by increasing confidence, reducing patient anxiety and improving treatment outcomes. Written information is extremely useful for preparing women for invasive procedures such as outpatient hysteroscopic investigation and associated surgical interventions, especially in a 'one-stop' situation, where no prior consultation with a gynaecologist may have taken place. In this 'see and treat' situation, it is important to demonstrate that patients have had adequate time to reflect preprocedurally upon likely treatment strategies. Where prior consultation has occurred, patient-friendly leaflets can reinforce, clarify and remind patients of important verbal information on which they can reflect. Furthermore, procedural aspects can be addressed such as when to arrive and how to prepare for particular procedures. The use of other formats such as websites for patients, audio-tape and video are likely to be increasingly employed to enhance communication.

Production of patient information leaflets involves carefully undertaking several stages, namely planning, writing, consultation, printing and distribution. Information sources and templates are available to aid production of high-quality information leaflets:

- NHS Direct Online (www.nhsdirect.nhs.uk)
- The Centre for Health Information Quality (CHIQ) (www.hfht.org/chiq)
- Department of Health. *Toolkit for Producing Patient Information*. Department of Health, 2003. Available at www.nhsidentity.nhs.uk/patientinformationtoolkit

Example

Let's take the example of a 56-year-old high-risk diabetic and hypertensive patient with a body mass index of 40 presenting with postmenopausal bleeding. Such a patient requires investigations to exclude endometrial pathology particularly endometrial carcinoma. A detailed history and examination are required. The options for investigations are:

- ultrasound scan of the pelvis to measure endometrial thickness and to exclude ovarian pathology;
- undergo outpatient ambulatory hysteroscopy and endometrial biopsy;
- inpatient hysteroscopy, dilatation and curettage.

Evidence-based practice would recommend ultrasound being the gatekeeper to determine the best investigative pathway according to the flowchart (see Fig. 6.4). If the patient is, however, brought in directly for inpatient general anaesthetic hysteroscopy and curettage, a possible breach of duty may result, particularly if complications occur. One could argue that, if ambulatory service does not exist in a hospital, then a patient could not be offered anything else other than inpatient diagnostic modalities. One could also present a case that a reasonable body of gynaecologists would also have done the same in similar circumstances. However, if it makes logical sense to try and avoid general anaesthesia because of the high-risk medical conditions, then good clinical practice dictates that outpatient local anaesthetic diagnosis should prevail. Such a patient could highlight the case to present to develop ambulatory services, as it can be argued along the basis of following good clinical practice guidelines, patient safety, clinical governance aspects, choice for patients and medicolegal issues. This can be a powerful method of persuading managers to develop new services on the basis of providing effective as well as cost-effective hospital services (Chapter 2).

Consent in the outpatient setting

VERBAL CONSENT

As the patient is conscious, some may argue that written consent is not required when invasive procedures with minimal complication rates are contemplated, e.g. diagnostic hysteroscopy. Patients can give immediate feedback and can object to the intervention at any point in the proceedings. Verbal consent is, however, essential prior to undertaking such procedures. In order to avoid dissatisfaction and complaints it is important to maintain privacy and identify and introduce all personnel present. Women should be made aware of what the proposed procedure entails, including the use of the lithotomy position. For hysteroscopic intervention, the woman should be prewarned that during the procedure she may feel:

- pain – usually period-like cramps, especially if an endometrial biopsy is taken. Such discomfort may last for a few hours following the procedure but is self-limiting and usually controlled with simple analgesia
- wet – if a fluid medium is being used, fluid can leak back from the uterus into the vagina.

WRITTEN CONSENT

As the invasiveness of procedures increases, so generally do potentially adverse effects. This applies to the outpatient setting as much as to the inpatient setting. In view of the unpredictable nature of the 'see and treat' approach and in light of the current litigious climate, good practice dictates that written informed consent should be obtained preprocedure in all patients. This is aided by the distribution of a clearly written patient information leaflet outlining what 'see and treat' hysteroscopy entails prior to the appointment. It is best to outline the risks and benefits of all potential therapies (e.g. polypectomy, insertion of levonorgestrel intra-uterine system (LNG-IUS), etc.) in advance. Some women may prefer time to reflect on new information, although most will opt for the convenience of immediate treatment, tailored by the preceding diagnosis. Most women will feel disempowered and vulnerable when exposed in the lithotomy position and so it is wholly inappropriate to discuss potential treatments opportunistically at this time.

In general, there are good reasons to suppose that gynaecological interventions in the conscious patient are safer compared with the unconscious patient. This is because risks of general anaesthesia are avoided, procedures are limited by feasibility and immediate patient feedback, which may protect against untoward adverse events such as perforations.

KEY POINTS

- Training in diagnostic and therapeutic outpatient hysteroscopy is necessary to optimize clinical practice and set up efficient services.

- Theoretical knowledge needs to be acquired in addition to practical training. This handbook is aimed at the needs of the modern outpatient hysteroscopist, providing relevant information to the trainee and acting as a reference for more experienced operators.

- Competence in diagnostic hysteroscopy should be secured before moving on to operative intervention.

- Practical training courses are available.

- Meticulous attention to pre-, peri- and postoperative care will minimize adverse outcomes.

- Women should be offered a choice regarding the need for local or general anaesthesia and the setting for intervention.

- Hysteroscopic treatment in the conscious patient confers significant safety advantages compared with that in the unconscious patient.

- Dissatisfaction and complaints are minimized by employing an empathetic and inclusive approach. Clear explanations and comprehensive information should be provided and the patient actively involved in decision-making regarding treatment.

- Written and verbal consent must be obtained and good documentation is a prerequisite.

FURTHER READING AND COURSES

Bolam v Friern Hospital Management Committee (1957) 1 W.L.R. 582.

Bolitho (deceased) v City and Hackney Health Authority (1987) 4 All E R 771.

Chapron C, Devroey P, Dubuisson JB, Pouly JL, Vercellini P. ESHRE guidelines for training, accreditation and monitoring in gynaecological endoscopy. *Hum Reprod* 1997;**12**:867–8.

Department of Health. *Good practice in consent implementation guide: consent to examination or treatment 2001.* (Available at http://www.dh.gov.uk/assetRoot/04/01/90/61/04019061.pdf)

Maynard v W Midlands Regional Health Authority (1984) 1 W.L.R. 634.

Course

- See and treat hysteroscopy workshop. Royal College of Obstetricians and Gynaecologists (RCOG), London. Sponsored by Gynecare Worldwide and run in conjunction with the RCOG and the British Society of Gynaecological Endoscopy.

Index

Colour Plates

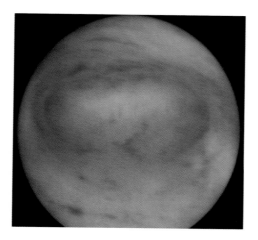

Plate 1 *Uterine cavity: hysteroscopic view.*

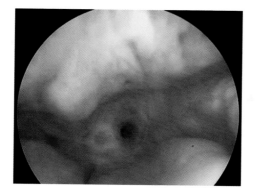

Plate 2 *Cervical canal (hysteroscopy). The endocervical canal may appear narrowed in postmenopausal women, making identification more difficult.*

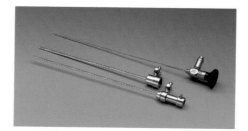

Plate 3 *Diagnostic hysteroscopy. The telescope is placed within the single flow irrigation sheath that is used for examination purposes. Housing the system within a perforated outflow sheath creates a continuous flow system if required. (© Karl Storz – Endoscope, Germany.)*

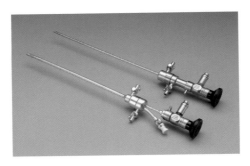

Plate 4 *Operative hysteroscopy: Bettocchi system. Continuous flow systems are necessary to maintain visualization when performing operative procedures. Semirigid ancillary instruments are passed down a specially designed working channel (© Karl Storz – Endoskope, Germany).*

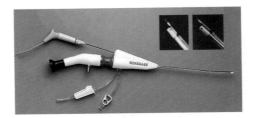

Plate 5 *Operative hysteroscopy: Versascope system. This disposable micro-system employs a deflected inflow sheath to allow peripheral viewing with a 0° semi-rigid hysteroscope. A collapsible working channel provides assess for instrumentation and fluid outflow (Courtesy of Gynecare, USA).*

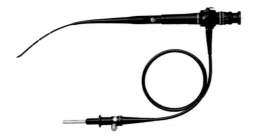

Plate 6 *Flexible hysteroscope HYF-XP (Olympus). This 0° flexible micro-hysteroscope has an outer diameter of 3.1 mm. The distal end can be deflected 100° in an upward or downward direction and employs a 1.2 mm irrigation channel. (Courtesy of Olympus, USA.)*

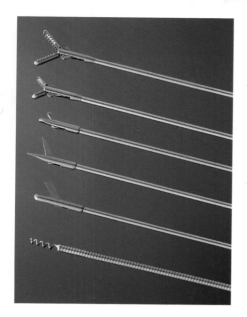

Plate 7 *Ancillary instruments: mechanical. A myoma fixations instrument and a selection of scissors, grasping forceps and biopsy forceps are shown (© Karl Storz – Endoskope, Germany).*

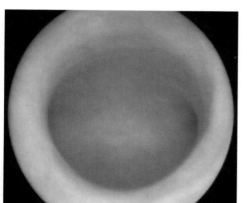

Plate 8 *Proliferative phase endometrium. Hysteroscopic view of a normal endometrial cavity. The endometrium is smooth and white-pink, compatible with the proliferative phase. The backward tilt of the uterus (0° lens) suggests that it is retroflexed.*

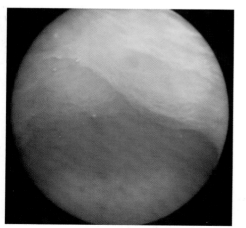

Plate 9 *Secretory phase endometrium. The endometrium appears pink, thick and irregular.*

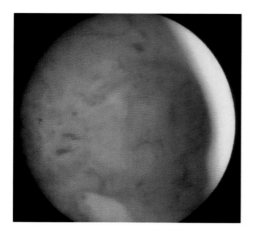

Plate 10 *Atrophic endometrium. The exposed myometrium and stroma impart a trabeculated or ridged appearance.*

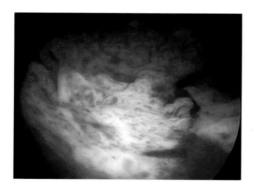

Plate 11 *Abnormal endometrium. The endometrium is focally thickened, irregular and vascular suggestive of a hyperplastic or malignant process. Histology confirmed an endometrial cancer. (Courtesy of P Wilson.)*

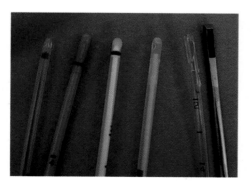

Plate 12 *Miniature endometrial biopsy devices. Flexible, disposable plastic aspiration devices and a miniature curette are shown. Global endometrial biopsy is an important diagnostic tool to be used alongside diagnostic hysteroscopy.*

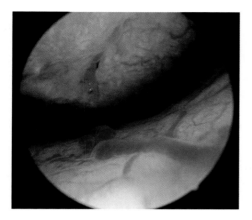

Plate 13 *Tamoxifen-induced endometrial changes as seen on hysteroscopy ('glandulocystic atrophy'). The endometrium is atrophic and highly vascular. Characteristic cystic changes were visible at higher magnification.*

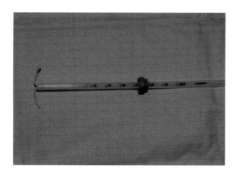

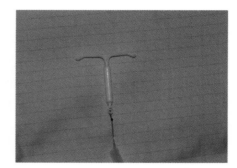

Plate 14 *Mirena (Schering, Germany): Levonorgestrel Intrauterine System.*

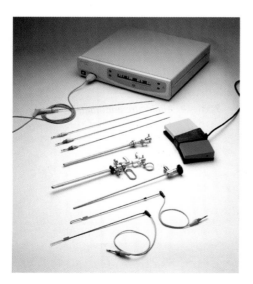

Plate 15 *The bipolar intrauterine system (Versapoint). The system consists of a dedicated bipolar generator, a reusable hand piece and connector cable to which is attached one of a choice of three single use, disposable coaxial electrodes. (Courtesy of Gynecare, USA.)*

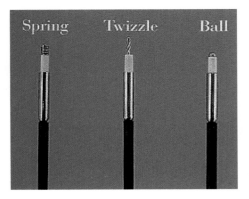

Plate 16 *Bipolar (Versapoint) electrodes. The flexible, coaxial electrodes comprise a distal active and proximal return electrodes separated by ceramic insulation. There are three types of electrode available: ball, spring and twizzle (thin wire). The different tip configurations provide a range of tissue effects – vaporize, cut and desiccate. (Courtesy of Gynecare, USA.)*

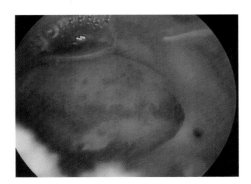

Plate 17 *Endometrial polyp. A polyp is seen on hysteroscopy as a discrete projection of endometrium, attached by a pedicle, which moves with the flow of the distension medium. This benign polyp is pedunculated and the thick overlying glandular mucosa obscures the delicate vascular network within. Malignant change within a polyp should be suspected if polyps are irregular, vascular, friable or necrotic, especially when seen in postmenopausal women.*

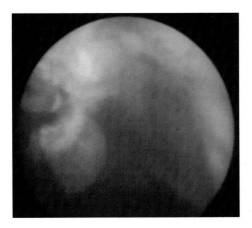

Plate 18 *Hysteroscopic (Versapoint) polypectomy.*

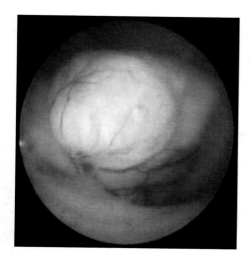

Plate 19 *Diagnosis of submucous fibroids: hysteroscopy (pedunculated). The superficial blood vessels are easily visible through the overlying stretched endometrium.*

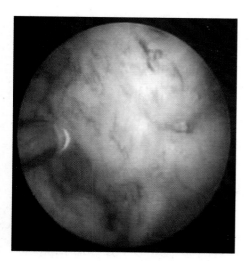

Plate 20 *Hysteroscopic (Versapoint) myomectomy. The attachment of the fibroid to the uterine wall is identified and a single cleavage plane created using bipolar diathermy.*

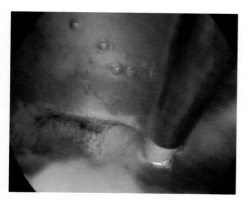

Plate 21 *Hysteroscopic septoplasty using Versapoint electrosurgery.*

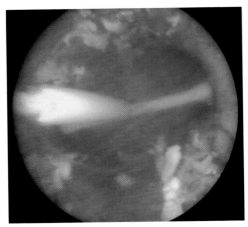

Plate 22 *Hysteroscopic retrieval of 'lost' Mirena. The intrauterine contraceptive system (IUCS) is seen within the uterine cavity. The strings are identified, grasped with hysteroscopic forceps and the IUCS removed. The side-arms of the device can be grasped if the strings have eroded (shown below).*

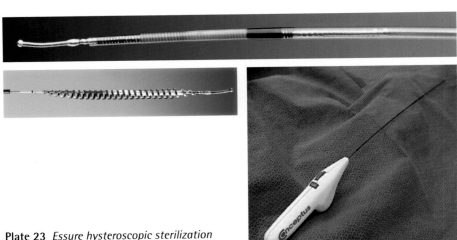

Plate 23 *Essure hysteroscopic sterilization system: guidewire, catheter and micro-insert. (Courtesy of Conceptus Inc. CA, USA.)*

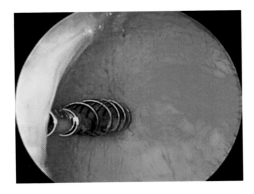

Plate 24 *Hysteroscopic view of tubal placement of Essure micro-insert. If between three and eight device 'coils' are visible within the uterus, placement is optimal. The device should be removed if the visible trailing length is >20 coils.*